HEALTH, ILLNESS, AND FAMILIES

A Life-Span Perspective

WILEY SERIES ON
HEALTH PSYCHOLOGY/BEHAVIORAL MEDICINE

Thomas J. Boll, Series Editor

THE PSYCHOLOGIST AS EXPERT WITNESS
    by Theodore H. Blau

HEALTH, ILLNESS, AND FAMILIES: A LIFE-SPAN PERSPECTIVE
    edited by Dennis C. Turk and Robert D. Kerns

MEASUREMENT STRATEGIES IN HEALTH PSYCHOLOGY
    edited by Paul Karoly

HEALTH, ILLNESS, AND FAMILIES

A Life-Span Perspective

Edited by

Dennis C. Turk
Yale University

Robert D. Kerns
West Haven Veterans Administration Medical Center
and
Yale University School of Medicine

A Wiley-Interscience Publication
JOHN WILEY & SONS
New York / Chichester / Brisbane / Toronto / Singapore

Library of Congress Cataloging in Publication Data:
Main entry under title:

Health, illness, and families.

(Wiley series on health psychology/behavioral
medicine)
"A Wiley-Interscience publication."
Includes index.
1. Medicine and psychology.   2. Sick—Psychology.
3. Sick—Family relationships.   4. Sick children—Family
relationships.   I. Turk, Dennis C.   II. Kerns, Robert D.,
1950–   III. Series.   [DNLM: 1. Attitude to Health.
2. Behavior.   3. Behavioral Medicine.   4. Family.
5. Life Change Events.   6. Sick Role.   WB 110 H4345]

R726.5.H433   1985   362.1'01'9   84-25655
ISBN 0-471-89200-9

Printed in the United States of America

10 9 8 7 6 5 4 3 2 1

List of Contributors

Tom Baranowski, Ph.D.
Department of Preventive
Medicine and Community Health
Department of Pediatrics
University of Texas Medical Branch
Galveston, Texas

Lori C. Bohm, Ph.D.
Department of Psychology
New York University
New York, New York

Joseph Paul Bush, Ph.D.
Department of Psychology
Virginia Commonwealth University
Richmond, Virginia

Alison D. Curley, M.A.
Department of Psychology
State University of New York at
Stony Brook
Stony Brook, New York

Herta Flor, Ph.D.
Psychologisches Institut der
Universitat Bonn
Bonn, Federal Republic of
Germany

David S. Gochman, Ph.D.
Raymond A. Kent School of Social
Work
University of Louisville
Louisville, Kentucky

Selby C. Jacobs, M.D., M.P.H.
Department of Psychiatry
Yale University School of Medicine
New Haven, Connecticut

Suzanne Bennett Johnson, Ph.D.
Departments of Psychiatry,
Pediatrics, and Clinical Psychology
University of Florida
Gainesville, Florida

STANISLAV V. KASL, PH.D.
Department of Epidemiology
Yale University School of Medicine
New Haven, Connecticut

ROBERT D. KERNS
West Haven Veterans
Administration Medical Center
and Yale University School
of Medicine
New Haven, Connecticut

THOMAS R. KOSTEN, M.D.
Department of Psychiatry
Yale University School of Medicine
New Haven, Connecticut

ELAINE A. LEVENTHAL, PH.D.
Department of Psychology
Madison, Wisconsin

HOWARD LEVENTHAL, PH.D.
Department of Psychology
Madison, Wisconsin

BARBARA G. MELAMED, PH.D.
Department of Clinical Psychology
University of Florida
Gainesville, Florida

PHILIP R. NADER, M.D.
Division of General Pediatrics
University of California Medical
Center
San Diego, California

JUDITH RODIN, PH.D.
Department of Psychology
Yale University
New Haven, Connecticut

DENNIS C. TURK
Department of Psychology
Yale University
New Haven, Connecticut

TRI VAN NGUYEN, PH.D.
Department of Sociology
Cornell University
Ithaca, New York

To all the families who have taught me so much about health and illness, especially the Turks: Lorraine, Kenneth, Katharine, Rose, and Irving, and the Meichenbaums: Donald, Marianne, Lauren, Michelle, David, Danny, and Florence

DENNIS C. TURK

To my daughter, Brandon, who has given the word "family" new meaning for me, and to my wife, Victoria, my parents, Robert and Altha, my brother, Daniel, and my sister, Susan

ROBERT D. KERNS

Series Preface

This series is addressed to clinicians and scientists who are interested in human behavior relevant to the promotion and maintenance of health and the prevention and treatment of illness. *Health psychology* and *behavioral medicine* are terms that refer to both the scientific investigation and interdisciplinary integration of behavioral and biomedical knowledge and technology to prevention, diagnosis, treatment, and rehabilitation.

The major and purposely somewhat general areas of both health psychology and behavioral medicine which will receive greatest emphasis in this series are: theoretical issues of bio-psycho-social function, diagnosis, treatment, and maintenance; issues of organizational impact on human performance and an individual's impact on organizational functioning; development and implementation of technology for understanding, enhancing, or remediating human behavior and its impact on health and function; and clinical considerations with children and adults, alone, in groups, or in families that contribute to the scientific and practical/clinical knowledge of those charged with the care of patients.

The series encompasses considerations as intellectually broad as psychology and as numerous as the multitude of areas of evaluation treatment and prevention and maintenance that make up the field of medicine. It is the aim of the series to provide a vehicle which will focus attention on both the breadth and the interrelated nature of the sciences and practices making up health psychology and behavioral medicine.

THOMAS J. BOLL

The University of Alabama in Birmingham
Birmingham, Alabama

Preface

The definition of behavioral medicine presented at the National Academy of Sciences meeting in April 1978 stated that "Behavioral Medicine is the interdisciplinary field concerned with the development of behavioral and biomedical science knowledge and techniques relevant to the understanding of health and illness and the application of this knowledge and these techniques to prevention, diagnosis, treatment and rehabilitation." Since its inception the field of behavioral medicine has grown exponentially. It is our opinion that much of the impetus for the growth of behavioral medicine has been the emphasis on the interdisciplinary nature of health and illness. Proliferation of interdisciplinary research is apparent in established medical, psychological, rehabilitation, sociological, and other journals. *The Journal of Behavioral Medicine* was first published in 1978 followed by *Behavioral Medicine Abstracts* and *Behavioral Medicine Update*. A Society of Behavioral Medicine and an Academy of Behavioral Medicine Research have been created. Further evidence of the growth of the field is the number of books that continue to be published. People who work in this broad field can hardly open their mailboxes without receiving an advertisement for a newly edited book in the area. Obviously, behavioral medicine is being seen as filling a void, a field whose time has come.

Having worked in the area of behavioral medicine since the mid-1970s, we have noted an interesting development. Although primary theoretical models for research in the area typically emphasize a *systems* approach, most edited books continue to focus on specific health problems and the *individual's* role in the development or maintenance of the problem or the *individual's* response to his or her plight. Papers have not focused on the importance of the family or other close support systems. This is not to suggest that research on the role of families in issues related to health and illness does not exist. In fact, there is an excellent tradition of family concerns in medical sociology and psychosomatic medicine. But it seems apparent from current books being edited that knowledge acquired in these areas is not being brought into the mainstream of behavioral medicine.

The lack of emphasis on the family is somewhat surprising to us. In our own work on coping with chronic illnesses, we have experienced an increasing concern for the family, both for its role in the development and maintenance of health and illness behaviors and for its role in treatment and rehabilitation efforts. As our interest in the central role of families has increased, we have noted that others in a number of areas are coming to similar conclusions. Thus we believe that a book on health, illness, and families that is addressed to the field of behavioral medicine is both important and timely. A book in this area can serve as an important addition in the evolution of the field.

Besides emphasis on the interdisciplinary nature of the field and important theoretical models derived from family theory, the present volume is designed to provide a developmental learning approach to understanding issues related to all stages of health and illness. The book takes a life-span approach including chapters on development of conceptions of health and health-promoting behaviors through the impact of acute, chronic, and terminal illness, to problems of aging. To ensure continuity across topics, each chapter includes a common format and covers four central themes. These include a historical perspective, current state of knowledge, research and methodological issues, and future directions.

We believe that each chapter included serves an important heuristic function both by underscoring the present state of knowledge and by pointing to important future clinical and research directions. We hope that this volume will stimulate interdisciplinary research on the family by those who work within the main disciplines that are included under the general rubric of behavioral medicine.

A number of individuals and resources were instrumental in helping us formulate the ideas for this book. We wish to acknowledge Yale University and the West Haven Veterans Administration Medical Center for providing stimulating and supportive environments in which to work. More specifically, we wish to thank our many academic and professional colleagues and students, especially participants in the Family Health Psychology

Seminar at the V.A., and the following individuals: Fran Berstein, Arnold Holzman, Jacob Levine, Mary Napp, and William Yellig. We are especially indebted to the many families who have been our teachers as well as our patients.

DENNIS C. TURK
ROBERT D. KERNS

New Haven, Connecticut
West Haven, Connecticut
February 1985

Contents

HEALTH, ILLNESS, AND FAMILIES

A Life-Span Perspective

1

The Family
in Health and Illness

Dennis C. Turk
Robert D. Kerns

How an individual behaves is a direct result of his or her definition of the situation. Each individual functions within a uniquely conceived reality based largely on prior experience. All human beings rely largely on their past experience to "make sense" of the world around them and to select behaviors appropriate to their interpretation of their situation. For example, each develops conceptions of what it means to be healthy or sick. To understand how individuals attempt to maintain health, cope with stress, and respond to illness, attention needs to be paid to their own conceptions of these relevant constructs.

Many of the conceptions that guide experience are developed within the context of the family. The family also comes to share conceptions with

Support for the completion of this manuscript was provided by Veterans Administration Merit Review Grants.

each of the individual members (e.g., Reiss, 1982). Thus both the individual's and the family's conceptions of health and illness are relevant when we try to understand the associations among health, illness, and the family.

Recently, two general areas, behavioral medicine and health psychology, have evolved that emphasize the importance of psychological factors as contributors to health and illness. Interestingly, these areas have tended to adopt the conventional medical model that focuses upon the individual. Examination shows that the authors of the many books on behavioral medicine have organized their texts along classic disease lines. That is, the chapters usually contain topics such as cardiovascular disorders, cancer, asthma, and so forth. Within such chapters there appears to be little attention given to the major context in which illness occurs and health is maintained. That is, the family context.

Although there is a large body of research on the impact of illness on various family members and conversely the role of the family on the maintenance of health and the response to illness, this knowledge has not been incorporated into the mainstream of the evolving disciplines; rather it has remained largely isolated in such relevant but peripheral areas as public health, psychosomatic medicine, and medical sociology. Furthermore, the research and conceptualizations of family theorists have received little attention in behavioral medicine and health psychology. Most recently, however, investigators in these areas have become more sensitive to the importance of the family context, and a body of empirical research is accumulating that should contribute to expanded views of health, illness, and the importance of the family. The major purpose of this volume is to bring together a number of investigators who have conducted research on the role of the family on the maintenance of health and the response to illness across the life span. Each chapter is designed to review the current state of knowledge in the relevant areas and to point toward future research directions.

Our major purposes in this chapter are to highlight the range of topics that have been considered, to examine characteristics of families that are important in all phases of health and illness, and to describe several of the family theories that may be of value in considering the associations among health, illness, and families. It is our intent to set the stage for the chapters that follow.

A PERSPECTIVE ON FAMILIES

Before considering the relationship among health, illness, and families, we need to present our perspective on families. In our view, families are groups composed of members who have mutual obligations to provide a broad range of emotional and material support (Dean, Lin, & Ensel, 1981).

Note from our definition that no attempt is made to suggest that families necessarily consist of blood relatives nor is it assumed that members live together; rather, the operative phrase is "mutual obligations." Furthermore, families within our perspective have (a) structure, (b) functions and assigned roles, (c) modes of interacting, (d) resources, (e) a life cycle, (f) a history, and (g) a set of individual members with unique histories. Each of these components of families needs to be considered when discussing health, illness, and families.

The *structure* or configuration of a family refers to characteristics of the individual members that make up the family unit including gender, age distribution, spacing, and size or number of members. *Function* refers to the tasks the family performs for society and its members (such as education, economic, reproductive). *Assigned roles* concern the prescribed responsibilities, expectations, and rights of the individual members (e.g., Nye & Berardo, 1973; Quick & Jacob, 1973). Thus one family member may be designated the role of breadwinner, another overseer of health care, and still another the manager of household operations. Roles do not have to be mutually exclusive and they seldom are. For example, Mechanic (1965) has noted that in most families the mother is the custodian of health as well as the manager of the household. Roles always have responsibilities with behavioral referents. *Mode of interaction* relates to the style adopted by the family members to deal with the environment and with one another in both problem solving and decision making (see discussion of this topic below when the works of Minuchin, Pratt, and Reiss are presented).

Resources include general health of the family members, social support and skills, personality characteristics, and financial support. These resources will influence the way that the family interprets events (e.g., Hill, 1949; Turk, 1979). *Family history* refers to sociocultural factors as well as prior history of illness and modes of coping with stress. As was the case for resources, the history of the family will affect the ways families interpret and respond to various events. Families also have a *life cycle* that changes over time. In brief, the family progresses through a reasonably well-defined set of phases of development beginning with a courtship phase and ending with the death of parents or parent figures. Each phase is associated with certain developmental tasks in which the successful completion leads to somewhat different levels of family functioning (e.g., Geyman & Tupin, 1980; Rakel, 1977).

Finally, families are comprised of *individual members* who have unique experiences beyond the family. Thus they have their own unique conceptions and behavioral repertoires that account for a substantial portion of what is observed within the family contexts. Some family theorists tend to lose sight of individual uniqueness. For example, children engage in a number of circumstances and experiences in school and in interactions with peers (see Gochman, Chapter 2, and Baranowski and Nader, Chapters 3 and 4, this volume). Considerable information is acquired by both children and adults from peers, coworkers, the media, and so forth. Thus it should not be assumed that the family comprises all the individuals' experiences or is the exclusive shaper of individuals' conceptions of themselves and the world. The unique characteristics of individual family members need to be considered in our thinking about families and family functioning.

We assume that all the family characteristics that we have noted, including the unique contributions of the individual family members, will influence a variety of important health and illness issues over the entire life span. For example, it is hypothesized that the family will play an important and necessary role in the development of the individual's health-related attitudes and behaviors. To determine how families transmit attitudes about health, symptoms, and illness, it is necessary to consider each of these characteristics of families. It is this complexity that makes studying families so difficult and why so much of the available data is so difficult to interpret.

The research on the ways that the health of an individual, as a member of a family, is affected by the family and vice versa is extensive and impressive, despite the fact that it has not been incorporated within current thinking in behavioral medicine and health psychology. One primary area of investigation refers to the family as the primary unit of health care (Litman, 1974). For example, a number of investigators have reported that the performance of a variety of health-promoting or inhibiting behaviors by children is associated with parental modeling (see Baranowski and Nader, Chapter 3, this volume, for a review of this literature). Many investigators have found that a person defines his or her symptoms by consulting family members (e.g., Picken & Ireland, 1968; Suchman, 1965; Vincent, 1963). Research studies indicate that 70–90% of all sickness episodes are handled outside the formal health care system, and self-treatment within the family provides a considerable proportion of health care (e.g., Hulka et al, 1972; Pratt, 1976). Even when professional help is sought and therapy prescribed, families still retain the responsibilities for making decisions about the management of therapies within the confines of the home. Moreover, mothers appear to evaluate symptoms of their children by relating them to previous symptoms of other family members (Turk, Litt, Salovey, & Walker, in press). Family attitudes have been shown to be a major factor in patient compliance (e.g., Ferguson & Bole, 1979; Heinzelmann & Bagley, 1970; Oakes, Ward, Gray, Klauber, & Moody, 1970; O'Brien, 1980; see Baranowski and Nader, Chapter 4, this volume).

Another major area of investigation has focused on the impact of illness on other family members. For example, several authors have noted that siblings of children with illnesses may be adversely affected (e.g., Crain, Sussman, & Weil, 1966; Lask & Matthew, 1979; Lavigne & Ryan, 1979; see Johnson, Chapter 6, and Kerns & Curley, Chapter 8, this volume). Vance,

Fazan, Satterwhite, and Pless (1980) found that the clinically healthy siblings of children with nephrotic syndromes reported that their own health was significantly worse than the siblings of health children. Langer and Michael (1963) observed that children of parents with psychosomatic symptoms were more likely to have psychosomatic symptoms themselves, such as asthma, ulcerative colitis, and hay fever. And Teiramaa (1979) found that 62% of asthmatic children had family models with asthma or other respiratory problems as compared to the control children who in only 30% of the cases had a family member with a respiratory problem.

The influence of illness modeling does not seem limited to parent–child interactions. For example, Stern and Pascale (1979) reported that in 26% of the families of post-MI (myocardial infarction) patients the wives had symptoms that mimicked those of their husbands (such as dizziness, shortness of breath, chest pain) despite the absence of pathology in the wives. Moreover, several investigators have indicated that spouses of chronically ill patients reported as much or more indications of stress than the patients themselves (Kerns & Turk, 1984; Shambaugh & Kanter, 1969). In addition, as has been frequently noted (see Flor and Turk, Chapter 9, this volume), if a family member has an illness, there is physical and financial strain on all family members. Regardless of the nature of the patient's difficulties, adjustment seems not to be solely a result of his or her individual characteristics but also a product of the family interactions.

One caveat that we wish to mention is that a great deal of the literature that focuses on the impact of illness on both individuals and families has emphasized the extremely negative impact of various diseases. Much less attention has been given to the large proportion of families and individuals who respond and adapt in a satisfactory if not exceptional way (Turk, 1979). Here, however, we are anticipating ourselves and we return to this important point and discuss it in more detail later in this chapter.

Conversely, stressful and maladaptive familial situations have been implicated in the etiology and course of a variety of both acute and chronic diseases. Meyer and Haggerty (1962), for example, followed for 12 months a set of families with two or more children and recorded life events that were distressing to the family or to particular family members. In addition, they collected throat cultures every three weeks, analyzed them for evidence of streptococcal infection, and had staff members conduct examinations to detect clinical signs of streptococcal respiratory illness. Among family members, a greater degree of family-related stress occurred during the two-week interval before both the documented and clinical acute respiratory illness than occurred during the two-week interval after such infection and clinical disease appeared. Quite apart from etiological considerations, Boyce, Jensen, Cassel, Collier, Smith, and Ramsay (1977) have linked stressful family situations to the duration of respiratory illness in young children. Minuchin and his colleagues (Minuchin, 1974; Minuchin et al. 1975) have written extensively about the role of families during the course of several chronic conditions including asthma, diabetes mellitus, and anorexia nervosa. We will discuss the work of Minuchin's group in more detail below.

Despite the emphasis of medical care on the individual who manifests the physical symptoms, and therefore "the patient," the important role of the family in the development and the maintenance of health as well as in the expression and response to somatic illness has long been known intuitively by health care providers. Largely inspired by Richardson's (1945) now classic book, a new subspecialty has emerged in medicine—family medicine. The distinguishing feature of family medicine is the insistence upon the need to enlarge the conceptual field within which a physician attempts to understand the pathology of the considered individual. This enlargement of perspective includes not only the patient holistically but also as a biological and social member of an intimate social group—the family (Carmichael, 1976).

The theoretical underpinnings of family medicine have been based on family theories that tend to emphasize the family as a discrete entity rather than as a collection of individuals. As such the family is viewed as being capable of experiencing its own distress, disruption, and dysfunction beyond that of the individual patient (Carmichael, 1976). In a sense, for family theorists, the family is considered as *the* patient and thus the family, rather than any individual member, becomes the focus of prevention or treatment. Part of this emphasis on the family as the focus of treatment derives from early work conducted by family therapists who worked with families of psychiatric patients (e.g., Ferreira, 1963; Watzlawick, Beavin, & Jackson, 1967). In the remainder of this chapter we will examine some of the basic tenets of several theoretical models that have been elaborated and adopted for considering a wider range of health-related issues. Although we discuss these different theories in separate sections, the reader will become aware that they are intricately related. We discuss them separately for convenience and to enhance clarity rather than because we view them as unique.

FAMILY SYSTEMS THEORY

The family meets the two basic requirements of a system established by Buckley (1967). The members are related to one another in a network of interactions. The four basic characteristics of a family system are (a) it is an open, rather than a closed, system and has a continuous interchange with the external social and physical environment; (b) it is complex with an intricate organizational structure; (c) it is self-regulating, in the sense of containing homeostatic mechanisms to restore balance; and (d) it is capable of transformation. The family system, confronted with continuous internal and external demand for change, may be able to respond with growth, flexibility, and structural evolution (Shapiro, 1983). Consequently, the family is a powerful determinant of behavior and can foster adaptive as well as maladaptive activities.

Proponents of family systems theory consider the family to function as a set of objects together with their attributes (Ferreira, 1963; Jackson, 1957; Watzlawick *et al.*, 1967). According to this perspective, what is important is the relationship or interaction between the family members rather than the actual content of the relationship of the members themselves. Emphasis is placed on the modes of communicating and the position of different family members in the family system rather than on specific information contained in the communication. Family systems theory postulates that individuals can be understood as members of a larger social context and that their behavior and specific concepts are formed through interaction with their family environment. Within family systems theory, the concept of linear causation of A resulting in B is supplanted by a circularity of cause and effect in which many interacting variables are taken into consideration. For family systems theorists, the emphasis is on the dynamics of the whole family, whereas observations of the component parts and their attributes are given less importance and attention.

As noted earlier, a major property of a system is the need to maintain a steady state. Jackson (1957) postulated that the family attempts to maintain an equilibrium of the dynamic forces between the family members called family homeostasis. He also suggested that a change in any family member makes it necessary for all other family members to adapt to the change. Jackson observed that families of psychiatric patients showed repercussions when the patient improved. He suggests that the patient's illness served as a homeostatic mechanism that kept the disturbed system in delicate balance (for an excellent illustration of this process, see Sheehan, 1982). The assumption here is that the family will try to maintain a constant state even if it is maladaptive or dysfunctional. Thus the family has a vested interest in restoring the recovering patient to his or her former "sick" state.

Minuchin and his colleagues (Minuchin, 1974; Minuchin et al., 1975) have suggested that physical illness in a child might serve as a stabilizing function in the family. The sick child may become a focus of attention and thus may serve to prevent marital conflicts. In this case, the "sick" child fulfills the role of maintaining family stability and equilibrium.

Another property of family systems is that families operate with a set of fairly well-defined beliefs shared by each family member. These beliefs, called "family myths" or "family paradigms", concern each member and the mutual interactions of each one in the family. The myth refers to the identified roles of family members (Ferreira, 1963). The role for the psychiatric patient noted above is that of "patient." When an event threatens to make inoperative the family myth, the perceptual context in which family behaviors occur changes, for the myth provides the explication of the rules that govern the relationships. The family struggles to maintain the myth so that it can function at a steady state.

Minuchin and his colleagues (Minuchin, 1974; Minuchin et al., 1975) have focused on the modes of family interaction and the way in which maladaptive modes may have an etiological or facilitative role in disease and symptoms of children. Minuchin (1974) believes that the functions of families are twofold. First, the family provides psychosocial protection for its members. Second, it accommodates to a culture and provides for the transmission of that culture. In order to carry out the family's functions, it is imperative that each family member has an identity to which he or she belongs and how that member is separate from the family both as an individual and as a component of the family unit. Because the family is a system, it operates within a set of functional demands that organize the ways in which family members interact. Essential to the family structure are boundaries that determine who participates and how. These boundaries preserve the identities of the family members. According to Minuchin, disease of adaption depends on how rigid or diffuse the boundaries are when a stressor occurs. Setting new boundaries means acquiring new family roles.

Grolnick (1972) has reported that the families with greater rigidity in structure more frequently develop psychosomatic illnesses that become chronic. He believes that psychosomatic illness results from the constant stress the family perceives when it is unable to adapt to the new situation because members are unable to change.

Minuchin and his colleagues (1975) have theorized extensively about family factors that are related to the etiology of disease and the exacerbation of symptoms in children specifically with three chronic conditions (diabetes mellitus, asthma, and anorexia nervosa). The five characteristics of family interaction found to be more prevalent in "psychosomatic families" are enmeshment, overprotectiveness, rigidity, lack of conflict resolution, and involvement of the sick child in parental conflict. Enmeshment, at its extreme, refers to a high degree of involvement and responsiveness among family members. There is a strong interdependence of relationships and poorly differentiated perception of self and other family members when there is a great amount of enmeshment. In addition, there is extreme sensitivity between family members and minor upsets are rapidly responded to with closeness and closing of ranks. There are also shifting alliances between family members that detract from real affiliation and individuation.

Overprotectiveness seen in the psychosomatic families refers to an overly high degree of concern that family members show for each other. As a result, individual competence and autonomy are retarded and personal control and problem solving are inhibited. The rigidity that these families demonstrate shows a marked tendency to maintain the status quo.

They also demonstrate low tolerance for conflict, and conflicts never tend to be addressed and resolved but are rather avoided.

According to Minuchin (1974), the child can become involved in parental conflict in three ways: (a) the child is put in a position to side with one or the other parent; (b) the child is in a stable coalition with one parent in which the child is always aligned with that parent against the other; and (c) the child becomes the focus of parental concern, and is either nurtured or criticized as the parents cease their conflict. Minuchin suggests that the presence of the characteristic patterns of a psychosomatic family, in combination with a real or apparent vulnerability of the child and a family organization and a set of beliefs that encourage a somatic expression of distress, will cause a child to develop an illness or will exacerbate an existing one.

In contrast to Minuchin and Grolnick, Pratt (1976) has examined the other side of the coin. She suggests that certain types of families, by virtue of structural or interactional patterns, can handle illness experiences without any major disruption. She has labeled this group as "energized families." Energized families are characterized by (a) varied and frequent intrafamily interactions; (b) established community ties; (c) encouragement of autonomy; (d) creative problem solving utilizing family skills and objectives; and (e) ability to adjust to role changes within the family.

A family system may promote a healthy condition or, conversely, it may constitute the condition sufficient to precipitate illness. It may act as a predisposing influence by increasing susceptibility or as fostering maladaptive response to stress (e.g., alcohol abuse). The family system also helps determine the course and outcome of acute diseases (e.g., Boyce et al., 1977; Meyer & Haggerty, 1962) and chronic diseases (e.g., Minuchin et al., 1975).

FAMILY STRESS THEORY

Of all the institutions in society, it is the family that is most likely to act as a buffer to absorb the strains and stresses its members experience. Yet a great variation in response has been noted among families coping with the identical stressful situation (Hansen & Hill, 1964). According to traditional family stress theory (Hill, 1949), this familial variation in response to the same potentially stressful event can be attributed to differing features of the event that may be selectively approached. Thus, in family stress theory it is the interaction between the family's resources and the objective event that determines the degree of stress. Within this model, family resources are seen as important factors aiding adaptation to crisis situations. Resources include financial (economic well-being), educational (contributing to cognitive ability that facilitates realistic stress perception and problem-solving skills), health (physical well-being), and psychological resources (e.g., personality characteristics).

Reiss (1981) has suggested that families may be distinguished according to their characteristic modes of perceiving and interacting with the social world. He refers to the differing characteristics as family paradigms or "sets of assumptions, convictions, or beliefs each family member holds about its environment . . . which guides its understanding of action in the world" (Reiss, 1982, p. 1413). These assumptions direct the family to sample or to attend to certain segments of its world and to ignore others, to view situations as threats or challenges, as malignant or benign.

According to Reiss (1981, 1982) the family's paradigm influences how families go about problem solving that will in turn affect how they go about coping with stressors such as the presence of an illness in one of the family members. Reiss postulates that families vary along three orthogonal dimensions: (a) "configuration," (b) "coordination," and (c) "closure." Configuration is the belief that the social environment is either ordered and capable of being mastered or as chaotic and uncontrollable. In a sense it is a belief held by the family regarding the solvability of a problem, independent of specific family skills or resources. Coordination is the family's perception of itself as either a collection of individuals or as a single unit. Families high on this dimension place a greater value on the solidarity of the family group in responding to the environment in contrast to viewing the environment as interacting separately with each individual. The individual has more or less autonomy depending on the degree of family cohesiveness. The third dimension postulated is closure. Closure refers to whether the environment is viewed as novel, which is interpreted largely through current experience in the context of the family, or whether it is viewed as familiar and is interpreted from past experience (Oliveri & Reiss, 1982).

ROLE THEORIES

Role theory conceptualizations of the family also emphasize the consideration of individuals within the family context. Each family member's preferences and expectations, however, are considered along with the interactional workings of the family (e.g., Nye & Berardo, 1973; Quick & Jacob, 1973).

The impact of a family member's illness on the health and functioning of the family appears to be related to the roles that members play in the family and the previous global level of health (Hill, 1965). For example, the mother or mother figure appears to play a crucial role in determining family decision-making styles, the utilization of health care services, and health beliefs held by the family (Litman, 1974). Moreover, the mother appears to play a major role in the health care and health practices of the family (e.g., Findlay, Smith, Graves, & Linton, 1969), whereas the husband is the financial supporter (e.g., Hornung & McCullough, 1981). A major illness in the mother is likely to have a direct impact on the stability of the family. If the role of caretaker, usually filled by the mother, is not filled due to her illness, then some family member who is unfamiliar with this role must take it over. This will likely lead to some disorganization of the family and will take the form of disruption of home activities, decreased mobility, and inability to pursue usual activities (Litman, 1974). If the father is the traditional individual to fulfill the role of financial provider, then his illness, for an extended period of time, will result in some other family member fulfilling his usual role. From traditional role theory, alteration of roles should almost always produce some disruption.

Baric (1970) has proposed a role theory for couples based upon activities and decision making. He suggests three role types: (a) "cooperative" roles where the husband participates in family activities but the wife makes the majority of the family decisions; (b) "merged " roles where joint decisions for the family and activities outweigh the individual decisions and activities of the husband and wife; and (c) "divergent" roles where the husband's and wife's activities and decisions are independent of each other. Baric reported that wives whose marital situation could be characterized as having cooperative roles were more likely to participate in a cervical smear test than wives whose conjugal roles were either merged or divergent.

This depiction of the family as an isolated nuclear structure with job specialization and traditional divisions of labor along gender lines has been challenged by sociologists (e.g., Yorburg, 1975). Yorburg argues that traditional divisions of labor are not adhered to in current families and suggests that rigid roles may never actually have been the norm. Pratt (1976) would suggest that one factor that would characterize those families who are able to adjust to an illness from those who have difficulty is the flexibility of role shift (a defining feature of the energized or resilient family).

As we noted, family systems theorists (e.g., Minuchin) have emphasized that an identified patient may serve a role by becoming the focus of attention and thereby prevent other family conflicts from becoming focal. In addition to prescribed family roles, the presence of a disease or an illness has been related to the performance of a set of behaviors that have been characterized as "sick–role" behaviors (Parsons & Fox, 1952). The sick–role behavior includes prescribed responsibilities and also includes the relinquishing of some previous role responsibilities. Family members are important in the processes of defining whether a member is sick and thereby they influence whether a person enters the sick role and how long he or she remains in that role. How an individual acts in the sick role will to some extent be related to the family expectations.

The sick-role model might be challenged for its passive depiction of the family. In a sense, the family is viewed as a victim of illness. Contrary to this model, stress and crisis are usually managed surprisingly well (e.g., Turk, 1979). This approach can be contrasted with Hill's (1949) emphasis on family coping described earlier. Parsons and Fox contend that an illness promotes a crisis. Parsons' and Fox's model gives no attention to active coping attempts. In contrast, Hill suggests that there are mitigating factors that influence the process and may, in fact, promote noncrisis or crisis management. These mitigating factors include the family's resources (financial, health, coping repertoire) in which all influence the appraisal of potential threat.

Finally, roles that are assumed by the different family members in response to crisis may lead to conflict (Young, 1983). For instance, problems can arise within a family relationship when one family member, for example, the father who, by withholding displays of emotion following the death of his child, is viewed as responding in an "inappropriate way." Conflict arises because others view that he *should* feel and respond in the same way as the grieving mother.

A TRANSACTIONAL MODEL

In a sense, the family theories described above conceptualize the family as primarily passive and reactive. That is, they focus on the family's response to information concerning health or to illness. Based on preexisting patterns of communication, assigned roles, or characteristics of a disease, families are predicted to respond in specified ways, with the ultimate goal of the family being maintenance of a homeostatic state. An alternative way to conceptualize the relationship between health, illness, the family, and individual family members is to view both the family and the individual members as active information processors who (a) seek out information and evaluate the features and characteristics of the information or of specific sources of stress and disruption (e.g., disease); (b) evaluate resources available for responding to the threat; (c) act on the environment and after responding; (d) evaluate the adequacy of the response (e.g., Hansen & Hill, 1965; Hill, 1949). In short, a transactional model emphasizes the active interactions among family members and their environment.

This transactional model extends Hill's family stress model and Reiss' family paradigm model as well as the various role theories. Families do develop myths or schemata about the world and themselves that are based on the history of the family and the individual. These schemata and available resources of the family for coping will influence the family's mode of responding. Moreover, the individual family member who experiences symptoms does contribute to the family's appraisal of the degree and nature of threat. And, finally, structural features of the family and stage in the family life cycle will differentially affect the nature of response and mode of adaptation. We believe that additional attention needs to be given to individuals within the family as well as to the family per se.

The transactional model highlights the nature of the (mis) fit among an individual, the family, and environmental demands. The discrepancy between the demands impinging on the family as well as on the individual members constitutes stress. Those demands can be internal or external, challenges or threats, and the way the family perceives its potential responses to these demands can result in the experience of stress. Within a transactional model, it is the family's perception of the stressfulness of the event and the appraisal of its ability to cope that ultimately defines stress (Hill, 1965; Lazarus & Launier, 1978; Turk, Meichenbaum, & Genest, 1983). Thus how the family interprets an environmental stimulus, the resources for responding to the demand, the configuration of the family, and the stage of the family life cycle, among other variables, rather than the stimulus or response per se determine the stressfulness of the stimulus. Our emphasis on the appraisal process may explain the findings of many studies (e.g., Davis, 1963; Fife, 1980; Venters, 1981) that demonstrate that neither the characteristics of the disease nor any dispositional pattern are consistently successful predictors of the family's response, stability, or disruption.

Within such a transactional model, one must immediately consider the nature of the coping processes, for coping is the other side of the coin from stress. Because physical and environmental demands are ubiquitous, what distinguishes one family from another is its ability to cope with the demands that are based on the host of the family and the individual factors that we have outlined.

Roskies and Lazarus (1980) have noted that coping is not simply a response to an event that has happened, but instead is an active process in shaping what has happened and what will happen. In short, a transactional model is established whereby the family is both the recipient and the perpetrator of stress, whereby the family's response is a reaction to demands and also a shaper of experience. Thus a solicitous spouse or other family member may be a beneficial support or a resource in coping with a problem or symptom. However, this may not always be the case. For example, an overprotective spouse may discourage participation in parts of a rehabilitation program and may usurp activities prescribed for the patient (Turk et al., 1983). Moreover, the family may reinforce excessive sick–role behavior and prolong recovery. Finally, it is important not only to consider the extent of familial support on an objective basis but also the patient's perception of the support. It may not be the actual support provided that is important but the individual patient's perception of and preference for support (Kerns & Turk, in press; Taylor, Wood, & Lichtman, 1983; Wortman & Dunkel-Schetter, 1979).

It is important to recognize that coping with stress is not limited to intrapsychic cognitive processes. For example, Lazarus and Launier (1978) define coping "as efforts, both action-oriented and intrapsychic, to manage (i.e., master, tolerate, reduce, or minimize) environmental and internal demands and conflicts which tax or exceed a person's resources." In some instances, an adequate coping response may be to change the situation for the better, if one can, or to escape from an intolerable one. In other situations in which one cannot alter or avoid the situation, he or she (or the family) may use what Lazarus and Launier call palliative modes of coping (i.e., methods of responding that make the individual or family feel better in the face of threat or harm without resolving the problem per se). Under certain conditions, such responses as intellectualizing, maintaining detachment, or avoiding thinking about certain matters may indeed represent the most appropriate means of coping. Successful coping in a given situation will not always involve mastery over the environment.

Pearlin and Schooler (1978) pointed out that the protective function of coping behavior can be exercised in three ways: "by eliminating or modifying conditions giving rise to problems; by perceptually controlling the meaning of experience in a manner that neutralizes its problematic character; and by keeping emotional consequences of problems within manageable bounds" (p. 2). We would expect that Pratt's (1976) energized families would demonstrate such adaptive forms of coping.

In addition to being somewhat deterministic and reactive, family theories focus almost exclusively on the family as a unit. The individual family members are given relatively little attention beyond that of serving a function within the family. That is, the experiences of the individual family members are rarely considered. When individuals are considered it is more likely that the impact of the individual on the unit will be examined, but how that one individual affects any other individual is given attention only in passing. Conversely, the impact of the family on a specific member is viewed as being of major importance, but the effect of one member on another is rarely discussed.

The transactional model that we described allocates attention to both the family as a unit and the characteristics of each family member. In the case of physical illness, although it is true that the occurrence of the illness in one family member influences the family unit, it is also true that different family members will have a unique set of responses as well as a set of responses in common with other family members. Conversely, although it is true that the family will affect the identified patient's responses, different family members may have differential impacts. It is also important to acknowledge that the physical symptoms of a patient can be directly experienced only by the patient. Either surgery or cancer, to mention only two disparate examples, will have an impact on the family unit; however, only the individual who has the surgery or cancer experiences the sensory phenomena that accompany them. What we are suggesting is that current family theories, in response to more individually oriented approaches, may have moved too far in the direction of giving preeminence to the family (e.g., Russell, Olson, Sprenkle, & Atilano, 1983).

IMPACT OF ILLNESS ON THE FAMILY

Few health professionals or family scholars challenge the proposition that illness or impairment in a family member has adverse effects on family functioning. Most agree that families of ill people generally function more poorly than families in which all the members are healthy. With the onset of an illness, the family's social life contracts and becomes primarily family centered. Within this circumscribed existence, the patient often becomes the focus of the family, with other family members forced into the background (Chowanec & Binik, 1982). Furthermore, most agree that the more severe and long lasting the illness or impairment, the greater the potential for family disruption. However reasonable these propositions, empirical data to support them are slim and far from compelling.

Only a handful of studies have specifically examined the relation of the degree of illness or disability to family characteristics such as marital satisfaction, family functioning, and decision-making patterns. These studies have produced somewhat ambiguous results. Litman (1974) claimed that the impact of illness on family solidarity was greater according to the extent that the illness was perceived as being more severe, but he insisted that families were brought together as often as they were pushed apart. Other studies (e.g., Klein, Dean, & Bogdonoff, 1968; Zahn, 1973) concluded that severely disabled persons enjoyed greater marital satisfaction and better family relations than did moderately disabled persons and attributed this to the lesser role ambiguity of the severely disabled. In contrast, Pless and Satterwhite (1973) failed to find any relation between severity of illness of a child and the family's overall functioning. In several other studies (e.g., Brown, Rawlinson, & Hardin, 1982; Fengler & Goodrich, 1979; Gibson & Ludwig, 1968; Kerns & Turk in press), no relation was found between the degree of disability of a spouse and marital satisfaction. Croog and Levine (1977) reported that the health level of patients recovering from a heart attack was unrelated to role changes in the family, to shifts in authority structure, to extent of marital consensus, or degree of marital happiness. They concluded that the effect of illness on family life was minimal.

How are we to understand such mixed results? It is likely that the impact of an illness on a family differs in intensity depending on the disease (e.g., its nature, time since onset, degree of disability involved, degree of stigma attached), several patient variables (e.g., gender, age), and many family-related variables, such as overall health of various family members, socioeconomic status, the age and stage of the family life cycle at which the disease occurred, and the status and position of the victim within the family constellation. Another way to view these results is to consider them as challenging the notion that disease impacts negatively on all families. These two sets of explanations are, of course, not mutually exclusive.

We do not yet clearly understand how, to what extent, and under what conditions specific health and illness variables affect or are affected by specific family variables (Brown *et al.*, 1982). Moreover, there is some evidence that some families may function more appropriately when there is a sick family member, as if mobilized to adaptive responding (e.g., Brown *et al.*, 1982; Venters, 1981). Much more work is needed to explicate the complex interrelationship among family factors and health and illness phenomena.

THE BASIS OF FAMILY MEDICINE: SOME UNANSWERED QUESTIONS

The assumptions of a family approach to health are that (a) the course and outcome of health or a given illness are influenced by the way the family members interact with each other; (b) the psychosocial and environmental context affects individual's responses; and (c) change in context can produce positive changes in health patterns or in an individual's adaptation to disease. A good deal of empirical evidence, reviewed throughout this volume, supports the important association between health, illness, and the family. However, unequivocal support for these assumptions is unfounded given the inconsistencies in the literature (see Gochman, Chapter 2, this volume for an extended discussion of the impact of families on the health attitudes and behaviors of children). Most of the empirical data has focused on individual patients and the responses of various family members. The notion that providing medical care to the entire family is inherently better in regard to efficacy, economy, and outcome has received considerable attention but relatively little empirical support. Even in the area of psychosomatic illness, empirical evidence to support the assumption that family treatment can affect the course of morbidity is lacking (Lask, 1979). Marinker (1976) has called for a more scholarly and rigorous approach to the study of the family by describing the present state-of-the-art as "a mishmash of vague sentimental yearnings, mythologies, and traditions about family life."

Part of the problem in the various family theories and consequently family medicine is that few of the relevant constructs have been defined or operationalized. Often assessment has relied on global, clinical impressions or has been based on interview procedures with little attention given to the subjective nature and reliability of these procedures. Moreover, when instruments to assess families are employed, they are often unidimensional and fail to examine the range of family factors that we have identified (e.g., point in the family life cycle, structural composition of the family). Several authors have concluded that with our lack of available instruments, there is currently no satisfactory method for assessing the impact of illness on families or for measuring the outcome of any intervention (Graves & Pless, 1976; Moore, 1975).

What are the characteristics of family health and "unhealth"? What tools are available to assess and diagnose families as functional or dysfunctional? What psychometrically appropriate instruments are available to measure family interaction patterns? Fundamental questions such as these need to be addressed if we hope to demonstrate the efficacy of family medicine and family therapy.

One problem with much of the family research is the failure to follow rigorous methodological designs. Many papers rely on anecdotal evidence. Other papers describe characteristics of dysfunctional families without demonstrating that these patterns are unique (e.g., Minuchin, 1975; Minuchin et al., 1976). Is it only families of children with diabetes that demonstrate a particular maladaptive pattern of interacting? Do all diabetic families demonstrate this interaction pattern? Part of the problem with this research is the failure to include control groups that are relevant. Additionally, the sample sizes used are often quite small and subject-selection criteria are unspecified.

Many family theorists have focused on identifying typologies of interacting or responding (e.g., Minuchin, 1974; Reiss, 1982). A problem with identifying typologies is that they reinforce the notion that there is a limited set of stereotypic modes rather than a wide diversity of ways of dealing with any circumstance. Moreover, there is an assumption that the characteristic patterns or styles are relatively rigid and will be consistently displayed across a range of situations or in a similar situation at a different time. The actual consistency of such patterns has not been given adequate attention in the family literature.

Much of the work in the various family theories described have focused on negative events and dysfunctional patterns of interacting and responding. The emphasis has been on the description of the tremendous adjustment problems of both the family and the patient. Very little attention has been directed toward understanding how these patients and families restructure their lives, how some develop effective ways of responding to the illness and the life circumstances that confront them and others do not, and how patients and families meet the challenges of chronic disease or disability (Seime & Zimmerman, 1983; Turk, 1979). When results do suggest that patients and families are doing well, these conclusions are often disregarded with the suggestion that the scores are the result of denial or that true pathology is only masked (e.g., Flannery, 1978; Glassman & Siegal, 1970).

Part of the reason for this emphasis on dysfunction stems from the fact that much of the family research and especially the family systems research has been conducted by clinical psychologists and psychiatrists. By the nature of their work, mental health professionals tend to see only those individuals and families who are having difficulty adjusting to their plight (i.e., patients and families who are most distressed and incapacitated). For example, Friedrich (1977) noted that much of the early clinical literature on parents of handicapped children focused on families who did not adjust very well. As a result, the maladaptive and pathological attitudes of a small minority came to be seen as normative for all parents and families with handicapped children. Relatively small percentages of patients with chronic diseases come to the attention of mental health professionals or are included in research studies. It is hazardous to generalize from such restricted and potentially unrepresentative samples.

Another concern with much of the research on families and family medicine is the reliance on cross-sectional data. This approach does not permit us to understand the changing demands and modes of responding and adjusting over time. Moreover, examination of maintenance of health and adjustment to chronic illnesses that may span many decades is a dynamic process that changes with the life cycle of the family as well as structural and functional characteristics of the family.

Examination of the family health literature leads one to conclude that the emphasis is on the mother's role in affecting health (e.g., Oakes, Ward, Klauber, & Moody, 1970). Few studies have attempted to examine the role of the husband or father on the health of family members. Yet, in the limited research available, fathers appear to play an important role (e.g., Mattson & Gross, 1966).

Another issue in this literature is the confusion between "cause–effect" relationships in examining family influences on health. The theoretical position that families are interacting systems, coupled with the substantial literature showing that illness impacts on the entire family, makes the conceptual study of family influence on health tenuous. The need for prospective field studies or experimental study is paramount. The causal direction of the family-health association must be explicit in the study design. Retrospective and cross-sectional designs that characterize this literature are inadequate for permitting the determination of the causal relationship between health and family.

In this chapter we have tried to underscore the range of influences that families have on health and illness. We described some of the relevant characteristics of families that are important. We reviewed several perspectives on family functioning and related these to the maintenance of health, illness onset and course, and the impact of disease on a family. We concluded by suggesting a number of questions that need to be addressed in the family medicine and behavioral medicine literatures. The remaining chapters will provide much more detailed coverage of many of the topics that we have mentioned and will each come to terms conceptually and empirically with the questions raised in our explication.

REFERENCES

Baric, L. (1970). Conjugal roles as indicators of family influence on health directed action. *International Journal of Health Education, 13*, 58–65.

Boyce, W. T., Jensen, E. W., Cassell, J. C., Collier, A. M., Smith, A. H., & Ramsey, C. T. (1977). Influence of life events and family routines on childhood respiratory tract illness. *Pediatrics, 60*, 609–615.

Brown, J. S., Rawlinson, M. E., & Hardin, D. M. (1982). Family functioning and health status. *Journal of Family Issues, 3*, 91–110.

Buckley, W. (1967). *Sociology and modern systems theory.* Englewood Cliffs, NJ: Prentice-Hall.

Carmichael, L. P. (1976) The family in medicine: Process or entity? *Journal of Family Practice, 3*, 562–571.

Chowanec, G. D., & Binik, Y. M. (1982). End state renal disease (ESRD) and the marital dyad. A literature review and critique. *Social Science & Medicine, 16*, 1551–1558.

Crain, A., Sussman, W., & Weil, W. (1966). Family interaction, diabetes, and sibling relationships. *International Journal of Social Psychiatry, 11*, 35–43.

Croog, S. H., & Levine, S. (1977). *The heart patient recovers.* New York: Human Sciences Press.

Davis, F. (1963). *Passages through crisis: Polio victims and their families.* Indianapolis: Bobbs-Merrill.

Dean, A., Lin, N., & Ensel, W. M. (1981). The epidemiological significance of social support systems in depression. In R. G. Simmons (Ed.), *Research in community mental health: Vol. 2. A research annual* (pp. 77–109). Greenwich, CT: JAI Press.

Fengler, A. L., & Goodrich, N. (1979). Wives of elderly men: The hidden patients. *Gerontologist, 19*, 175–183.

Ferguson, K., & Bole, G. G. (1979). Family support, health beliefs, and therapeutic compliance in patients with rheumatoid arthritis. *Patient Counselling and Health Education, 3*, 101–105.

Ferreira, A. J. (1963). Family myth and homeostasis. *Archives of General Psychiatry, 9*, 457–463.

Fife, B. L. (1980). Childhood cancer is a family crisis: A review. *Journal of Psychiatric Nursing, 18*, 29–33.

Findlay, I. I., Smith, P., Graves, P. J., & Linton, N. J. (1969). Chronic disease in childhood: A study of family relations. *British Journal of Medical Education, 3*, 66–69.

Flannery, J. G. (1978). Adaptation to chronic renal failure. *Psychosomatics, 19*, 784–787.

Friedrich, W. N. (1977). Ameliorating the psychological impact of chronic physical disease in the child and family. *Journal of Pediatric Psychology, 2*, 26–31.

Geyman, J. P., & Tupin, J. P. (1980). Family development. In G. M. Rosen, J. P. Geyman, and R. H. Layton (Eds.), *Behavioral science in family practice* (pp. 67–93). New York: Appleton-Century-Crofts.

Gibson, G., & Ludwig, E. G. (1968). Family structure in a disabled population. *Journal of Marriage and the Family, 30*, 54–63.

Glassman, B. M., & Siegel, A. (1970). Personality correlates of survival in long-term hemodialysis program. *Archives of General Psychiatry, 72*, 629–637.

Graves, G. D., & Pless, I. B. (Eds.) (1976). *Chronic childhood illness: Assessment of outcome.* (DHEW Publication No. NIH 76–877). Washington, DC: U.S. Government Printing Office.

Grolnick, L. (1972) A family perspective of psychosomatic factors in illness: A review of the literature. *Family Process, 11*, 457–486.

Hansen, D., & Hill, R. (1964). Families under stress. In H. Christiansen (Ed.), *Handbook of marriage and the family* (pp. 3–41). Chicago: Rand McNally.

Heinzelmann, R., & Bagley, R. W. (1970). Responses to physical activity programs and their effects on health behavior. *Public Health Reports, 85*, 905–911.

Hill, R. (1949). *Families under stress.* New York: Harper & Row.

Hill, R. (1965). Generic features of families under stress. In H. J. Parad (Ed.), *Crisis intervention* (pp. 32–52). New York: Family Service Association of America.

Hornung, C. A., & McCullough, B. C. (1981). Status relationships in dual-employment marriages: Consequences for psychological well-being. *Journal of Marriage and the Family, 43*, 125–141.

Hulka, B. S., Kupper, L. L., & Cassel, J. C. (1972). Determinants of physician utilization. *Medical Care, 10*, 300–309.

Jackson, D. D. (1957). The question of family homeostasis. *Psychiatric Quarterly, 31*, 79–90.

Kantor, D., & Lehr, W. (1976). *Inside the family.* San Francisco: Jossey-Bass.

Kerns, R. D., & Turk, D. C. (in press). Depression and chronic pain: The mediating role of the spouse. *Journal of Marriage and the Family.*

Klein, R. F., Dean, A., & Bogdonoff, M. D. (1968). The impact of illness upon the spouse. *Journal of Chronic Diseases, 20*, 241–248.

Langer, T., & Michael, S. (1963). *The mid-town Manhattan study of mental health.* New York: McGraw-Hill.

Lask, B. (1979) Family therapy outcome research 1972–1978. *Journal of Family Therapy, 1*, 87–91.

Lask, B., & Matthew, D. (1979). Childhood asthma: A controlled trial of family psychotherapy. *Archives of Disorders of Childhood, 54*, 116–119.

Lavigne, J., & Ryan, M. (1979). Psychological adjustment of siblings of children with chronic illness. *Pediatrics, 63*, 616–627.

Lazarus, R. S., & Launier, R. (1978). Stress-related transactions between persons and environment. In L. A. Pervin & M. Lewis (Eds.), *Perspectives in interactional psychology* (pp. 139–174). New York: Plenum Press.

Litman, T. J. (1974). The family as a basic unit in health and medical care: A social behavioral overview. *Social Science & Medicine, 8*, 495–419.

Marinker, M. (1976). Albert Wanderer Lecture: The family in medicine. *Proceedings of the Royal Society of Medicine, 69*, 115–117.

Mattson, A., & Gross, S. (1966). Adaptational and defensive behavior in young hemophiliacs and their parents. *American Journal of Psychiatry, 122*, 1349–1356.

Mechanic, D. (1965). Perception of parental response to illness. *Journal of Health and Human Behavior, 253*, 6–19.

Meyer, R. J., & Haggerty, R. J. (1962). Streptococcal infections in families. *Pediatrics, 29*, 534–549.

Minuchin, S. (1974). *Families and family therapy.* Cambridge, MA: Harvard University Press.

Minuchin, S., Baker, L., Roseman, B., Liebman, T., Milman, L., & Todd, T. (1975). A conceptual model of psychosomatic illness in children. *Archives of General Psychiatry, 32*, 1031–1038.

Moore, T. D. (Ed.). (1975). *The care of children with chronic illness.* Columbus, OH: Ross Laboratories.

Nye, F. I., & Berardo, F. M. (1973). *The family, its structure and interactions.* New York: Macmillan.

Oakes, T. W., Ward, J. R., Gray, R. W., Klauber, M. R., & Moody, R. M. (1970). Family expectations and arthritis patient compliance to a hand resting splint regimen. *Journal of Chronic Diseases, 22*, 757–764.

O'Brien, M. E. (1980) Hemodialysis regimen compliance and social environment: A panel analysis. *Nursing Research, 29*, 250–255.

Oliveri, M. E., & Reiss, D. (1982). Families' schemata of social relationships. *Family Process, 21*, 295–311.

Parsons, T., & Fox, R. (1952). Illness, therapy, and the American family. *Journal of Social Issues, 8*, 31–44.

Pearlin, L. I., & Schooler, C. (1978). The structure of coping. *Journal of Health and Social Behavior, 19*, 2–21.

Picken, I. B., & Ireland, G. (1969). Family patterns of medical care utilization. *Journal of Chronic Diseases, 22*, 181–191.

Pless, I. B., & Satterwhite, B. (1973). A measure of family functioning and its applications. *Social Science & Medicine, 7*, 613–621.

Pratt, L. (1976). *Family structure and effective health behavior. The energized family.* Boston: Houghton-Mifflin.

Quick, E., & Jacob, T. (1973). Marital disturbance in relation to role theory and relationship theory. *Journal of Abnormal Psychology, 82*, 399–412.

Rakel, R. (1977). *Principles of family medicine.* Philadelphia: Saunders.

Reiss, D. (1981). *The family's construction of reality.* Cambridge, MA: Harvard University Press.

Reiss, D. (1982) The working family: A researcher's view of health in the household. *American Journal of Psychiatry, 139*, 1412–1420.

Richardson, H. (1945). *Patients have families.* New York: Commonwealth Fund.

Roskies, E., & Lazarus, R. S. (1980). Coping theory and the teaching of coping skills. In P. O. Davidson & S. M. Davidson (Eds.), *Behavioral medicine: Changing health lifestyles* (pp. 184–205). New York: Brunner/Mazel.

Russell, C. S., Olson, D. H., Sprenkle, D. H., & Atilano, R. B. (1983). From family symptom to family system. Review of family therapy research. *American Journal of Family Therapy, 11*, 3–14.

Seime, R. J., & Zimmerman, J. (1983). Dialysis: A unique challenge. In E. J. Callahan & K. A. McClusky (Eds.) *Life-span developmental psychology* (pp. 281–304). New York: Academic Press.

Shambaugh, P. W., & Kanter, S. S. (1969). Spouses under stress: Group meetings with spouses of patients on hemodialysis. *American Journal of Psychiatry, 125*, 931–936.

Shapiro, J. (1983). Family reactions and coping strategies in response to the physically ill or handicapped child: A review. *Social Science and Medicine, 17*, 913–931.

Sheehan, S. (1982). *Is there no place on earth for me?* New York: Vintage Books.

Stern, M. J., & Pascale, L. (1979). Psychosocial adaptation post-myocardial infarction: The spouse's dilemma. *Journal of Psychosomatic Research, 23*, 83–87.

Suchman, E. (1965). Social patterns of illness and medical care. *Journal of Health and Human Behavior, 6*, 2–15.

Taylor, S. E., Wood, J. V., & Lichtman, R. R. (1983). It could be worse: Selective evaluation as a response to victimization. *Journal of Social Issues, 39*, 19–40.

Teiramma, E. (1979). Psychic factors and the inception of asthma. *Journal of Psychosomatic Research, 23*, 253–262.

Turk, D. C. (1979). Factors influencing the adaptive process with chronic illness. In I. G. Sarason & C. D. Spielberger (Eds.), *Stress and anxiety* (Vol. 6) (pp. 291–311). Washington, D.C.: Hemisphere.

Turk, D. C., Litt, M. D., Salovey, P., & Walker, J. (in press). Seeking pediatric care: Factors contributing to frequency, delay, and appropriateness. *Health Psychology.*

Turk, D. C., Meichenbaum, D., & Genest, M. (1983). *Pain and behavioral medicine: A cognitive-behavioral perspective.* New York: Guilford Press.

Vance, J. C., Fazan, L. E., Satterwhite, B., & Pless, I. B. (1980). Effects of nephrotic syndrome on the family: A controlled study. *Pediatrics, 65*, 948–955.

Venters, M. (1981). Familial coping with chronic and severe childhood illness: The case of cystic fibrosis. *Social Science & Medicine, 15,* 289–298.

Vincent, C. E. (1963). The family in health and illness. Some neglected areas. *Annals of the American Academy of Political and Social Sciences, 346,* 109–116.

Watzlawick, P., Beavin, J. H., & Jackson, D. C. (1967). *Pragmatics of human communication: A study of interactional patterns, pathologies, and paradoxes.* New York: Norton.

Wortman, C. B., & Dunkel-Schetter, C. (1979). Interpersonal relationships and cancer: A theoretical analysis. *Journal of Social Issues, 35,* 120–155.

Yorburg, B. (1975). The nuclear and the extended family: An area of conceptual confusion. *Journal of Comparative Family Studies, 6,* 6–13.

Young, R. F. (1983). The family-illness intermesh: Theoretical aspects and their application. *Social Science and Medicine, 17,* 395–398.

Zahn, M. A. (1973). Incapacity, impotence and invisible impairment: Their effects upon interpersonal relations. *Journal of Health and Social Behavior, 14,* 115–123.

2

Family Determinants of Children's Concepts of Health and Illness

David S. Gochman

Although strong consensus exists across behavioral and social science disciplines, and in the real world of lay persons as well, that the family is a major—perhaps *the* major—socializer of the child, the manner in which the family determines the child's concepts of health and illness remains virtually unexplored. Although it might be comfortably assumed that children's definitions of health and illness and their health-related beliefs, expectations, attitudes, and motives all reflect the impact of family characteristics, systematic research to date has been scanty. Relatively few scientifically sound reports are available, data are scarce, and appreciable bodies of knowledge have not accumulated in any area within this broad domain.

This chapter begins with some definitions and establishes the major focuses. It continues with an historical perspective, an examination of current knowledge, and an assessment of research and methodological issues, and concludes with a discussion of future directions for research.

THE DOMAIN

Children's Concepts of Health and Illness

The investigation of children's concepts of health and illness is a relatively new and emerging area. There is no abundance of clear-cut, agreed-upon definitions, or a history replete with definitional debate. The domain can be defined narrowly or broadly. Strict construction would limit consideration to how youngsters define health and illness, and to what they believe health and illness to mean, either in the abstract or in terms of their own lives and experiences. A broader construction would allow consideration of a variety of health-relevant concepts or cognitions including—but not limited to—youngsters' expectations about encountering health problems, their beliefs about how much control they have over their health, their reactions to illness experiences, their assessments of their own health status, and the value they attach to health. Such breadth is more appropriate for this chapter. It widens the still-limited range of research available for inclusion and provides a more representative view of research into children's concepts of health and illness. For convenience and simplicity these will be referred to as children's health concepts.

Family

In striking contrast, the domain of the family has long been subject to well-argued definitional analysis (e.g., Christensen, 1964a,b). Although research on the family's determination of children's health-relevant beliefs embraces multiple perspectives of what is meant by "family," the few studies of how families determine children's health concepts devote scant attention to definitional concerns. Instead, family factors are incorporated in varied ways. Some studies consider the family only insofar as it endows the child with socioeconomic status or with other social or demographic characteristics. Others examine relationships between the child's health concepts and characteristics of selected family members, for example, the mother or a sibling. Rarely is the family treated as an interactive entity or as a dynamic social group or system. Again, because available data are scarce, broad construction will better serve this chapter, and "family" will include any of these definitions or considerations.

Focus

This chapter is primarily concerned with the intersection of these two domains: (1) the relationships between family characteristics—whether these be solely demographic, or attributes of specific family members, or attributes of the family as an integral social group—and (2) children's health concepts—whether these be solely definitional, or more broadly construed. Because this intersection is represented by limited knowledge, some discussion will include research on children's health concepts where no family determinants were involved and research on family determinants of adult health concepts and behaviors where children have not been a focus. In this way, research and methodological issues and future directions can be better delineated.

Areas that will *not* be addressed are the family's contributions to children's health status, responses to treatment, overt compliance with, or acceptance of, medical regimens, and psychogenically determined illnesses.

HISTORICAL PERSPECTIVES

In such a young field of study, the distinction between "historical" and "current" is artificial. For convenience, however, this section will describe selected lines of research to provide relevant and representative background material.

The three major areas in this section are children's health concepts, the family and adult health behavior, and the family and children's health concepts. The next section will define what is currently known and not known.

Children's Health Concepts

The discussion of children's health concepts is organized topically rather than theoretically or conceptually. The topics, representing major lines of research, are beliefs about causes of illnesses, beliefs about hospitalization, beliefs about body parts, definitions of health and illness, perceived vulnerability to health problems, health motivation, beliefs about internal control, and socioeconomic effects.

Beliefs About Causes of Illnesses. Among the earliest studies of children's health concepts are those of Nagy (1951, 1953) who systematically explored beliefs about germs, contagion, and the causes of illness in samples of Hungarian, British, and American children in school settings. Using a variety of techniques, including having respondents draw pictures and write brief essays, and controlling comparisons appropriately, Nagy observed that beliefs about causes of illness changed with age: Very young respondents, those younger than five, seemed incapable of grasping the real origins of illness; those six and older appeared to be able to apply the concepts of infection with a precision that increased developmentally. Nagy's conclusions, however, are not based on statistical analysis.

Beliefs About Hospitalization.   Another early line of research, most of it based on case histories, were the psychoanalytically oriented observations of hospitalized children. This literature suggests that children's beliefs and perceptions about their illnesses and conditions, and about the medical and surgical procedures to which they were subjected, were markedly different from those of adults (e.g., Chapman, Loeb, & Gibbons, 1956; Deutsch, 1942). Children often view hospitalization as reflecting rejection, abandonment, and/or punishment (e.g., Jessner, Blom, & Waldfogel, 1952; Vernon, Foley, Sipowicz, & Schulman, 1965, chap. 8).

Beliefs About Body Parts.   Gellert (1962, 1978), noting the dearth of investigations of how children view their bodies, devised a standardized questionnaire technique, the Gellert Index of Body Knowledge, to explore this area rigorously and systematically. In a pilot study based on individual interviews of 96 youngsters ranging in age from four years and nine months to 16 years and 11 months—all but four of whom were hospitalized—Gellert (1962, p. 387) observed certain tentative developmental trends. As children grow older, their reality orientation predictably increases and they acquire more valid, more accurate notions of how their bodies and component organs function. More important, from a theoretical perspective, Gellert observed that egocentrism and concreteness tended to be more characteristic of the way in which younger children—in contrast to older ones—viewed their bodies. Older children tended to demonstrate greater degrees of articulation of parts of the various body systems and increased conceptions of permanent as opposed to fluid structures (e.g., materials ingested or egested) than did younger ones. Gellert noted the congruence between these observations and a Piagetian conception of development. Moreover, Gellert's (1962) data suggest that the modal age for "correct"—or adult-type responses—was either nine to ten or 11 to 12. Such data are considered "strong evidence that knowledge about the body increases sharply around the age of 9 years." (p. 388) Gellert's thorough presentation of data did not, however, include systematic statistical analyses of these developmental changes. The trends are inferred from tabular presentation of percentages.

Definitions of Health and Illness.   Complementing these studies of children's concepts of their bodies and of the disease process is Rashkis' (1965) work on children's conceptions of health and of the correlates of these conceptions. Based on play-period interviews with 54 elementary schoolchildren, ranging in age from four years nine months to eight years nine months and representing a wide range of socioeconomic backgrounds, Rashkis' data revealed, among other findings, that although the modal response to the question "What is it like to be well?" was "Not sick," there were no statistically significant differences between this and other responses for the total sample. However, there were statistically significant grade-related differences in the frequency of *pleasant* responses in that older youngsters more often than younger ones equated being well with positive, pleasant states. Younger ones more than older ones tended to respond either that they did not know or in terms of not being sick. Rashkis interprets these and other observations as reflecting the inability of younger children, that is, those below age seven, to integrate their health-related feelings and experiences into a clear, conscious conception of health as a positive state. At all grade levels, youngsters reveal an awareness that personal and social factors set limits upon maintaining health, that other persons have the ability to keep the children healthy, and that actions undertaken by others in relation to the youngster's health were more likely to be protections against illness than acts of physical care. Furthermore, although the study did not relate family factors to how health is defined, it did reveal that physicians, more so than family members, are more likely to be seen as the persons responsible for health. This difference was statistically significant among the oldest subjects and increasing confidence in physicians was directly and significantly related to age. Regardless of whether physicians or parents (who mediate the interaction with the physicians) are responsible, Rashkis' data support the view that the child maintains a protective image of adults, which is interpreted as a generalized expectancy arising from the child's continued positive contact with parents.

In similar fashion, Natapoff's (1978) study of first, fourth, and seventh graders, who represented a variety of socioeconomic backgrounds, demonstrated that in general youngsters primarily equated being healthy with—in order of preference—feeling good, their ability to do things they wanted to do, and not being sick. They were least likely to equate being healthy with being happy or having a strong body. They equated not being healthy with being sick and not being able to do things. Natapoff interprets age–group data as suggesting that older children demonstrate greater analytic processes, greater levels of abstraction in their thinking, and greater ability to see part–whole relationships than do younger ones. Natapoff (1982) uses Piagetian developmental stages to interpret these and other relevant data: Children's health concepts move from the preoperational, egocentric, syncretistic functioning of those younger than seven or eight, through the concrete operational functioning of the eight-to-ten-year-olds, to the formal operational functioning of those older than ten.

Simeonsson, Buckley, and Monson (1979) report similar findings in their study of conceptions of health and illness from a Piagetian perspective in a group of 60 hospitalized youngsters aged four through nine.

Perceived Vulnerability to Health Problems. The observations of youngsters' beliefs that there are limiting conditions to health maintenance (Rashkis, 1965) are especially relevant to research dealing with youngsters' perceptions of vulnerability to health problems, much of which is derived from the health-belief model (e.g., Becker, 1974; Maiman & Becker, 1974; Rosenstock, 1974). In an essentially cognitive paradigm, the model postulated—in its original form—that perceptions of being susceptible to some condition, the perceived severity of that condition, and perceptions of the availability of behaviors that prevent or treat the condition are all positively related to the likelihood that a person will engage in some specific preventive health behavior. According to Green (1974), reference is made to this model in "virtually every dissertation related to health behavior." (p. 324)

Guided by the model, Gochman developed a series of studies of perceived susceptibility in young populations (e.g., Gochman, 1970a, 1971a, 1972a, 1977, 1981a,b). Youngsters in varied settings—scout troops, YW-YMCA activities, a summer camp, and classrooms in a large, industrial city—were asked a series of questions about the likelihood of their encountering selected health problems. Samples ranged in size from 108 to 686. In the original form of the health-belief model, perceived susceptibility dealt with beliefs or expectancies about a single health problem. Gochman's work expanded this to reflect the degree to which children believe or expect they are likely to encounter a variety of health problems, illnesses, or accidents. The term *perceived vulnerability* was used to designate this broader, more general concept. In its final form, the Gochman Perceived Vulnerability Scale is made up of 15 items. The question form is "What chance is there of your getting the flu during this next year"? And the responses are "no chance," "almost no chance," "a small chance," "a medium chance," "a good chance," "almost certain," and "certain," scored from one to seven. The other 14 health problem expectancies are a bad accident, a rash, a fever, having a tooth pulled, a sore throat, a toothache, a cold, bleeding gums, an upset stomach, missing a week of school because of sickness, a cavity, a bad headache, breaking or cracking a tooth, and cutting a finger accidentally.

Repeated analyses have shown perceived vulnerability to be consistent within individuals as well as across groups of individuals. Youngsters who have relatively high (low) expectations of encountering one health problem usually have relatively high (low) expectations of encountering others (e.g., Gochman, 1970a, 1971a; Gochman, Bagramian, & Sheiham, 1972; Gochman & Saucier, 1982). Moreover, regardless of age, sex, socioeconomic status, race, or nationality, the ranking of mean expectancy scores for each health problem across several demographic subgroups remains relatively invariant (e.g., Gochman, 1970a, 1971a; Gochman, Bagramian, & Sheiham, 1972; Gochman & Sheiham, 1978).

Although perceived vulnerability demonstrates some significant linkage to age, its developmental changes are complexly mediated by sex and socioeconomic levels (e.g., Gochman, 1972, 1981a; Gochman & Saucier, 1982). Moreover, although perceived vulnerability increases between ages eight and 13 and decreases after that, the mean values for all ages—eight to 15 and older—hover fairly close to "4," the midpoint of the scale, a point of neutrality. Children and young adults do not perceive themselves to be generally vulnerable to health problems. In natural environments where no specific attempts are made to alter them, these beliefs do not change appreciably by themselves (Gochman, 1981a).

Perceived vulnerability thus emerges as a stable, consistent personality characteristic. Evidence shows it to be negatively related to self-concept or self-esteem (e.g., Gochman, 1977; Gochman & Saucier, 1982); more closely related to self-concept than to prior traumatic experiences (Gochman, 1977); and directly related to anxiety (Gochman & Saucier, 1982). To date, perceived vulnerability perhaps remains the most systematically examined health concept in young populations. However, its origins in family, peer, media, and experiential factors remain to be studied.

Health Motivation. Concomitant with studying perceived vulnerability, Gochman explored health-related motivation in youngsters. From pictorial tasks, for example, the Health Ideation Pictures (Gochman, 1970b) and the Mouth-Appearance Pictures (e.g., Gochman, 192b, 1975, 1982a) evidence accrued that health in itself is not an especially important motive, value, or priority for youngsters, except for those younger than nine. The strength of health as a motive, in relation to appearance or cosmetic concerns, decreases markedly between ages eight and 15 (Gochman, 1975, 1982a). Admittedly, this measure is an exceptionally simple one in relation to the complexity of the full range of human motives. Comparisons of the strength of health with other motives have not been made, and the possibility exists that the observed relative weakness of health as a motive, as well as its development decrease, may not generalize to other comparisons. As is true of perceived vulnerability, the origins of health-germane motivation remain unexplored.

Beliefs About Control. An alternative frame of reference for understanding children's health beliefs—beliefs about internal versus external locus of controls—derives from Rotter's social learning theory (e.g., Wallston & Wallston, 1978). Beliefs about internal control are considered important precursors of a person's estimate of the likelihood that a given behavior will have a given outcome. Parcel and Meyer (1978) have developed a reliable, internally consistent instrument to assess health locus of control in children. Their measure, the Children's Health Locus of Control Scale, correlates appreciably with the Nowicki–Strickland Children's Locus of Control Scale. Its items cluster heavily around three major factors: (1) a powerful others control subscale; (2) an internal control subscale; and (3) a chance control subscale.

The measure is currently being used to determine the impact of health education interventions on preschoolers (Bruhn & Parcel, 1982b), but the results and other correlates of the scale and subscales have not yet entered the literature. Additional use of this instrument may facilitate research into the formation and development of children's health concepts and the manner in which family factors determine these.

Socioeconomic Effects.   In analyses of socioeconomic effects upon health concepts, researchers observed that in youngsters younger than 12 socioeconomic status was directly related to levels of perceived vulnerability and inversely related to levels of health motivation (Gochman, 1975, 1981a; Gochman & Saucier, 1982). Youngsters under 12 from inner city neighborhoods or from areas with relatively low levels of parental income and education had lower levels of perceived vulnerability and higher levels of health motivation than did their counterparts in suburban neighborhoods or areas with higher levels of parental income and education. However, despite assumptions made about the potency of socioeconomic status, no such differences were observed for youngsters 12 and older. Moreover, socioeconomic effects were not readily found for other health concepts such as beliefs about the health benefits of selected health actions (Gochman, 1984). This raises a question about the overall importance of socioeconomic factors as determinants of children's health concepts. To the degree that socialization within the family reflects socioeconomic status, where such status is not a determinant of children's health concepts, it follows that differential family effects are less likely to be found.

Family Structure and Health

The relationships between the family and health are discussed in terms of the following approaches: cosmopolitanism-parochialism, social integration, and the "energized" family.

Cosmopolitanism-Parochialism.   A seminal work on social organization, family structure and personal health, and medical orientations was Suchman's (1965) large-scale attempt to show how the patterns by which families link to their community, organize their social life, and observe traditional authority are related to the medical beliefs of family members. In a random sample of 1883 adults in the Washington Heights section of New York City, Suchman observed that a "parochial" group structure—defined as a constellation of high levels of ethnic exclusivity, friendship solidarity, and adherence to custom and traditional male authority within the family—was associated with (1) nonscientific or "popular" health orientations as exemplified by lower levels of medical or health knowledge; (2) greater skepticism about medical care; and (3) greater dependency in illness. Conversely, "cosmopolitanism"—reflecting lower levels of ethnic exclusivity, friendship solidarity, and adherence to tradition and authority—was associated with (1) a scientific or technological medical orientation as exemplified by greater medical knowledge; (2) less skepticism about medical care; and (3) less dependency in illness. Suchman further observed that the three components within both the cosmopolitan-parochial and the lay-scientific medical orientations were empirically interrelated, and that relationships between cosmopolitanism-parochialism and individual medical orientations were held independently of socioeconomic status, even though socioeconomic status was clearly related to cosmopolitanism-parochialism.

Geertsen, Klauber, Rindflesh, Kane, and Gray (1978) attempted to replicate Suchman's work on a comparable sample of Mormons in Salt Lake City. The data revealed that neither cosmopolitanism-parochialism nor lay-scientific medical orientations were empirically unified dimensions. Furthermore, the components of the former did not predict the latter in the manner observed by Suchman. For example, high adherence to family authority and strong friendship solidarity were related to greater medical knowledge as well as to low skepticism; ethnic exclusivity was not related to any of the medical orientation components. Geertsen and his colleagues thus take issue with the generalizability of Suchman's findings and explanations. They propose an alternative model that identifies the family as the key social group in determining health beliefs and practices and that also further takes into account an understanding of cultural and subcultural beliefs.

Social Integration. Moody and Gray (1972) additionally articulated concepts related to those that Suchman investigated, and observed in a sample of 959 mothers that social integration—measured in terms of both social participation and alienation scales—was a better predictor of engaging in a preventive health behavior (acceptance of oral polio vaccine) than was socioeconomic status. Mothers who were involved to a greater degree in voluntary community activities, and who did not feel socially isolated, were more likely to accept the polio vaccine than those who participated less in community activities and who felt socially isolated. Socioeconomic status did not prove to be an independent predictor of preventive behaviors when the effects of social participation and alienation were controlled.

The "Energized" Family. A final paradigm linking family structure and health is that proposed by Pratt (e.g., 1973, 1976). Pratt's model deals with the degree to which families are "energized," that is, the degree to which their "members interact with each other regularly in a variety of contexts . . . maintain varied and active contacts with other groups and organizations . . . to advance family members' interests . . . attempt to cope and master their lives. . . . The energized family tends to be fluid in internal organization. Role relationships are flexible. . . . Power is shared. . . . Relationships among members tend to support personal growth and to be responsive and tolerant. Members have a high degree of autonomy within the family" (Pratt, 1976, pp. 3–4).

In what must be considered a pioneer study of the effects of methods of socialization on children's health behavior, Pratt (1973) observed, for example, that parents' use of "developmental" methods of child rearing (implicit in the concept of the energized family)—by emphasizing rewards for good behavior, using reasons and explanations, and the granting of autonomy—was associated with a greater level of desirable health behavior among children (personal cleanliness, dental care, and/or regularity of elimination) than using traditional disciplinary methods based on punishment, lack of instructions, and attempts to retain control over the child. Pratt noted that the granting of autonomy was the most important of these predictors. Among numerous findings Pratt (1976) further observed, for example, that sound health practices within the family were related to regular interaction between husband and wife, between parents and child (p. 93), and to the extent in which the family participated in social and community activities (p. 95) and also to the flexibility and egalitarianism in roles and power (p. 95).

Family and Children's Health Concepts

Although the preceding discussion provides a perspective on the two major focal points of this chapter, it becomes clear that the major lines of research in each domain do not systematically embrace one another. There are, however, some studies that do. These include analyses of determinants of beliefs about hospitalization, maternal characteristics, parental health beliefs, and sibling effects.

Maternal Characteristics.   Jessner's, Blom's, and Woldfogel's (1952) psychoanalytically derived assessments of children's responses to surgery suggest that maternal anxiety is imparted to the child and that hostile or ambivalent parent–child relationships lead the child to equate hospitalization and surgery with being sent away or punished. Such intriguing data are, however, empirically soft.

In a more rigorous study of 350 mother–child pairs representing varied backgrounds, Mechanic (1964) attempted to relate maternal characteristics to youngsters' willingness to report symptoms, risk-taking attitudes, views of their own health, attitudes about the denial of pain, and perceptions of when a physician is necessary. According to Mechanic, the data showed few relationships. Very little of the variance in the children's responses could be explained by the maternal characteristics studied—the interests she had in her child's symptoms and the degree to which she responded attentively to these. Sixteen years later, in a follow-up study of 91% of these youngsters to identify educational variables associated with health behaviors, Mechanic (1980) further noted that maternal education did not contribute to predicting health behaviors when the respondent's own education and degrees of perceived parental interest were examined and controlled.

Congruent with this observed absence of an appreciable number of meaningful relationships between maternal characteristics and children's health-related concepts, Campbell's (1975a,b, 1978) study of 264 hospitalized children revealed that maternal judgments of whether specific symptoms were signs of illness were not significant predictors of their children's judgments about these symptoms (1975a), and that a mother's general tendency to attribute illness either to herself or to her children was not significantly predictive of the child's general tendency to attribute illness (1975a). On the other hand, Campbell (1978) did observe that some of a family's demographic characteristics—maternal education and paternal socioeconomic status (based on education and occupation)—were related to children's reports of their conceptions of sick role. Children whose mothers had higher levels of education tended to be stoic and less emotional about illness than children whose mothers were not well educated, but these relationships were mediated by the child's age and gender. Maternal education and paternal socioeconomic status were both observed to be positively related to a child's likelihood of rejecting sick role. Other family characteristics such as maternal religious affiliation and the degree of maternal employment were less clearly related to the child's conception of the sick role.

More important were Campbell's (1978) observations that maternal values of self-direction versus conformity and self-assertiveness versus attentiveness to others interacted significantly with the child's age in determining aspects of the child's conception of sick role. For example, only among older children was the degree to which mothers valued self-direction in the child negatively related to the degree to which the children perceived themselves to be emotional in sick role; the degree to which mothers valued attentiveness to others in the child was tied to the child's tendency to reject the sick role; and both of these maternal values were related to the child's initiation of sick-role identification.

Because so few studies have been conducted relating maternal characteristics to children's health concepts, it is difficult to weave these fragmented findings into unequivocal, convincing conclusions. Although maternal education does seem to offer some promise as a predictor of some health concepts, further research is necessary to clarify its role and how its effects are mediated and obtained.

Parental Health Beliefs.   Dielman, Leech, Becker, Rosenstock, and Horvath (1982), noting that attempts to relate parental and youngsters' health beliefs and behaviors have been "relatively rare," systematically investigated the way in which parental beliefs about susceptibility to illness and other characteristics were related to children's beliefs. Their data did not show any strong convincing relationships: "Child health beliefs are scarcely influenced by parental characteristics." (p. 63)

Sibling Effects. Focusing on sibling influences rather than on parental ones and employing both a "systems" and a Piagetian framework, Caradang, Folkins, Hines, and Steward (1979), in a well-controlled study of 36 siblings of diabetics and 36 comparison subjects, noted that the presumed stress of dealing with a sibling's illness was reflected in decreased ability to conceptualize the causes and treatment of illness at the same level of cognitive maturity demonstrated by those who presumably are not faced with such stress.

CURRENT STATE OF KNOWLEDGE

Reviews of the developmental literature (Kalnins & Love, 1982; Natapoff, 1982) report convergent, consistent findings for the small number of health concepts investigated. As children grow older, beliefs about health and illness become less concrete and more abstract (e.g., Campbell, 1975a,b, 1978); less egocentric (e.g., Natapoff, 1978); less likely to be solely determined by external cues or the responses of others (e.g., Neuhauser, Amsterdam, Hines, & Steward, 1978); less likely to overgeneralize the concept of contagion and employ concepts of immanent justice (e.g., Kister & Patterson, 1980); increasingly differentiated (e.g., Gochman, 1971c, 1972a); and increasingly consistent (e.g., Gochman, 1971a). These findings are interpretable through either a Piagetian or a Lewinian developmental perspective; they do not differentially support one over the other. The results are congruent in large measure with both.

Despite these inferences, most available evidence suggests that youngsters' health concepts can be seen as relatively stable. Although levels of health knowledge and understanding about health, illness, and medicine predictably increase with age and general cognitive development, appreciable changes of a more "psychological" nature, that is, changes in attitudes, perceptions, beliefs (of course, one can claim that "factual knowledge" itself represents a set of beliefs), and expectations are not readily observed. With the exception of dramatic developmental decreases in health motivation in relation to appearance motivation (Gochman, 1975, 1982a), available data—limited as they may be—about other beliefs, such as perceptions of the health benefits of dental visits and brushing teeth and attitudes toward prevention, do not show clear-cut developmental progressions. Developmental changes are often either nonlinear, nonexistent, nondescribable, or appreciably modified by sex and socioeconomic factors (Gochman, 1984). Even the statistically significant changes that occur in perceived vulnerability are nonlinear and nonappreciable (Gochman, 1972a, 1981a; Gochman & Saucier, 1982). Furthermore, Stone (1976) has demonstrated the difficulty of modifying children's levels of perceived vulnerability. Thus children's health concepts often show a natural "conservatism." They may, in large measure, be part of what Rokeach (1960) terms a person's central, "primitive" belief system, that is, beliefs that are established very early in life, are markedly stable and highly unlikely to change in later childhood or adulthood. If health concepts are truly stable during childhood, a relevant question then is "To what degree do family influences engender such stability?"

In addition, very little is known about health-germane motivation. Broadly defined, this includes all motives or values that foster health behaviors, not only health per se, as a motive or value. Apparently no studies have examined how family factors generate any such motivation.

Furthermore, with few exceptions (e.g., Gochman, 1977), very little is known about how children's health concepts are related to one another, and whether family factors determine the nature of these relationships.

Where developmental changes in selected concepts of health and illness are observable, the determinants of these concepts and their development remain unknown. A clear consensus emerges from literature reviews (Blos, 1978; Kalnins & Love, 1982; Natapoff, 1982), state-of-the-art conferences (Bruhn, Williams, & Fitzsimmons, 1980; Bruhn & Parcel, 1982a), and a special state-of-the-art volume of *Health Education Quarterly* devoted to children's health beliefs and health behavior (Gochman & Parcel, 1982): Children's concepts of health and illness have been rarely studied in rigorous fashion, and there is a dearth of research in this increasingly important area. Blos (1978) in examining the more abundant literature on the emotional effect of hospitalization, surgery, and chronic illness reports that cognitive research—research on children's knowledge and concepts about their bodies and illness—"is sparse and hard to find" (p. 2); and that "children's health beliefs and their development have rarely been studied" (p. 6). Kalnins and Love (1982) in reviewing the literature on children's concepts of health and illness assert that there is "a dearth of knowledge about what children really think about *health*, how they perceive the relationship between health and illness, and their own role in maintaining health" (p. 18).

Moreover, there is currently little convincing evidence of large-scale, important relationships between the family and children's health beliefs. A variety of research and methodological issues must be confronted and resolved before more conclusive, comprehensive relationships can be either definitively established or categorically denied. It remains for future research to accomplish this. For the present the few studies that attempt to generate such data deal with relatively small segments of the family, and these attempts do not yet yield strong support for relationships between these two domains.

Possibly, the failure to observe such relationships is attributable to the stability—and thus lack of variability of the health concepts. If exploration of a wider range of health concepts coupled with increased precision in measurement demonstrates that this stability is more apparent than real, family determinants may be more readily found.

From available data, the *possibility* must be entertained—despite deeply held assumptions to the contrary—that family factors may *not* be primary determinants of children's health concepts. Current knowledge, approaches, and methods do not themselves encourage optimism about establishing an appreciable number of such determinants in the near future.

RESEARCH AND METHODOLOGICAL ISSUES

The difference between research issues and methodological ones is difficult to establish. At the risk of appearing arbitrary, however, these issues are clustered under two rubrics: (1) the former comprising issues related to theories, concepts, and research perspectives and (2) the latter comprising issues of specific procedures for deriving empirical data and for increasing external validity or generalizability.

Research Issues

The two major research issues that must be addressed in the continued exploration of how, and in what way, families determine children's concepts of health and illness are conceptual clarity and theoretical alternatives.

Conceptual Clarity.   There is urgent need for increased conceptual clarity. Few of the studies have systematically derived their variables from carefully constructed theoretical concepts. There are virtually no instances— Pratt's work (1976) being a rare exception—where the concept of "family" received careful theoretical elaboration and where "family" is used to refer to more than selected personal characteristics of individual members. Although there is no consensus that any one model of the family is the single most appropriate one, such agreement is not a prerequisite for increasing conceptual clarity. Researchers can select among several theoretical models. They can choose to focus, for example, on the family as a set of roles and role relations, a pattern of communication and interaction, a socializing agent, a source of modeling effects for social learning, a social system, a reflection of broader societal and cultural institutions, a socioeconomic unit that locates its members within a stratification system, a linkage between its members and the larger community, a social grouping that experiences developmental changes, or combinations of these.

Regardless, the definition must be clearly made and the family must be studied as an integral unit, not simply as the discrete characteristics of some of its members. The concept of the family must not be thought of only in terms of parental influences upon the child, but it must also embrace siblings and must allow for multilateral influences. Siblings must be studied as important components in the formation of health-related concepts (Caradang, Folkins, & Steward, 1979). Adolescent family members have roles as potential gatekeepers of health information and thus as determinants of health education and of health-related decision making within families (Nader et al., 1982). Viewing youngsters as agents of change suggests that reciprocity may exist in the formulation of health-related concepts and that the role of the younger generation as determinants of parental conceptual systems might be worth exploring.

Closely related is the need for increased conceptual clarity about what is meant by beliefs about health and illness. A task force on children's health concepts (Bruhn & Parcel, 1982a) reports that "In the entire area of cognitive systems, concepts need to be sharper and clearer and they need to be integrated with theory" (p. 151).

With few exceptions (e.g., Campbell, 1975a, Gochman, 1971c; Neuhauser, Amsterdam, Hines, & Steward, 1978; Simeonsson, Buckley, & Monson, 1979), as Bibace and Walsh (1981) and Crider (1981) note, research on children's health concepts has not been systematically derived from theoretical models of development. The potential breadth of this area must be recognized. It represents the varied way in which youngsters (and adults as well) relate themselves to the manifold dimensions of health (and/or illness) that impinge upon them. In abstracting further from Bruhn and Parcel (1982a), concepts of health and illness can be seen to embrace what persons know as well as how they organize this knowledge; how they evaluate health, that is, their attitudes, values, and their feelings about health; their health-related beliefs (whether veridical or not) and the organizational structure of these beliefs; their body images; and how they process and/or deal with health-relevant stimuli or data (Bruhn & Parcel, 1982a, pp. 149–153). Variables within this broad range should be clearly defined conceptually in addition to being capable of being measured operationally, and—to the degree possible—clearly and systematically related to some theory, model, or paradigm. In this way there would be hope for meaningful comparisons between, and replications of, findings. Currently, different researchers may use a single term, such as perceived vulnerability, to refer to entirely different concepts (e.g., Gochman, 1977; Lewis & Lewis, 1982).

Moreover, increased conceptual clarity would vitiate tendencies to fuse concepts inappropriately. The original health-belief model, for example, imputed motivational characteristics to high levels of perceived susceptibility and perceived severity together with perceptions of available actions or benefits (Maiman & Becker, 1974; Rosenstock, 1974). This equated expectations, beliefs, and perceptions with motivation. Motivation has a well-defined place in psychological theory (e.g., Birney, 1968; O'Kelly, 1968). It implies priorities that energize and organize behaviors. Research that measured health motivation and perceived vulnerability separately (e.g., Gochman, 1972b, 1977) has shown them to be empirically independent. Such data support the position that motivation is not to be inferred from other cognitions. Motives are distinctly different psychological characteristics. Confusing such characteristics presents problems for research development as well as for health professionals who inappropriately assume that target populations possess selected psychological characteristics.

Factor analysis may have some value in developing such clarification. Parcel and Meyer's (1978) factor analysis of the Children's Health Locus of Control Scale suggests that the locus of control concept is multidimensional. Children's general beliefs about the degree to which they exercise control over their own health are not unequivocally or linearly related to their beliefs that health and illness are determined by luck or chance, or to their beliefs that powerful agents such as physicians and nurses determine health and illness outcomes. Such findings augment understanding of what "locus of control" means in young populations, have the potential to increase the precision with which the concept is used, and offer opportunities to develop and test differential predictions for the three subscales.

Dielman, Leech, Becker, Rosenstock, and Horvath's (1980) factor analysis of an assortment of health beliefs demonstrates that items that assess perceived susceptibility (vulnerability) to specific conditions (e.g., "How much of a chance do you think there is—in the next few months—that you might have a pain in your stomach?") are factorially distinct from those that assess general and specific health concerns (e.g., "When you are sick, how much do you worry about it?"). Such findings strengthen the position that perceived susceptibility (vulnerability) is distinct from worry about health or appraisals of health status, measures of which have at times been used as indices of perceived susceptibility (e.g., Lewis & Lewis, 1982). Although Dielman, Leech, Becker, Rosenstock, and Horvath (1980) also suggest that perceived susceptibility itself may not be unidimensional, the final factor structure that they present does not argue convincingly for this multidimensionality. The susceptibility items appear to load on three factors: (1) perceived susceptibility—specific conditions; (2) perceived seriousness of and susceptibility to disease; and (3) perceived susceptibility—general; however, several of the items load nearly equally well on two of the three, thus diminishing the clarity of the proposed distinctiveness of the three factors. Similar careful analyses of larger amounts of conceptually derived responses should facilitate the clarification process.

Concomitant with increasing the conceptual clarity of both of the major domains under discussion is the need to apply increasing conceptual rigor to the socioenvironmental arena in which children's health concepts develop. Typical research that equates socioeconomic status with selected income and educational variables must be augmented by research that more comprehensively describes "class." Wright and Wright (1976), who elaborate on Kohn's refinement of class concepts, provide evidence that nonclass variables such as region, religion, and ethnicity are significant contributors to the prediction of personal values. There is, they assert, a need "to provide a conceptual model within which . . . nonclass effects are plausible. . . . It is not likely that our understanding of parental values will progress very far . . . until these tasks are accomplished" (p. 536).

Theoretical Alternatives. Although the health-belief model provides a highly productive theoretical formulation for the continued derivation of research, it is itself not a theory of psychological development. Alternative paradigms are needed. Piagetian and Lewinian models of cognitive development and social learning theory offer promise for future progress in the field. In addition, the cyclically emergent derivatives of Heider's (1958) balance theory such as attribution theory (Kelley, 1967) or behavioral intention theory (Fishbein & Ajzen, 1975) might prove to be productive.

Attribution theory "refers to the process of inferring or perceiving the dispositional properties of entities in the environment" (Kelley, 1967, p. 193). In allowing for "the allocation of causality between the environment and the self" (p. 196), it relates attribution of validity to information received from other persons to perceptions of these sources. In the area of children's health beliefs, attribution theory could offer a way of making predictions about the acceptability of health education programs and health-related messages from health professionals as well as from significant others, and ultimately about the changes in, or acquisitions of, health concepts.

Behavioral intention theory identifies the intention to engage in a specified behavior as the best predictor of a person's behavior (Fishbein & Ajzen, 1975, pp. 381–382). If interest in children's health concepts reflects a more ultimate interest in more overt health behavior or health action, then behavioral intention theory would urge that researchers investigate youngsters' intentions to engage in selected health and safety behaviors, and the theory provides models for doing this. Family factors ought then to be investigated as antecedents of these attributions and intentions.

Further elaboration of the linkages between beliefs and behaviors is also necessary. Weisenberg, Kegeles, and Lund (1980), summarizing the accumulated literature, conclude that causal relationships between beliefs and behaviors are "still cloudy." In a pioneer prospective study, investigating how youngsters' levels of perceived vulnerability were related to their acceptance of a preventive dental activity (mouth rinsing), they observed that perceived vulnerability was *inversely* related to acceptance of the activity. Weisenberg et al.'s suggestion that both beliefs and behaviors may reflect other independent factors in the child's experience, and different learning processes as well, cautions against simplistic interpretations of correlational linkages between them. These data and conclusions are congruent with the position that perceived vulnerability may have anxiety components (Gochman, 1981b; Gochman & Saucier, 1982) that reflect both cognitive and affective characteristics.

Crider (1981) in addressing children's concepts about parts of their bodies raises questions about whether cognitive development occurs at the same rate in relation to different parts. One might infer that cognitive development—whether considered in terms of Piagetian operations or Lewinian differentiation—might occur at different rates for different sets of health-related concepts.

Further development and clarification of theory is equally a prerequisite for identifying those family characteristics offering the greatest promise for increasing knowledge and understanding of children's health concepts (Bruhn & Parcel, 1982a, p. 148). A need also exists to develop and refine a theoretical model that would embrace both the child's concepts and the antecedent family characteristics that are likely to be determinants of these. Systems theory (e.g., Bertalanffy, 1950; Weiss, 1939) may offer one such alternative.

The existing paucity of data coupled with the lack of both conceptual clarity and articulated theory suggest that a major broad and innovative theoretical breakthrough may be somewhat distant. For the moment increasing conceptual clarity and rigorously obtaining larger amounts of data relevant to these concepts may be sufficient substitutes.

Methodological Issues

Three major methodological issues that underlie research into family determinants of children's health-related concepts are measurement, data bases, and procedures.

Measurement Issues.   Parallel with the absence of rigorously and clearly defined concepts is the lack of systematically and coherently derived measuring instruments. In both the domain of children's health concepts and the domain of the family, adequate measurement is a serious problem (e.g., Bruhn et al., 1980, p. 73; Bruhn & Parcel, 1982a, p. 151). Researchers have noted (Bruhn & Parcel, 1982a) that although some measures of children's health-related concepts are becoming more widely used and recognized, for example, the Gochman (1977) scale of perceived vulnerability and the (Parcel & Meyer, 1978) scale for health locus of control, there is an urgent need to develop new and improved measures. Additionally, in the area of the family, although some self-report and observational techniques can be identified, "the measurement of family interaction and other aspects of family functioning, however, is as yet in its infancy. . ." (Bruhn & Parcel, 1982a, p. 148).

Evidence that health problem expectancies are relatively stable and organized by age eight or so (Gochman, 1971a, 1981a) points critically to the importance of studying younger, preschool populations to increase understanding of the way in which these concepts emerge. It is likely during these formative years that family factors are themselves the most appreciable. Innovative, creative measures that would assess health-related concepts in children as young as two or three are thus particularly needed. Pictorial, manipulative, play and other approaches that minimize oral and verbal skills are also particularly needed.

The availability of improved and more precise measures at all ages further increases the chance of observing real developmental changes in children's health concepts that have previously gone undetected, which thus increases the likelihood that real family determinants of these changes will themselves be discovered.

Finally, if these measures are ultimately to achieve respectability in terms of construct validity, their development must proceed in tandem with the development of conceptual clarity.

Data Bases. Increased understanding of the relationships between family factors and children's health concepts ultimately requires an expanded data base. Research designs must be elaborated to go beyond readily available, sometimes-captive populations with the limits these place on generalizability. Obviously, there is a need to increase the age range studied. With the emergence of new measures, the responses of increasingly younger children could be incorporated into the body of available knowledge.

The importance of examining family life cycle in relation to health behaviors and decision making has already been demonstrated (Schafer & Keith, 1981). It is necessary to study a variety of health-related concepts throughout the life cycle—in late adolescence, early adulthood, middle years, and the years of increasing maturity—to determine whether, and in what way, they are linked to family factors. Such data would reveal the degree to which the family determinants interact with age, and might indicate when family factors are most potent.

Heterogeneity of social background and ethnic diversity must also be explored systematically. Although evidence exists that socioeconomic status by itself is not a significant determinant of selected health-related cognitions in older children (e.g., Gochman, 1972a, 1975, 1981a), there is a need to design studies to explore the relationships between family factors and children's health concepts while systematically controlling for a range of well-defined socioeconomic and sociocultural contexts.

It is additionally important to control health status and health history in the youngsters themselves and within their families. Although Brodie's (1974) work suggests that healthy children view illness differently from the way ill, hospitalized children do, very little research has attempted to compare, in some controlled way, the health beliefs of healthy and nonhealthy youngsters. The role played by health history or health status in the emergence of these concepts is ambiguous (e.g., Gochman, 1971b).

Procedural Issues. It is a truism that the study of factors that determine development requires combinations of cross-sectional and longitudinal procedures. Although cross-sectional research may itself be costly and time consuming if thoroughly conceptualized, properly conducted, and rigorously analyzed, the problems it presents are minimal compared with those of longitudinal study. There are many problems inherent in longitudinal research regardless of the topic. In a mobile society it is difficult—and sometimes impossible—to follow large numbers of intact families over a period of five to ten years. Even where previously stable target populations are identified, longitudinal study may encounter unforeseen problems, for example, when new school construction causes a redrafting of school districts (e.g., Gochman, 1981a) or when industries close. Furthermore, since the late 1960s, funding sources have become increasingly reluctant to make the commitment to underwrite long-term projects.

More specific to research in the domain under discussion are procedural problems arising from the source of data. More often than not, as Gorton, Doerfler, Hulka, and Tyroler (1979) observe, data relating to family determinants of children's health concepts are obtained from the mother. Gorton et al. demonstrate that when responses of family members about their perceptions of symptoms and their perceptions of relationships between these symptoms were obtained independently, the children's responses showed greater similarity to their fathers than to their mothers. Inferences are made that the father may be becoming a more critical role model for health-related behaviors and that maternally provided data that show contrary findings may reflect the bias of the mother's own perceptions. Such evidence raises important questions about the reliability of maternal reports about a family's health-related behaviors—of which health concepts are important components. Study designs that incorporate responses obtained independently from all family members, as Gorton and her colleagues (1979) have done, are a way of assuring against such bias. Perhaps as child-rearing and home-focused activities become more equally shared by women and men, the choice of the mother as a respondent simply because she is more generally available to interviewers during traditional work hours will become less habitual.

FUTURE DIRECTIONS

The directions of future activity in this area cannot be predicted with any certainty. But three frames of reference might lead to more fruitful and meaningful research: (1) a definition of health behavior, (2) systemic models, and (3) demedicalization and wellness.

Health Behavior

A Working Definition. The codifying of "behavioral medicine" (Schwartz & Weiss, 1978) and its now increased visibility have been exceptionally important steps in addressing health problems, and in reinforcing the ties between medicine and its technology on the one hand and knowledge and research methods from the social and behavioral sciences on the other. The findings emanating from behavioral medicine research are being in large measure translated into newer approaches to alleviate disorders. Behavioral medicine by itself is only one frame of reference relevant to the health area.

However, a definition more relevant to research in the area of the family's and children's health-related concepts is that proposed for health behavior. As a working definition, "health behavior" substantively denotes "those personal attributes such as beliefs, expectations, motives, values, and other cognitive elements; personality characteristics, including affective and emotional states and traits; and overt behavior patterns, actions, and habits that relate to health maintenance and wellness, to health restoration and to health improvement." (Gochman, 1982b, p. 169) The definition further denotes "that these personal attributes are influenced by, and otherwise reflect family structure and processes, peer group and social factors, and societal, institutional, and cultural determinants." (p. 169) Such a working definition stands independently of pathology, of specific disorders, and of the medical model. It embraces issues of health maintenance in general as well as behaviors related to specific disorders. It reflects a comprehensiveness that includes both mental and somatic health and recognizes their dynamic interplay, where behavioral medicine—with minor exception—excludes nonphysical problems. The definition thus includes the three distinct areas defined by Kasl and Cobb (1966): health behavior, illness behavior, and sick-role behavior.

Health behavior also has a directional aspect: Health behavior research is the interdisciplinary study of the phenomena included in the substantive definition. It is not the exclusive property of any one discipline or profession. Sociologists, anthropologists, psychologists, social workers, health educators and planners, physicians, nurses, and other health and human service professionals would be involved in a collegial way in fostering health behavior research. "Health behavior" thus defined would increase rigorous, interdisciplinary, collaborative, *basic* research on those personal attributes that mediate actions to maintain, restore, and improve health, "as well as on the family, peer group, societal, institutional, and cultural bases of the personal characteristics" (Gochman, 1982b, p. 170).

Health behavior as a research area would not be *primarily* concerned with treatment, with health education programs, with medical interventions, or with service delivery systems. Yet the solid, meaningful data it would generate would assuredly touch profoundly and productively upon each and all of these. Moreover, health behavior research would encourage the organization of accumulated data either conceptually or by levels of analysis (i.e., the person, the family, peer groups, etc.)—either individually or in combination—rather than by disease category, at-risk populations, or type of treatment/intervention.

Health-Germane Motivation. Among the important future tasks for health behavior researchers is identifying health-germane motivation in children (and adults as well). Although health as such may not appear to be a potent motive in young populations (e.g., Gochman, 1975, 1982a), other motives may be both potent and relevant in generating health behaviors. It is necessary to distinguish health—or the wish to possess good health—from other motives that might foster health maintenance, health restoration, and health improvement. These motives might include the youngster's wishes to be active physically and socially, to advance academically, and to succeed occupationally and vocationally. Once these have been identified, a related task would be the determination of how family factors enter into their emergence and development.

Taxonomy of Health Concepts. A second critical task, the taxonomy of health-related concepts, hinges on increased conceptual clarity and on the accumulation of rigorous data. There is a need for a comprehensive "catalog" of health-related beliefs, expectations, perceptions, motives, values, "understandings," and other cognitions along with their definitions, theoretical derivations, empirical measurements, and relationships—both theoretical and empirical—with other variables. Such a compendium would help define a universe of dependent variables against which the predictive value of family factors might be displayed.

Systemic Models

A second frame of reference, systemic models, was introduced earlier in this discussion and is implicit in the working definition of health behavior. Health-related concepts, as parts of health behavior, must be increasingly examined both as systems and as subsystems of larger systems. Evidence that beliefs about vulnerability to health problems themselves behave as systems (e.g., Gochman, 1973; Gochman & Sheiham, 1978) invites investigation of the systemic characteristics of other clusters of beliefs, such as perceived health locus of control, preventive attitudes, and perceptions of causality.

It follows from the systemic model, and the working definition of health behavior, that systems of health-related concepts exist within the larger systems of the person, the family, social groups, the community, and so forth. Possibly, health concepts are determined to a greater degree by proximal than by distal factors; possibly not. They have typically been studied without reference to any of these larger systems, and serendipitous findings may await future observers. Researchers might profitably explore the effects of larger systems on the emergence and development of health concepts.

Furthermore, systemic models (e.g., Bertalanffy, 1950; Weiss, 1939) suggest that certain common processes such as differentiation and interdependence—and the outcomes of these processes—can be observed in all living systems, and that the way in which systems are structured or organized has implications for the way in which these systems behave or function. Perceived vulnerability, for example, shows developmental increases in differentiation (Gochman, 1972a) and interdependence or consistency (Gochman, 1971a). Pratt's (1976) work adapts such concepts for examining the family as it relates to children's health practices. Future research embracing systemic dimensions might demonstrate that variability in differentiation and interdependence within the family are related to variability in differentiation and interdependence with a youngster's health concepts. Systemic concepts have thus already proven their value in this area.

A systemic perspective would properly locate the family in a social and cultural context and view it as both an independent and intervening determinant. This would encourage research into how the family mediates between the larger social, community, institutional, societal, and cultural systems and the manner in which youngsters develop health concepts. Possibly the family's mediation of the impact of these larger systems may be its most critical act as a determinant of children's health concepts.

Finally, a systemic frame of reference would both encourage and be consistent with the interdisciplinary efforts that are inherent in the working definition of health behavior. The collaboration of researchers from several disciplinary backgrounds would provide the most productive arrangement for the identification of appropriate common dimensions and for the translation of systemic concepts at the relevant levels.

Demedicalization and Wellness

The third direction for the future is also inherent in the working definition and relates as well to the content of the child's health concepts. Fox (1977), taking a serious look at the overmedicalization of contemporary American society, encourages a critical reconsideration of the overuse of the health–illness metaphor and detects trends toward demedicalization. Bruhn et al. (1980) also urge increased demedicalization and assumption of self-responsibility. One of the trends toward demedicalization is the "wellness" movement. Bruhn and Cordova (1977) define "wellness" in terms of the development of abilities to seek actively to change life situations so that persons can function at their capacity, including the development of competence to deal responsibly with their health.

"Demedicalization" and "wellness" are frames of reference that encourage movement away from the traditional medical model toward acceptance of greater personal responsibility for health. The wellness perspective, in particular, recognizes that skills, coping mechanisms, and adaptive and proactive capacity exist independently of the health–illness continuum. It also recognizes the importance of systematically educating people, from their earliest years, to develop competent coping strategies. A number of social systems, including the family, can be viewed as either inhibiting or facilitating the acquisition of wellness skills (Bruhn & Cordova, 1977; Bruhn, Cordova, Williams, & Fuentes 1977; Bruhn et al., 1980).

Most research on children's health concepts has been derived implicitly from the medical model and has dealt with medically defined problems and presumably valid treatments or regimens. Demedicalization and wellness may generate a different range of health-related concepts than can be currently identified. Some examples of these might be youngsters' beliefs about how well they generally cope with demands and challenges including those of remaining healthy and safe; the priority they assign to personal and social functioning; their ability to distinguish between what might be identified as behavior problems and what might be more justifiably termed illnesses; and their overuse of the illness metaphor. These, although not traditionally identified as concepts of health and illness, can be defined as such within a demedicalized, wellness framework.

Harris and Guten (1979), noting that most research on health behavior selects medically approved behaviors such as direct contact with health professionals or compliance with medical regions, suggest an alternative strategy. They propose investigations of any behavior believed by an individual to protect, promote, or maintain health regardless of whether such behaviors are medically defined as effective. Lau and Hartman (1983) also provide a nonmedicalized approach in their research on common sense, subjective experiences, and representations of the causes, courses, and consequences of diseases.

These alternatives expand the realm of health concepts that might be explored in children. How the family instructs in, inculcates, or serves as a role model for the acquisition of these very nontraditional health concepts might become a major focus for future health behavior research.

REFERENCES

Becker, M. H. (Ed.). (1974). The Health belief model and personal health behavior. *Health Education Monographs, 2.*

Bertalanffy, L. von. (1950). The theory of open systems in physics and biology. *Science, 111,* 23–29.

Bibace, R., & Walsh, M. E. (1981). Children's conceptions of illness. In R. Bibace & M. E. Walsh (Eds.), Children's conceptions of health, illness, and bodily functions. *New directions in developmental psychology* (Vol. 14). San Francisco: Jossey-Bass.

Birney, R. C. (1968). Motivation: Human motivation. In D. L. Sills (Ed.), *International encyclopedia of the social sciences* (Vol. 10). New York: Macmillan and Free Press.

Blos, P., Jr. (1978). Children think about illness: Their concepts and beliefs. In E. Gellert (Ed.), *Psychosocial aspects of pediatric care.* New York: Grune & Stratton.

Brodie, B. (1974). Views of healthy children toward illness. *American Journal of Public Health, 64,* 1156–1159.

Bruhn, J. G., & Cordova, F. D. (1977). A developmental approach to learning wellness behavior: Part I. Infancy to early adolescence. *Health Values, 1,* 246–254.

Bruhn, J. G., Cordova, F. D., Williams, J. A., & Fuentes, R. G. (1977). The wellness process. *Journal of Community Health, 2,* 209–211.

Bruhn, J. G., & Parcel, G. S. (1982a). Current knowledge about the health behavior of young children. In D. S. Gochman & G. S. Parcel (Eds.), Children's health beliefs and health behaviors. *Health Education Quarterly, 9,* 142–166.

Bruhn, J. G., & Parcel, G. S. (1982b). Preschool health education program (PHEP): An analysis of baseline data. In D. S. Gochman and G. S. Parcel (Eds.), Children's health beliefs and health behaviors. *Health Education Quarterly, 9,* 20–33.

Bruhn, J. G., Williams, J. A., & Fitzsimmons, E. L. (1980). *Self-responsibility for health: Focus on the child and the family. Final report of a conference.* Galveston: University of Texas Medical Branch.

Campbell, J. D. (1975a). Attribution of illness: Another double standard. *Journal of Health and Social Behavior, 16,* 114–126.

Campbell, J. D. (1975b). Illness is a point of view: The development of children's concepts of illness. *Child Development, 46,* 92–100.

Campbell, J. D. (1978). The child in the sick role: Contribution of age, sex, parental status, and parental values. *Journal of Health and Social Behavior, 19,* 35–51.

Caradang, M. L. A., Folkins, C. H., Hines, P. A., & Steward, M. S. (1979). The role of cognitive level and sibling illness in children's conceptualization of illness. *American Journal of Orthopsychiatry, 49,* 474–481.

Chapman, A. H., Loeb, D. G., & Gibbons, M. J. (1956). Psychiatric aspects of hospitalizing children. *Archives of Pediatrics, 73,* 77–88.

Christensen, H. T. (1964a). Development of the family field of study. In H. T. Christensen (Ed.), *Handbook of marriage and the family.* Chicago: Rand-McNally.

Christensen, H. T. (Ed.). (1964b) *Handbook of marriage and the family.* Chicago: Rand-McNally.

Crider, C. (1981). Children's conceptions of the body interior. In R. Bibace and M. E. Walsh (Eds.), Children's conceptions of health, illness, and bodily functions. *New directions in developmental psychology* (Vol. 14). San Francisco: Jossey-Bass.

Deutsch, H. (1942). Some psychoanalytic observations in surgery. *Psychosomatic Medicine, 4,* 105–115.

Dielman, T. E., Leech, S. L., Becker, M. H., Rosenstock, I. M., & Horvath, W. J. (1980) Dimensions of children's health beliefs. *Health Education Quarterly, 7,* 219–238.

Dielman, T. E., Leech, S. L., Becker, M. H., Rosenstock, I. M., & Horvath, W. J. (1982). Parental and child health beliefs and behavior. In D. S. Gochman & G. S. Parcel (Eds.), Children's health beliefs and health behaviors. *Health Education Quarterly, 9,* 60–77.

Fishbein, M., & Ajzen, I. (1975). *Belief, attitude, intention, and behavior: An introduction to theory and research.* Reading, MA: Addison-Wesley.

Fox, R. (1977). The medicalization and demedicalization of American society. In J. H. Knowles (Ed.), *Doing better and feeling worse: Health in the United States.* New York: Norton.

Geertsen, H. R., Klauber, M. R., Rindflesh, M., Kane, R. L., & Gray, R. (1978). A reexamination of Suchman's view on social factors in health care. *Journal of Health and Social Behavior, 16,* 226–237.

Gellert, E. (1962). Children's conceptions of the content and functions of the human body. *Genetic Psychology Monographs, 61,* 293–405.

Gellert, E. (1978). What do I have inside me? How children view their bodies. In E. Gellert (Ed.), *Psychosocial aspects of pediatric care.* New York: Grune & Stratton, 1978.

Gochman, D. S. (1966). A systemic approach to adaptability. *Perceptual and Motor Skills, 23,* 759–769.

Gochman, D. S. (1970a). Children's perceptions of vulnerability to illness and accidents. *Public Health Reports, 85,* 69–73.

Gochman, D. S. (1970b). The health ideation pictures (HIP): Reliability and internal consistency. *Perceptual and Motor Skills,30,* 271–278.

Gochman, D. S. (1971a). Children's perceptions of vulnerability to illness and accidents. A replication, extension and refinement. *HSMHA Health Reports, 86,* 247–252.

Gochman, D. S. (1971b). Some correlates of children's health beliefs and potential health behavior. *Journal of Health and Social Behavior, 12,* 148–154.

Gochman, D. S. (1971c). Some steps toward a psychological matrix for health behavior, *Canadian Journal Behavioural Science, 3,* 88–101.

Gochman, D. S. (1972a). The development of health beliefs. *Psychological Reports, 31,* 259–266.

Gochman, D. S. (1972b). The organizing role of motivation in health beliefs and intentions. *Journal of Health and Social Behavior, 13,* 285–293.

Gochman, D. S. (1973). A context for dental health education. *International Journal of Health Education, 16,* 37–42.

Gochman, D. S. (1975). The measurement and development of dentally relevant motives. *Journal of Public Health Dentistry, 35,* 160–164.

Gochman, D. S. (1977). Perceived vulnerability and its psychosocial context. *Social Science and Medicine, 11,* 115–120.

Gochman, D. S. (1981a, August). *Development and demography of perceived vulnerability in youngsters.* Presented at the meeting of the American Psychological Association, Los Angeles.

Gochman, D. S. (1981b, August). *Sex, expectations of health problems and youngsters' preventive attitudes.* Presented at the meeting of the American Psychological Association, Los Angeles.

Gochman, D. S. (1982a, August). *Health motivation in youngsters: A longitudinal replication.* Paper presented at the meeting of the American Psychological Association, Washington, D.C.

Gochman, D. S. (1982b). Labels, systems and motives: Some perspectives for future research and programs. In D. S. Gochman & G. S. Parcel (Eds.), Children's health beliefs and health behavior. *Health Education Quarterly, 9,* 167–174.

Gochman, D. S. (1984, August). *Youngsters' health beliefs: Cross-sectional and longitudinal analyses.* Paper presented at the meeting of the American Psychological Association, Toronto.

Gochman, D. S., Bagramian, R. A., & Sheiham, A. (1972). Consistency in children's perceptions of vulnerability to health problems. *HSMHA Health Service reports, 87,* 282–288.

Gochman, D. S., & Parcel, G. S. (Eds.). (1982). Children's health beliefs and health behaviors. *Health Education Quarterly, 9* (Nos. 2–3).

Gochman, D. S., & Saucier, J-F. (1982). Perceived vulnerability in children and adolescents. In D. S. Gochman & G. S. Parcel (Eds.), Children's health beliefs and health behaviors. *Health Education Quarterly, 9,* 46–59.

Gochman, D. S., & Sheiham, A. (1978). Cross-national consistency in children's beliefs about vulnerability. *International Journal of Health Education, 21,* 188–193.

Gorton, T. A., Doerfler, D. L., Hulka, B. S., & Tyroler, H. A. (1979). Intrafamilial patterns of illness reports and physician visits in a community sample. *Journal of Health and Social Behavior, 20,* 37–44.

Green, L. W. (1974). Editorial. In M. H. Becker (Ed.), The health belief model and personal health behavior. *Health Education Monographs, 2,* 324.

Harris, D. M., & Guten, S. (1979). Health-protective behavior: An exploratory study. *Journal of Health and Social Behavior, 20,* 17–29.

Heider, F. (1958) *The psychology of interpersonal relations.* New York: Wiley.

Jessner, L., Blom, G. E., & Waldfogel, S. (1952). Emotional implications of tonsillectomy and adenoidectomy on children. In R. S. Eissler et al. (Eds.), *The psychoanalytic study of the child.* New York: International Universities Press.

Kalnins, I., & Love, R. (1982). Children's concepts of health and illness and implications for health education: An overview. In D. S. Gochman & G. S. Parcel (Eds.), Children's health beliefs and health behaviors. *Health Education Quarterly, 9,* 8–19.

Kasl, S. V., & Cobb, S. (1966). Health behavior, illness behavior and sick–role behavior. *Archives of Environmental Health. 12,* 246–266, 534–541.

Kelley, H. H. (1967). Attribution theory in social psychology. In D. Levin (Ed.), Current theory and research in motivation, *Nebraska symposium on motivation* (Vol. 15). Lincoln: University of Nebraska Press.

Kister, M. C., & Patterson, D. J. (1980). Children's conceptions of the causes of illness: Understanding of contagion and use of imminent justice. *Child Development, 51,* 839–846.

Lau, R. R., & Hartman, K. A. (1983). Common sense representations of common illness. *Health Psychology, 2,* 167–185.

Lewin, K. (1935). *A dynamic theory of personality: Selected papers.* New York: McGraw-Hill.

Lewis, D. E., & Lewis, M. A. (1982). Children's health related decision making. In D. S. Gochman & G. S. Parcel (Eds.), Health beliefs and health behaviors. *Health Education Quarterly, 9,* 129–141.

Maiman, L. A., & Becker, M. H. (1974). The health belief model: Origins and correlates in psychological theory. In M. H. Becker (Ed.), The health belief model and personal health behavior. *Health Education Monographs, 2,* 336–353.

Mechanic, D. (1964). The influence of mothers on their children's health attitudes and behavior. *Pediatrics, 39,* 444–453.

Mechanic, D. (1980). Education, parental interest, and health perceptions and behavior. *Inquiry, 17,* 331–338.

Moody, P. M., & Gray, R. M. (1972). Social class, social integration, and the use of preventive health services. In G. Jaco (Ed.), *Patients, physicians and illness* (Chap. 19). New York: Free Press.

Nader, P. R., Perry, C., Maccoby, N., Solomon, D., Killen, J., Telch, M., & Alexander, J. K. (1982). Adolescent perceptions of family health behavior: A tenth grade educational activity to increase family awareness of a community cardiovascular risk reduction program. *Journal of School Health, 52,* 372–377.

Nagy, M. H. (1951). Children's ideas on the origin of illness. *Health Education Journal, 9,* 6–12.

Nagy, M. H. (1953). The representation of "germs" by children. *Journal of Genetic Psychology, 83,* 227–240.

Natapoff, J. N. (1978). Children's views of health: A developmental study. *American Journal of Public Health, 68,* 995–1000.

Natapoff, J. N. (1982). A developmental analysis of children's ideas of health. In D. S. Gochman & G. S. Parcel (Eds.), Children's health beliefs and health behaviors. *Health Education Quarterly, 9,* 34–45.

Neuhauser, D., Amsterdam, B., Hines, P., & Steward, M. (1978). Children's concepts of healing: Cognitive development and locus of control factors. *American Journal of Orthopsychiatry, 48,* 335–341.

O'Kelly, L. I. (1968). Motivation: The concept. In D. L. Sills (Ed.), *International encyclopedia of the social sciences* (Vol. 10). New York: Macmillan and Free Press.

Parcel, G. S., & Meyer, M. P. Development of an instrument to measure children's locus of control. In B. A. Wallston & K. A. Wallston (Eds.), Health locus of control. *Health Education Monographs, 6,* 149–159.

Pratt, L. (1973). Child rearing methods and children's health behavior. *Journal of Health and Social Behavior, 14,* 61–69.

Pratt, L. (1976). *Family structure and effective health behavior: The energized family.* Boston: Houghton-Mifflin.

Rashkis, S. R. (1965). Child's understanding of health. *A.M.A. Archives of General Psychiatry, 12,* 10–17.

Rokeach, M. *The open and closed mind.* (1960). New York: Basic Books.

Rosenstock, I. M. (1974). Historical origins of the health–belief model. In M. H. Becker (Ed.), The health belief model and personal health behavior. *Health Education Monographs, 2,* 328–335.

Schafer, R. B., & Keith, P. M. (1981). Influences on food decisions across the family life cycle. *Journal of American Dietary Association, 78,* 144–148.

Schwartz, G. E., & Weiss, S. M. (Eds.). (1978). *Proceedings of the Yale conference on behavioral medicine.* DHEW Publication, No. NIH, 78–1424.

Simeonsson, R. J., Buckley, L., & Monson, L. (1979). Conceptions of illness causality in hospitalized children. *Journal of Pediatric Psychology, 4,* 77–84.

Stone, E. J. (1976). *The effects of a health–education curriculum on locus of control, perceived vulnerability, and health attitudes of fifth grade students.* Unpublished doctoral dissertation, University of New Mexico.

Suchman, E. A. (1965). Social patterns of illness and medical care. *Journal of Health and Human Behavior, 6,* 2–16.

Vernon, D. T. A., Foley, J. H., Sipowicz, R. P., & Schulman, J. L. (1965). *The psychological responses of children to hospitalization and illness: A review of the literature.* Springfield, IL: Charles C Thomas.

Wallston, B. S., & Wallston, K. A. (1978). Locus of control and health: A review of the literature. In B. S. Wallston & K. A. Wallston (Eds.), Health locus of control. *Health Education Monographs, 6,* 107–117.

Weiss, P. (1939). *Principles of Development.* New York: Holt, Rinehart & Winston.

Weisenberg, M., Kegeles, S. S., & Lund, A. K. (1980). Children's health beliefs and acceptance of a preventive activity. *Journal of Health and Social Behavior, 21,* 59–74.

Wright, J. D., & Wright, S. R. (1976). Social class and parental values for children: A partial replication and extension of the Kohn thesis. *American Sociological Review, 41,* 527–537.

3

Family Health Behavior

Tom Baranowski

Philip R. Nader

People engage in an enormous variety of behaviors, for example, playing, working, teaching, and studying. Some of these behaviors, for example, dietary, smoking, or exercising, have been a particular focus of scientific concern because a person's performance or nonperformance of these behaviors has been shown to be related to a person's health and length of life (Berkman & Breslow, 1983). The discipline of public health has generated a variety of concepts that provide a structure within which to understand relationships between behavior, health, and length of life.

Certain *behaviors* (e.g., eating a lot of saturated fat) will lead to certain

Support in part during the writing of this chapter is acknowledged by grants for "The Family Health Project" from the W. T. Grant Foundation (Nader & Baranowski), the W. L. Moody Foundation (Nader & Baranowski), and the Preventive Cardiology Division of the National Heart, Lung and Blood Institute of the National Institutes of Health (Baranowski).

51

physiological states called *risks* (e.g., hypercholesterolemia, having too much cholesterol in the blood). Although not considered diseases themselves, these "risks" or "risk factors" signal the high probability of the development of *disease* (e.g., atherosclerosis, the hardening of the arteries), which in turn lead to *complications* of the disease process (e.g., heart attacks or kidney failure) and utlimately to *death*.

We can further categorize these health-related behaviors into primary, secondary, and tertiary preventive behaviors (Smith, 1979). Primary prevention includes those activities (including, but not limited to, human self-care behaviors) that prevent the onset of disease. Secondary prevention includes those activities that lead to the early detection of disease. Tertiary prevention includes those activities that prevent the development of complications that result from having the disease. For example, the conduct of a blood pressure screening program in order to detect new cases of hypertension (high blood pressure) would be classified as secondary prevention. Healthy people changing their diet and exercise habits to prevent high blood pressure from ever developing would be considered cases of primary prevention. If the same dietary and exercise changes are implemented by hypertensive patients to control their blood pressure, these would be considered cases of tertiary prevention, that is, to prevent the likely complications of heart attacks, strokes, and kidney disease.

An extensive amount of research has been conducted to identify which behaviors are likely to lead to disease (Lauer & Shekelle, 1980). This chapter will focus on some of the behaviors that have been identified as risk factors for a number of different diseases. Certain behaviors (e.g., diet or smoking) may lead to many different disease processes. The focus here is limited to primary and tertiary prevention because secondary prevention usually concerns using professional services of one sort or another. The distinction between primary and tertiary prevention behaviors is important in large part because of differences in the motivations of those instituting the changes, and the location in which training such behaviors is likely to take place.

Role of the Family

The family has a potentially important role to play in these general life style change (primary prevention) and regimen compliance (tertiary prevention) events. What do we know about how any family member might go about altering maladaptive behavioral patterns such as eating foods high in salt and saturated fats or not adhere to a medical regimen? The rest of this chapter is organized around one question: What do we know about families in relation to health-related behaviors?

The importance of the family in life style change and regimen compliance makes intuitive sense. Children learn many things from parents, and probably learn health behaviors (see Gochman, Chapter 2, this volume).

Family members are also interdependent. A change in one person's diet, for example, requires changes in the purchasing, preparation, and eating patterns on the part of other familly members. Dietary changes by one person may challenge the tastes and preferences of other family members, who in turn may give the dieter a hard time, or even taunt or nag the dieter with the old favorites.

An enormous, albeit dispersed and obscure, amount of literature relates to these issues. We make no claim to having been comprehensive in accumulating the relevant literature because it is so large. Nor can we provide a theoretical integration for all this literature because it is so complex. Our goals instead are to point out the almost ignored but potentially important relation of the family to health behaviors; to summarize some of the findings; and to critique some of the methods, pointing to future research. Certain facets of the literature have been emphasized because more work has been done in these areas and answers could be more confidently stated. This chapter reports on studies in which the natural variation in family variables was explored in relation to some aspect of health behavior. In the next chapter we report on experiments promoting health behavior change in which family variables were either systematically varied or explored.

DEFINITION OF THE "FAMILY"

We must clarify what we mean by "family." Most people approaching the study of the family bring a concept that reflects either our nationally idealized structure of a nuclear family or the structure in which they themselves were raised. Many changes have occurred in family structures due to various social trends (Campbell et al., 1969). The nuclear family with original parents is no longer as predominant as it once was, and therefore does not provide the sole, nor even the primary, reference for the term *family*.

Most of the literature on family aspects of health behaviors has not provided any definition of what constitutes family for that research. We know in several studies reported that the title "family" included various structures of single parents and unrelated and related adults and children in every imaginable combination, often including multiple generations, joint custody, and other arrangements. Thus the traditional concept of the nuclear family does not apply to increasingly large numbers of what would ordinarily be considered a "family."

The definition of family will often vary to meet the particular needs of a study. For example, studies of the elderly will most likely focus on currently childless individuals or couples, and focus on the relation of these individuals to their independently housed offspring who may play some caretaker role (see Bohm & Rodin, Chapter 10, this volume). At the other end of the family continuum may be the pregnant or recently delivered teenage mother who shares responsibility with her parents for the care of the offspring. Somewhere in the middle are cases of families of divorced and remarried individuals who jointly share custody for children among several families because of a complex set of marriages among former couples who were good friends. Somewhere in the middle are also found common-law marriages, and couples who may not be bound legally but who have cohabited for an extended period of time, sharing a variety of household and other tasks.

Rather than explore all the intricacies of the definitional problems, for purposes of this chapter a family will most often be defined as two or more individuals who reside in the same household, who can identify some common emotional bond, and who are interrelated by performing some social tasks in common, for example, socialization of children or nourishment. What social tasks are included will have differing implications for whichever individuals in the same household are categorized as family. Even the concept of living in the same household can be too restrictive. Oilfield workers and certain fishermen are often gone for months at a time and yet would be considered as members of the family in which spouse and children reside. The definition of family accepted in a particular study can have enormous implications for the results and interpretation because health behaviors may more likely develop in some families than in others (Pratt, 1976).

The task of this chapter is to demonstrate that families or aspects of families are related to health behaviors. We do this by focusing on noninterventive studies (i.e., where the phenomenon of concern was the naturalistic occurrence of the behavior). These naturalistic studies will be reported first for primary preventive health behaviors and next for regimen compliance (tertiary preventive) behaviors. With these relationships documented, in the next chapter we will review the cases in which aspects of the family were taken into account in designing programs to promote primary or tertiary prevention.

PRIMARY PREVENTIVE HEALTH BEHAVIORS

It is important to note that people participating in one form of health behavior (e.g., controlling the amount of calories consumed) may not participate in other health-related behaviors (e.g., using a seat belt or stopping smoking) (Langlie, 1979; Steele & McBroom, 1972; Tapp & Goldenthal, 1982; Williams & Wechsler, 1972). This suggests that each behavior or type of behavior may have its own unique determinants and situational reinforcers and thus must be analyzed separately (Mechanic, 1979). Another way of stating this is that there does not appear to be a general or common "preventive health personality" (i.e., a type of person who is likely to engage in a broad variety of preventive health behaviors). At the next level of analysis, however, Pratt (1976) has provided data to support her contention that certain kinds of families are more likely to engage in a broad variety of health-related behaviors.

In particular, Pratt (1976) proposed a family type, the "energized family," in which the family is more likely to engage in a broad variety of health (particularly primary prevention) behaviors. Pratt restricted her analysis to dual parent middle-class families and characterized the energized family as having many "liberated" characteristics (e.g., flexible division of household tasks between husband and wife, egalitarian family decision making, joint husband–wife involvement in the raising of children, active problem solving as a coping strategy, emphasis on individual autonomy, and extensive contacts and involvement with community institutions). No ensuing research has been reported that verifies Pratt's findings.

When health-related behaviors and risk factors have been analyzed one at a time, a phenomenon called "familial aggregation" has been documented (Glueck et al., in press). Familial aggregation simply means that the similarity of the frequency or pattern of these behaviors or risks is greater within families than between families. The following risks or behaviors have been shown to be more common within than between families: utilization of health services (Gorton, Doerfler, Hulka, & Tyroler, 1979); blood pressure levels in hypertensives (Biron, Mongeau, & Bertrand, 1975; Klein, Hennekens, Jesse, Gourley, & Blumenthal, 1974); weight and overweight (Garn, Cole, & Bailey, 1976); eating habits and food preferences (Bryan & Lowenberg, 1958); smoking behavior (Borland & Rudolph, 1975); use of alcohol (Tennant & Detels, 1976); and aspects of coronary prone behavior between fathers and their adolescent sons (Butensky, Faralli, Heebner, & Waldron, 1976). This suggests that there is something about these behaviors or risks that are promoted within the family. These within family commonalities may be due to genetic factors and/or to aspects of the family environment. Several studies are worthy of more detailed description in relation to selected health behavior areas.

Eating Behaviors.   Researchers in the family and nutrition area have usually focused on maladaptive eating behavior patterns. One of the most common concerns has been with calorie overconsumption or obesity. Garn, Bailey, Solomon, and Hopkins (1981) studied the probability of one person in the family being obese given the obesity/leanness of other members of the family. If no other family member is obese, the index child has only a 3.2% (sons) or 5.4% (daughters) chance of being obese. If all the other members of the family are obese, the index child has a 27.5% (sons) and 24.1% (daughters) chance of being obese. Although these are dramatic differences, it is unclear whether they may be due to genetic or environmental influences. Hartz, Giefer, and Rimm (1977) studied 73,532 members of the TOPS (Take Off Pounds Sensibly) organization. From extended analysis of various subsets of this population, they concluded that any-where from 32 to 39% of the variation in obesity among children is due to numerous variables labeled family environment, whereas only 11% was due to genetic factors. These findings were supported by Khoury, Morri-son, Laskarzewski, and Glueck (1983) who demonstrated significant rela-tionships between the body mass of parents and their living-at-home children, but no such relationships between parents and their adult living-away-from-home children. The Khoury et al. (1983) data thus suggest that immediate family environment is the crucial component in predicting body mass.

Further support for the nongenetic influences of the family on obesity can be found in Kramer, Barr, Leduc, Boisjoly, and Pless (1983) who iden-tified several attitudinal and infant-feeding behaviors by which parents promote infant obesity. Eppright, Fox, Fryer, Lamkin, and Vivian (1969) identified behavioral aspects of eating that may influence obesity in older children. They reported that in a survey of 2000 households in 12 north-central states, 25% of the households used food as a reward and 10% in-volved food in punishment. They also reported that the family imposed a variety of emotional connotations on sweets. Foods, in general, and sweets, in particular, may thereby assume rewarding qualities and be used by the children themselves as rewards in a broad variety of situations.

Waxman and Stunkard (1980) reported the first observational study of meal behavior in families with one obese and one nonobese child. Al-though not primarily an analysis of family interaction patterns, the authors reported that mothers served their obese child far larger portions than they served their nonobese child. Klesges et al. (1983) reported a microanalysis of interactional patterns between parents and young children during meal-times in a sophisticated observational study. Despite a small sample (14 families), the study documented statistically significant correlations of the frequency of parental encouragements to eat ($r = .81$) and of the frequency of parental food prompts ($r = .82$) with the child's relative weight. In a subanalysis they documented that encouragement to eat, offers of food, and total food prompts were significantly more likely to occur within fam-ilies with overweight than normal weight children. Klesges, Malott, Boschee, and Weber (in press) replicated the relationship between encour-agements to eat and relative weight. This research clearly demonstrated that family members behave differently in regard to promoting eating be-tween obese and nonobese children, even within the same family. Al-though not establishing causality of obesity, increased consumption by obese children is maintained at least by different family interactional pat-terns that promote eating behavior.

Diet-related obesity is obviously not the only form of health-related eat-ing behavior. Lawrence (1980) reviewed the extensive health benefits from breastfeeding and the importance of breastfeeding over at least the first six months of the infant's life. Rassin, et al. (1984), however, have shown that relatively small proportions of various ethnic groups ever begin breast-feeding. Bentovim (1976) generated a conceptual systems model of the psychosocial factors influencing the decision to breastfeed. Social support was identified in that model as a necessary link in a complex chain of events ending in breastfeeding. Several articles reported factors that mothers considered to be influences on their decision to breast or bottle feed. Some of the sources of influence or support were from the husband (Bacon & Wylie, 1976; Bryant, 1982) and the mother of the index mother (Bryant, 1982; Mackey & Fried, 1981; Oseid et al., 1982). Baranowski et al. (1983) demonstrated that social support was important in the breastfeeding decision, and the most important source of support varied by ethnic group. Among Black Americans, support from a close friend was most important. Among Mexican Americans, support from the mother's mother was most important. Among Anglo Americans, support from the male partner was most important. The strengths of these relationships also varied by ethnic group.

Graham's (1980) report indicated that the maintenance or the non-maintenance of breastfeeding beyond the first month resulted from the mother attempting to manage and balance her responsibilities to the infant versus other members of her family, both of which can be quite time consuming and at times in conflict. Aspects of the family are important influences on the decision to perform a particular health-related behavior and maintaining that behavior over the duration of that behavior's effectiveness.

The family has been implicated in many other aspects of diet as well. An important teaching of nutritionists is to obtain a broad variety of necessary nutrients by consuming many different kinds of foods. Kintner, Boss, and Johnson (1981) studied the relationship of family factors to the adequate consumption of selected nutrients and food categories. Using a sample of 42 husband–wife pairs, they conducted an abbreviated dietary history and applied Moos and Moos (1981) Family Environment Scale (FES). The FES measures simultaneously ten facets of family functioning, classified into three categories: (1) relationships, (2) personal growth, and (3) system maintenance. Kintner and his colleagues reported statistically significant correlations between the various scales of the FES and their nutrient intake scores separately for women and for men. Although 16 of 90 correlations were statistically significant for women, only five of 90 were significant among men. The only consistent pattern showed family cohesion to be related to protein, calcium, iron, vitamin A, and fresh vegetable consumption among women. The authors made much ado about the statistically significant relationships between overall nutrient-consumption adequacy and family conflict and organization among men. They interpreted this latter finding to indicate that the negative aspects of family functioning (i.e., high conflict and high levels of organization) predisposed men to poor diets. Two major shortcomings of the study (i.e., low participation rate (42%) and likely Type I error—significant findings only by chance—vitiate any interpretations made.

Moving more into the dietary aspects of heart disease, Laskarzewski et al. (1980) demonstrated modest (highest $r = .319$) but statistically significant parent–child correlations for the consumption of total carbohydrates, saturated fats, polyunsaturated fats, and calories, but not for cholesterol. These authors interpreted their results to indicate that some proportion of the parent–child concordance in cardiovascular disease risk was due to a common diet.

Hertzler and Vaughan (1979) reviewed multiple studies documenting the influence of various aspects of the family (e.g., family organization and parental relationships) on the eating behavior of infants and young children. Hertzler (1983) identified other facets of family life (e.g., exposure, modeling, positive reinforcement, and discipline) that have been shown to be related to child food preferences. Robertson (1979) reviewed the literature on child influence on family purchasing patterns in general and food purchasing in particular in response to child-focused television advertising. One study typified this literature in reporting that parents yielded to 87% of a child's request for cereals, 63% for snack foods, and 42% for candy (Ward & Wackman, 1972). These reviews provide further support for the reciprocal influences of child and family in the development of food preferences, food purchasing, and food consumption in childhood. By implication these dietary behaviors lead to the risk factors of middle age. The relative importance of, or interrelationships among, these aspects of family in affecting food preferences and diet have not been determined.

The family and diet literature is difficult to synthesize or criticize. Rather than having been conducted to develop a coherent body of knowledge, most of these studies were undertaken for different, often specific applied, purposes. As a result, the conceptual foundations, the populations sampled, the measures, and the approaches to analysis vary. However, that family characteristics are related to diet is indisputable. Other more meaningful questions must be raised and systematically investigated in the future. Differing areas of investigation involve differing nutrients. Heart disease investigators are often concerned with sodium, potassium, saturated and polyunsaturated fats; cancer investigators are often concerned with total fat and fiber; obesity investigators are interested in total calories from foods low in major nutrients (low nutrient density foods). The nutrient focus of this research needs to be more clearly specified because relationships are likely to vary by nutrient or other food characteristics of concern (Baranowski et al., unpublished).

Measures of habitual consumption of the foods need to be developed and validated (Block, 1982; Baranowski et al., unpublished). Given the huge numbers of foods, accurate measurement becomes a major problem. With a specific dietary focus, emphasis needs to be placed on studies of the process of family influence. In this regard, the use of existing family theory may help elucidate which aspects of family process are the most related to food behavior. For example, do all children and the nonfood-preparing spouses simply eat the food served or in some families are there general discussions resulting in shared decision making, as proposed by Pratt (1976)? Do parents model appropriate dietary behaviors (Bandura, 1977), or does early exposure to certain foods create taste preferences that influence later habits (Hertzler, 1983)? What effect does using food as a positive reinforcer or its withdrawal as a negative reinforcer have on food preferences and behaviors?

There are many ways of analyzing family influence: from the macrofamily-functioning level (Kintner et al., 1980) down to the microlevel of mothers giving larger food portions to obese children (Klesges et al., 1983). What are the relationships between macro- and microlevel analyses of the same behaviors? Can we validate Pratt's findings by using more re-liable close-ended measurements? How do these patterns vary by ethnicity, family structure, and social class? Can we demonstrate these influences in prospective studies as opposed to the currently available retrospective or cross-sectional studies? Many meaningful questions remain to be asked and answered in the area of family and diet.

Exercise.   A recent national sample survey (Perrier, 1979) demonstrated that parental attitudes and interests in sports and fitness discriminated between active and nonactive children. The active adults also reported that they often pursued their activities while participating together with their own families. Griffiths and Payne (1976) found that although the children of obese parents in their study were no larger (in height, weight, or per-cent body fat) than children of normal parents, they had significantly lower average daily energy expenditure (334 Kcal per day less) and signif-icantly lower basal energy expenditure. The children of these obese par-ents had already begun a lack-of-exercise life style that promotes obesity. Dowell (1973) found that the parents' (mother or father) attitudes toward exercise were related significantly to those of their child. Ashton (1983) showed that the physical activity patterns of parents, and particularly those of the mother, correlated with the activity patterns of the children. Livingood, Goldwater, and Kurz (1981) reviewed several studies that doc-umented how parents socialized children into sports participation. They concluded that parents are more important socializers for girls than for boys.

Reversing this usual parent-to-child direction of socialization for exer-cise, Snyder and Purdy (1982) documented a variety of influences of the child in enhancing the parents' interest in sports. Butcher (1983) explored factors related to adolescent girls participating in several different kinds of physical activity or several different ways of measuring activity. Mother's socialization and father's socialization were the primary correlates of com-munity organized activity, but not interschool teams or school intramural activities. These relationships might have been enhanced if multiple-item instead of single-item scales of socialization had been employed. The work is important, however, in identifying the likely category of specific effect of parental influence.

Waxman and Stunkard (1980) reported an observational study of the activity patterns of obese and nonobese children. These authors reported that in the home the obese children were much less active than their nonobese siblings. Seventy-four percent of the obese children's time in the home was spent sitting, whereas the same observation for the nonobese children was 49% of the time. Similar, but less dramatic, differences were obtained outside the home. Klesges, Coates et al. (in press) developed and validated an observational protocol for recording the activity and concurrent family interaction patterns of young children. During 90 minutes of "typical" postdinner family interaction in the first of three studies, these authors demonstrated that an obese child was significantly less active than a nonobese child, and the nonobese child received three times as many encouragements to be active as the obese child. In the second study of 14 nonobese children, parental encouragements to be active correlated .53 with a composite activity index, and parental discouragements correlated − .48 with the same index. The activity index correlated − .55 with relative weight.

Klesges, Boschee, and Weber (in press) reported a replication study with 30 young children. The results revealed the same significant relationships between encouragements to be active and the composite activity index (r = .32) and relative weight (r = − .45), but they were not the same for the discouragements to be active. Subanalyses revealed that encouragements to be active were the most highly correlated with extreme levels of activity, but not for moderate or minimal activity. The extreme activity was correlated (r = − .50) with relative weight.

Because fewer studies have been conducted in this area, the family and exercise data are more difficult to critique. The same kinds of criticisms and questions can be leveled here. There are many facets of exercise behavior. Much recent attention has focused on aerobic activity, because this form of exercise seems to be protective of heart disease. Accurate methods for assessing aerobic activity need to be validated with the various age and sex groups of concern (Baranowski, Dworkin, Cieslik et al., in press). The specific kind of activity or exercise of interest must be clearly delineated.

Although the initially reported studies documented correlations between the activity behaviors and the attitudes of parents and children, the latter observational studies identified specific behaviors performed by parents that encourage or discourage activity. The latter thereby provide stronger support for the role of families in affecting the activity of children, but it is unlikely that these activities were aerobic. These observational results were obtained among young children (two- to four-year-olds). It is likely that more sophisticated influence for exercise techniques are employed as the child becomes older, and this influence is more likely to be reciprocal (at least for a time). This remains to be documented. We have found no literature on husband–wife exercise correspondence or influence techniques.

Cardiovascular Disease Risk-Related Behaviors.   Concordance within families of heart disease risk variables has also been documented. Deutscher, Epstein, and Kjelsberg (1966) is a classic on this issue. Similar to the pattern of findings of Khoury et al. (1983), Deutscher et al. (1966) found strong relationships between parents and children under 16 years of age on total serum cholesterol, systolic blood pressure, relative weight, and blood glucose after a standard glucose challenge. No such relationships were obtained between parents and their 16- to 40 year-old-children, but modest such relationships reappeared between parents and their 40+ year-old-children. The authors interpreted these findings to indicate that family environment variables were most important in the younger ages.

Barrett-Conner, Suarez, and Criqui (1982) reported on 2236 married spouse pairs from predominently white, upper middle-class older adults in southern California. They reported low, but statistically significant, correlations between spouses for total cholesterol (.05) and triglycerides (.07). Barrett-Connor et al. reported significant spouse concordance for relative weight, cigarette smoking, and egg and milk consumption in these same couples. The relative weight by itself explained most of the concordance in the cholesterol and triglyceride values. Bucher, Schrott, and Lauer (1982) extended these findings by demonstrating concordance between children selected to be in the highest 5%, the midrange, and the lowest 5% of plasma total cholesterol value groups and their first, second, and third degree relatives. Moll, Sing et al. (1983) obtained the same pattern of results in a similarly designed study, but also demonstrated that grandfathers under 65 years of age had a 2.5 times increased risk of death due to CHD if they were related to children in the high lipid group of children. These studies revealed that these cardiovascular risks are more common within families than between families. One of these studies accounted for a major portion of this concordance by a relationship with relative weight, which was shown earlier to be influenced by family variables. The last study related these elevated risk variables in children to increased likelihood of kin mortality.

Blood Pressure.   Changing the focus to blood pressure, Biron, Mongeau, and Bertrand (1975) found significant parent–child correlations for both systolic and diastolic blood pressure. Also studying blood pressure, Harburg et al. (1977) employed a family set method for separating the relative influences of genetic and environment on index residents of Detroit and four of their relatives. Their family set method is a statistical model that attributes to genetic or environmental influences the variance shared by the index person with blood versus nonblood relatives living in the same household and in other households with that of another individual living in the same neighborhood. They concluded that unspecified common environmental variables (e.g., diet, stress, geographic area) accounted for a major portion of the variance, whereas genetic influences accounted for almost none of the variance. Moll, Harburg, Burns, Schork, and Ozgoren (1983) reanalyzed these data employing multiple family set models within a maximum likelihood procedure and concluded that genetics do play a primary role, and that environmental variables are important among whites but not blacks. Annest, Sing, Biron, and Mongeau (1979) reconfirmed the family correlational results of Biron, Mongeau, and Bertrand (1975) and also showed that a greater proportion of this concordance was due to common family environment than to genetic variation.

Esler et al. (1977) documented that at least one form of hypertension (mild high-renin hypertension) is neurogenic in origin, and likely psychogenic. More recent studies have supported the idea that certain forms of anger and hostility (particularly unexpressed forms) are likely to lead to hypertension (Diamond, 1982). Baer et al. (1980) attempted to explain the family concordance findings by focusing on family sources of anger and hostility. Families with hypertensive, and others with nonhypertensive, fathers (all mothers and children were nonhypertensive) were given a conflict-laden role-playing task. The interaction was videotaped and analyzed for verbal and nonverbal interactions. They showed that although the fathers themselves did not differ significantly in their behavior in the structured interactions, families with hypertensive fathers displayed significantly more negative nonverbal behavior and less positive verbal behavior than families with normotensive fathers. There were no differences in negative verbal behavior or in positive nonverbal behavior. These differences were more likely to occur in families with male than with female children. The authors reported, "When conflict-laden tasks were imposed on the families, the families with the hypertensive fathers produced more negative behavior, that is, behavior that reflects hostility or interpersonal rejection" (p. I–75). Although these data do not establish causality, they provide a piece of evidence on what it is about families that may lead to elevated blood pressures.

Baer et al. (1983) reported three replications of the original Baer et al. (1980) research. When combined across all three studies, families with the hypertensive father were significantly more likely not to look at another family member (averted gaze) when talking. Averted gaze during speech was more likely among fathers, mothers, and children in families with the hypertensive father. Averted gaze was more likely to occur during incidents of negative verbalizations than among positive verbalizations. The authors interpreted their results to indicate that families with hypertensive fathers were more likely to avoid conflict than confront and resolve it. This conflict avoidance likely led to suppressed anger and hostility, which in turn has been shown to be related to high blood pressure.

Ewart, Burnett, and Taylor (1983) arrived at similar conclusions from a different research perspective. Within the context of marital behavioral counseling for improved communication, and using an A–B–A–B design, these authors demonstrated that the hypertensive husband's blood pressure rose much higher during periods of "usual" interaction than during periods when behavioral communication–clarification procedures were employed. Spouse interruption of communication was a high-frequency "usual" communicative behavior that exacerbated conflict. Ewart et al. (1983) evaluated the effect of a marital communication–behavior modification program for mild to moderate hypertensives and documented greater decreases in systolic blood pressure reactivity and lower basal systolic blood pressure at posttest and at four-month follow-up in their experimental group than in their control group.

Although these data do not establish causality, they support the contention that anger and hostility are related to high blood pressure, and that at least in part this higher anger and hostility are due to patterns of communication in the family such as negative verbal and nonverbal behaviors in general, and averted gaze and frequent interruptions in particular. Prospective research on family interaction patterns among families with individuals at high risk for hypertension (e.g., family history) would contribute to establishing the causality of family interaction patterns in relation to hypertenseion.

Smoking Behaviors and Attitudes. Within social psychology, attitudes are considered either to be predictive or reflective of behavior. In either interpretation we would expect that attitudes toward health behaviors and health risks would be more common within families than between. Attitudes toward smoking and smoking behaviors are particularly important because of the tremendous impact of smoking on health and disease. One group of investigators has explored family aspects of attitudes to smoking. Nolte, Smith, and O'Rourke (1983a) demonstrated that the absence of one parent (mother or father) in the family of 7th- to 12th-grade children made it less likely for a child to perceive smoking as a serious health problem, more likely to perceive family and friends as enjoying smoking, less likely to ask the permission of others to smoke, and much more likely to be a regular smoker. Nolte, Smith, and O'Rourke (1983b) proceeded to the relationship of parental attitudes and behaviors to the children's attitudes and behaviors. They reported that the children were twice as likely not to smoke if neither parent smoked, and almost twice as likely to smoke if both parents smoked. These effects remained the same for boys and girls separately. If either parent smoked, the proportion was in between; with the father alone a smoker it was perhaps more likely increasing the chances of sons smoking, and with the mother alone a smoker it was perhaps more likely increasing the chances of daughters smoking. Stronger effects, however, were detected in relation to parental attitudes. If neither parent was upset about the child smoking, the child was approximately five times more likely to smoke than if both parents were upset.

Spielberger, Jacobs, Crane, and Russell (1983) investigated the relationships between parent and child smoking and older sibling and child smoking in a sample of 955 college freshmen. They demonstrated a stronger relationship between older sibling and child smoking than that between parent and child smoking and found no evidence of same sex parental modeling of smoking behavior. Rantakallio (1983) took the next step in this research and investigated the relationship of father and child smoking of 10,937 14-year-olds in Finland within the context of a broader number of social and other variables. Using stepwise regression analysis, Rantakallio revealed that in her sample the 14 family variables accounted for only 6.5% of the variance in smoking habits among girls and 3.5% among boys. (These analyses only had the father smoking status as an actual smoking behavior.) Alternatively, an expanded set of 24 variables (including the 14 family variables) accounted for 55.7% of the variance among girls and 42.7% of the variance among boys. These analyses revealed that although family variables were significantly related to the smoking habit in early adolescent boys and girls, they were not the predominant influences.

Although Rantakallio's (1983) data demonstrate significant relationships between family variables and child smoking behavior, causality, of course, cannot be inferred. As suggested by Speilberger and his colleagues (1983) the stronger relationship between older sibling and child smoking than that between parent and child smoking is likely due to the age of these participants (mostly 19-year-old-college freshman) who are probably more susceptible to peer than to family influence. Their specific hypothesis was that parents may be more influential at the onset of smoking than in its maintenance. Their evidence for this would have been stronger if they had asked a question about the time the participants initiated smoking in their sample and cross tabulated this with parental and older sibling smoking practices. The analyses were also restricted to those with older siblings. What were the effects of parents on first born children? Was this different from later born children? It is unfortunate that Rantakallio did not have maternal smoking or older sibling smoking to test these effects as well. Given the age of the children (14 years) in the Rantakallio study most smokers should have been early smokers and according to the Spielberger hypothesis, the parent behaviors should have been more important than the older siblings.

Current parental smoking, however, may be a misleading variable. It is reasonable to believe that parental exsmokers may be more strident proselytizers against smoking than nonsmokers. It would be interesting to assess these differences in the nonsmoking parent population. This would also give us some insight into the processes that may occur within families. Is the effect of parental and older sibling smoking simply a question of modeling, or of sanctioning an otherwise socially undesirable behavior, or are more complex interactions occurring among parents, older children, and target children?

Summary

What has been reported in this section is a sampling of studies relating to the intrafamily concordance for health-related attitudes, behaviors, and risks. Family concordance has been shown for spouse pairs and parent–child pairs, for differing behaviors and risks. In many cases, a greater proportion of the concordance in the risk factors has been demonstrated to be due to family environment than to genetic variables. Although all the processes mediating these relationships have not been explicated, it is obvious that what health behaviors one family member performs are likely to be related to the attitudes, health behaviors, and risks of other family members. Little further research appears to be necessary to document family concordance. The focus must switch instead to delineating the family-related processes that promote this concordance. For example, do hypertensive families have generally more conflicts or do they not deal adequately with the problems they have? In what ways other than gaze aversion do they avoid these conflicts? How did they learn these conflict avoidance interactional strategies? Is there something adaptive in the conflict avoidance among hypertensive families (e.g., fewer divorces)? One might infer that a potentially important approach to changing these behaviors and risks would be to intervene with families. A clearer delineation of family-related mediating variables would provide clearer targets for family-based behavior change programs.

REGIMEN COMPLIANCE

Families also play an important role in the many aspects of compliance with medical regimens. Becker and Green (1975), for example, reviewed the literature on families and compliance that suggested that health-belief model variables (i.e., perceived seriousness of the illness and perceived susceptibility to aversive outcome) played an important role in mediating the acts of family members in promoting compliance. Within a different theoretical framework Gentry (1976) reviewed the literature demonstrating the ability to train parents to be behavior modifiers for regimen compliance among children with asthma. Most of the research on family aspects of compliance has been conducted with children, although some has been done with adults. They are reported separately.

Parent and Child Compliance

In pediatric care, the mother (and less frequently the father) is the major point of contact between the patient (the child) and the health care provider. The parent as a child caretaker therefore plays an important role in regimen compliance. Mechanic (1964) explored the concordance (and by implication the influence) of the mother and child in illness-related behaviors. He found little support for the hypothesis that the child's attention and response to symptoms reflected that of the mother's. Mechanic did find that mothers were more concerned with their child's health than with their own, and those mothers experiencing higher levels of stress were more likely to phone the doctor concerning their child's health. The parents' health-related behavior toward their child is not just a reflection of their self-care behavior.

Missing scheduled appointments is an important aspect of regimen noncompliance. Alpert (1964) reported that pediatric care appointment breakers were twice as likely as appointment keepers to come from broken homes and significantly more likely to come from a home in which the mother was working. This builds a picture of appointment breaking as one facet of the lives of families that are either more disorganized or overwhelmed with other responsibilities. Cooper and Lynch (1979) reinforced this picture by showing *no* relationship between attendance at a pediatric outpatient department and family size, but a much lower likelihood of attendance as the frequency of diffuse social problems affecting the family and number of medical problems increased.

An important program of research on family involvement in pediatric care regimen compliance was started by Korsch and her colleagues (Korsch, Gozzi, & Francis, 1968; Francis, Korsch, & Morris, 1969; Freemon, Negrete, Davis, & Korsch, 1971). This early work sparked a recent spate of articles (Arntson & Phillipsborn, 1982; Bogdan, Brown, & Foster, 1982; Linder-Pelz, 1982a,b; Pantell et al. 1982; Weinberger, Green, & Mamlin, 1981). In a large sample of 800 mostly middle-class mothers and children who were interviewed at two points after a visit to an emergency room clinic in Los Angeles, Korsch et al. (1968) demonstrated that the mother of the pediatric patient entered the physician's office with a variety of expectations (e.g., wanting to be told of the diagnosis and cause of the current problem) and a variety of fears or anxieties (e.g., Does this illness mean my child has cancer?). If the physician met this expectation, or quelled the anxiety, the parent was more likely to be satisfied with the care provided than if the physician did not. Francis et al. (1969) in turn demonstrated that dissatisfied parents were both less likely to comply with the prescribed regimen and more likely to seek other sources of medical care. These findings have been interpreted within a variety of theoretical frameworks (Baranowski & Parcel, 1984; Becker & Green, 1975; Linder-Pelz, 1982a,b; Parcel & Baranowski, 1981).

The Korsch and ensuing research considered primarily the parent as patient proxy in relation to the physician, ignoring other members of the family and other facets of family relationships. Several studies of child regimen compliance have gone to the next level of social complexity and empirically examined the relationship of family structure and process with compliance. In almost all these studies, the family variables were secondary, rather than primary, aspects of the research. Furthermore, the studies are difficult to compare because they deal with different diseases, which imply differing regimes and different patient populations. The studies are reported within categories of disease, and only the family-related aspects of these studies are reported.

Charney et al. (1967) studied compliance with otitis media (middle ear infections, the most common acute illness in younger children) regimens that primarily require three or four times daily administration of an antibiotic for ten days and return visit in ten days to two weeks to check on the efficacy of the regimen. These authors identified no statistically significant relationships between compliance and number of children in the family, position (birth order) of the child in the family, intercurrent illness in other family members, or education level of the parents. They did find a slight relationship between the physician's characterization of the mother's personality and compliance. In basic support of the Charney et al. findings, Becker, Drachman, and Kirscht (1972) also studied compliance with otitis media regimens and found no statistically significant relationships between compliance and age of the mother, marital status, education of the mother, number of persons in the home, or extent of family problems. Compliance was, however, negatively related to the mother's report of interference of the regimen with her social role. The family variables in both these studies were primarily structural and revealed little to no relationship. However, when the regimen interfered with the mother's daily activities compliance was less likely to occur.

Switching the focus slightly to compliance with a prophylactic (tertiary preventive) antibiotic regimen among children with rheumatic fever, Elling (1960) reported many interrelationships among compliance variables. He reported (but provided little data to support) that compliance was most likely to occur among families who were upwardly mobile, without any serious relationship problems, and geographically stable. These were also the families who had an adequate concept of rheumatic fever and who had a positive "reactive self-concept" (i.e., felt positively evaluated by clinic doctors). Elling proposed that the "reactive self-concept" was the key mediating variable in determining utilization and medication compliance.

In a study of compliance with any regimen specifying an antibiotic, Arnhold et al. (1970) reported no statistically significant relationships between compliance and number of children in the family, whether the mother worked, and mother's or father's education. On the other hand, Ehmke, Stehbens, and Young (1980) found significant negative relationships between rheumatic fever regimen compliance (also involving antibiotics) and number of children in the family and parent's rating of the child's conduct. A confusing aspect of this research is the finding of a positive relationship between compliance and maternal educational level in a retrospective study but a negative such relationship between these variables in an interventive study.

Also studying rheumatic fever regimens, MacDonald, Hagberg, and Grossman (1963) found no statistical relationship between compliance and household composition, size of household, persons per room, parental concern about housing, employment of parents, family income, or parental evaluation of income. They found significant relationships with concurrent illness in other family members, relationship of father and child, and relationship of mother and child. To further muddle the rheumatic fever regimen compliance literature, Gordis, Markowitz, and Lilienfield (1969) found no significant relationships between compliance and position (birth order) of child in the family, number of parents in the household, self-report of cohesiveness of family unit, self-report of family problems, mother administered versus child administered medication, self-report scale of family tension and instability, and frequency of illness in the family or presence of chronic illness in the family. They did find negative relationships with number of children in the family and family history of rheumatic fever, and positive relationships with child being accompanied by a parent at every clinic visit and hospitalization for previous acute rheumatic fever attack.

In cases of compliance with kidney transplantation regimens, Korsch et al. (1978) found negative relationships between compliance and fatherless household, the patient tending to be closest to someone outside the family, mother and child having difficulty talking to the father, mother seeing herself as having less of a voice in family decision making, mother tending to be more easily angered now than before the illness, the person perceived by the mother as being most helpful during the illness was someone other than the physician, and parental friction and quarrels increasing during the year after the transplant. Family income was positively related to compliance.

The relationships between family variables and compliance in these studies have varied. In general, aspects of family and social structure (e.g., single versus double parent family, number of children, education of parents, employment of head of household) were less likely to be related to compliance, whereas aspects of family process (e.g., family cohesiveness, interference of regimen with social role tasks) were more likely to be related. Because there is a decisional aspect of compliance and because compliance decisions are made within the context of family relationships, it is likely that family process variables rather than family structure would affect compliance. Compliance with more severe problems, however, may be responsive even to variations in family structure. The first set of regimens reviewed was of relatively minor medical problems with only inexpensive or modestly expensive regimens. Kidney transplantation and its attendant regimen is the only severe illness and regimen reviewed. It was in the latter in which father absence was significantly related to compliance. The regimen in these cases may be so overwhelming (procedurally, financially, and emotionally) that the absence of the father may significantly impair the resources available within the family to cope with all the problems, one of which is regimen compliance.

It is also interesting to note that it was more often the negative aspects of family structure and process (e.g., interference with social role tasks, parent's rating of child's conduct, fatherless household, mother tending to be more easily angered, parental friction and quarrels increasing after the transplant) that related to compliance. This may indicate that compliance is not accorded a high priority in the family. As a result, there may be no aspects of family life that maximize compliance, but many aspects that inhibit and detract from compliance.

Along these lines, but focusing on another disease process, Schafer, Glasgow, McCaul, and Dreher (1983) explored the relationships between two sets of family process variables and compliance with diabetic regimens among children attending a diabetic camp. Of particular note they compared the predictive power of Moos and Moos (1981) Family Environment Scale (FES), a self-report inventory of aspects of family functioning, with a Family Behavior Checklist (FBC) developed within a social learning framework based on earlier work in hypertension regimen compliance (Baranowski, Chapin, & Evans, 1982). Only the conflict scale from the FES was negatively related with the number of daily glucose tests. The father's negative support on the FBC was negatively related to the number of daily glucose tests. Because only the scales indicating some family discord were related to compliance, it appears that disharmony in the family has greater implications for juvenile diabetic regimen compliance than aspects of positive family functioning (see Johnson, Chapter 8, this volume).

Anderson and Auslander (1980) reviewed the literature on juvenile diabetic regimen compliance conducted within a family system theory framework. In their review the negative aspects of family functioning were clearly related to poor disease control. It is not clear whether this was because of some direct effect of family discord on physiological variables or because more poorly functioning families may have more disoriented behavior patterns with a greater likelihood of noncompliance. Anderson and Auslander, however, pointed to severe methodological limitations in this literature, for example, small sample sizes, inadequate measurement, and no control groups.

It is difficult to summarize the family and child regimen compliance literature. It appears that family structure variables are less likely to be related, whereas family process variables are more likely related to compliance. Among the family process variables, aspects of negative family interactions, or problems in the family, appear to provide a more fruitful approach to understanding family aspects of pediatric regimen compliance. Other conceptual frameworks (e.g., family systems and stress theory), however, should be explored.

Any theoretical formulation must be judiciously applied to a particular aspect of regimen compliance. The demands placed on a child and the family will vary by disease, the form of the disease, the severity of the disease, and the stage in the disease process at which the child is found. More work must be done to define precisely the tasks (a task analysis) that have to be performed for each disease, form and stage of the disease, and the problems that families are likely to encounter in performing these tasks (Schwartz & Gottman, 1976; Windsor, Roseman, Gartseff, & Kirk, 1981; Windsor, Baranowski, Cutter, & Clark, 1984). Such work will give clearer guidance to the design of programs for involving families and a clearer context within which to place or apply family theories of compliance. Work may in fact be done on identifying the common regimen tasks and problems across diseases, which would identify common types of diseases to which a single family theory should apply.

Just as the demands of the regimen will vary with disease, the problems in compliance will vary with the age of the child, sex of the child, and the family ethnicity. For example, the mother is the primary contact between the child and the physician for children seven years of age or less, whereas the adolescent requires no intermediary. Characteristics of the mother should be more predictive of compliance among the younger children, whereas characteristics of family functioning or peer pressures should be more predictive of compliance among the adolescents. Because dietary practices vary by ethnicity (Brittin & Zinn, 1977), regimens with a dietary component will make differing demands across different ethnicity groups. To the extent that other family practices that are impinged upon by a regimen vary by ethnicity, ethnicity will be an important variable in studying regimen compliance. Future research must delineate and select particular age, sex, and ethnicity groupings for intensive analyses of family with compliance relationships.

Within these disease, age, sex, and ethnicity groups, initial work should include more intense analyses of interaction patterns because of the primitive state of our knowledge of how family functioning is most likely to be relevant. This more open-ended data collection should, however, be supplemented with responses to more standard instruments for assessing family functioning, both to validate the initial impressionistic data and to provide some quantitative basis for statistical analyses.

Models for Future Research.   Virtually all the reported studies have been cross-sectional. This leads to several problems of causal inference. The common current conception inferred from this literature is that family functioning affects compliance, which in turn affects disease control (see model in Figure 3.1a). It is just as possible that family functioning directly affects disease control (e.g., through emotional or stress-related mediating variables) as well as compliance (as depicted in the model in Figure 3.lb). Because we are dealing in many cases with chronic degenerative diseases, another possibility for explaining the documented cross-sectional correlations is that poor disease control leads to additional problems to be faced by the family, which in turn leads to poorer family functioning and reduced compliance (as depicted in Figure 3.lc). Furthermore, the poor disease control may require more difficult regimens and pose other emotional problems for family functioning, and the compliance may cause problems in family functioning, which in turn exacerbate problems of disease control (as depicted in Figure 3.ld). Of course, these potential explanations are not

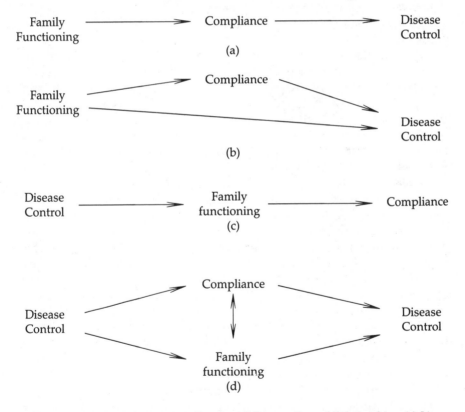

FIGURE 3.1 Models of Family, Compliance, and Disease Control Relationships. (a) Linear sequential model from family functioning to compliance to disease control. (b) Parallel influence model with compliance-disease control interaction. (c) Linear sequential model from disease control to family functioning to compliance. (d) Double parallel influence model with compliance and family functioning interaction.

mutually exclusive. There may be an element of truth to each. These models, however, provide alternative frameworks that should guide future prospective research attempting to explicate the relationships among family characteristics and regimen compliance.

Adult Compliance. Compliance among adults poses a variety of differing concerns. Adults are more likely to have personal responsibility for compliance. They go through differing phases of development. The chronic illnesses they experience are different, thus imposing differing regimens. Adults are more likely to have spouses as potential compliance collaborators instead of parents. A separate literature on family aspects of adult regimen compliance has developed.

Among a group of 82 chronically ill senior citizens recently discharged from a public ward in a Boston hospital, Donabedian and Rosenfeld (1964) reported that patients with someone at home upon return from the hospital were more likely to comply, whereas 4% of the self-stated reasons for failure to comply were due to noncooperative families. They reported the lack of relationship with their marital status or living arrangements before admission.

In a rare theory-based (role theory) study of families in adult compliance, Baric (1970) demonstrated that women were more likely to attend a pap smear test if the invitation were sent to the husband and the husband–wife relationship were characterized by "cooperative" conjugal roles (i.e., the husband participated in family activities, but the wife made most of the family activity decisions). This cooperative role structure was more likely found among families with nonmanual workers, (i.e., middle to upper class).

Oakes, Ward, Gray, Klauber, and Moody (1970) demonstrated that arthritis patients were much more likely to use a prescribed overnight hand resting splint when family members expected them to wear it than when family members did not. This effect was stronger for women, older, and middle- to upper-class people, but was detected in all these groups when controlling for social class, sex, and age. The importance of family expectations may vary over time. O'Brien (1980) reported the stronger influence of expectations of family and friends on compliance over those of health care professionals in the first year of dialysis. The influence of the health care professionals, however, was more important three years into dialysis. In support of Oakes et al. (1970), subanalyses within social class categories revealed that this reverse relationship over time was primarily true of middle- to upper-class families. In lower-class families, the expectations of health care providers were more important at both times.

Home hemodialysis places severe demands on a family. Extensive dietary changes are required and patients must be physically linked to a dialysis machine for long periods of time several times a week. These regimen requirements have led to concern about the dependency of the patient on the spouse to fulfill basic needs with the attendant likelihood of severe marital disruption. In a study of 16 previously stable marital pairs, Streltzer et al. (1976) showed that home hemodialysis failures occurred only in cases where the spouse was overly dependent on the patient prior to home hemodialysis. In an ensuing study of 23 chronic hemodialysis patients (home or center based) Steidl et al. (1980) demonstrated that six of ten ratings of family functioning significantly correlated with an index of overall compliance. Compliers were more likely to come from families who efficiently solved problems, where strong coalitions were formed between parents rather than between parent–child pairs, where clear parent–child boundaries were maintained, where family members were open and responsive to the opinions and feelings of others, in which marital partners shared power and negotiated, and in which family members assumed responsibility for their own behaviors.

Little work has been done on compliance in families of ethnic minorities. Lecca and McNeil (1982) reported a survey of compliance factors in a sample of elderly Mexican-American hypertensive patients. They reported statistically significant relations between compliance and family assistance (receiving and giving more assistance to one another) and family integration. No comparisons were made, however, with other ethnic groups.

There are too few naturalistic studies of the relationships of compliance to family variables among adults from which to draw any definite conclusions. Aspects of the family have been shown to relate to compliance; but these relationships may vary by illness, regimen, time since initiation of regimen, ethnicity, and a variety of other variables. No single investigator has mounted a program of research on families and adult compliance that systematically investigates variables over a series of studies and attempts to maintain some comparability across studies. As with the literature on children, it would appear to be more valuable for future research to emphasize family process as opposed to family structure variables. Of course, an infusion of family theory would be welcome in order to specify more clearly alternative hypotheses on how family variables promote or inhibit compliance. The existing reports have studied family variables at differing levels of theoretical interest.

Several of the studies have investigated sociological or macrolevel family functioning and marital status variables (e.g., marital happiness, power relationships in task-related decision making, family integration), whereas others have investigated more behavioral or microlevel interaction variables (e.g., providing assistance to one another in accomplishing the regimen's task, family expectations for regimen compliance). These sets of variables are obviously relevant to differing levels of family theory, and may be subject to differing sources of influence. It would be helpful for a model to be generated that describes some sequence of relationships from the more sociological family interaction variables to the more behavioral regimen-related family variables to regimen compliance. For example, do the types of family supportive behaviors vary from high cohesiveness to low cohesiveness families? Reciprocal directions of influence should also be assessed (e.g., how does a particular regimen affect the various levels of family relationships?). At a more practical level, documenting the reactions of families to particular regimens would be enormously useful in making judgments about the suitability or acceptability of alternative regimens when several regimens are available for treating a particular illness. There are many practically important and theoretically exciting possibilities for naturalistic research on the relationship of family characteristics to adult regimen compliance behaviors.

CONCLUSION

We have reviewed the literature on family aspects of various primary and tertiary preventive health behaviors. The empirical results clearly demonstrate relationships between various aspects of family functioning and these behaviors. Future research must begin to specify more clearly the relationships by identifying what aspects of family functioning and family interaction promote or retard the desired behaviors. This will require an infusion of theory and also a creative adaptation of theories to these new areas of interest. The challenge poses many exciting possibilities.

REFERENCES

Alpert, J. J. (1964). Broken appointments. *Pediatrics, 30*, 127–131.

Anderson, B. J., & Auslander, W. F. (1980). Research on diabetes management and the family: A critique. *Diabetes Care, 3*, 696–702.

Annest, J. L., Sing, S. F., Biron, R., & Mongeau, J. G. (1979). Familial aggregation of blood pressure and weight in adoptive families. II. Estimation of the relative contributions of genetic and common environmental factors to blood pressure correlations between family members. *American Journal of Epidemiology, 110*, 492–503.

Arnhold, R. G., Adelbonojo, F. O., Callas, E. R., Callas, J., Carte, J., & Stein, R. C. (1970). Patients and prescriptions. Comprehension and compliance with medical instructions in a suburban pediatric practice. *Clinical Pediatrics, 9*, 648–651.

Arnston, P. H., & Phillipsborn, H. F. (1982). Pediatrician–parent communication in a continuity-of-care setting. *Clinical Pediatrics, 21*, 302–307.

Ashton, N. J. (1983). *Relationship of chronic physical activity levels to physiological and anthropometric variables in 9–10 year old girls.* Paper presented to the annual meeting of the American College of Sports Medicine, Montreal.

Bacon, C. J., & Wylie, J. M. (1976). Mother's attitudes to infant feeding at Newcastle General Hospital in Summer, 1975. *British Medical Journal, 1*, 308–09.

Baer, P. E., Reed, J., Bartlett, P. C., Vincent, J. P., Williams, B. J., & Bourianoff, G. G. (1983). Studies of gaze during induced conflict in families with a hypertensive father. *Psychosomatic Medicine, 45*, 233–242.

Baer, P. E., Vincent, J. P., Williams, B. J., Bourianoff, G. G., & Bartlet, P. C. (1980). Behavioral response to induced conflict in families with a hypertensive father. *Hypertension* (2, Suppl.), I-70–I-77.

Bandura, A. (1977). *Social learning theory*. Englewood Cliffs, NJ: Prentice-Hall.

Baranowski, T., Bee, D., Rassin, D., Richardson, C. J., Brown, J., Guenther, N., & Nader, P. R. (1983). Social support, social influence, ethnicity, and the breastfeeding decision. *Social Science & Medicine*, 17: A, 1599–1611.

Baranowski, T., Chapin, J., & Evans, M. (1982). *Dimensions of social support for hypertension regimen compliance*. Galveston: University of Texas Medical Branch.

Baranowski, T., Dworkin, R. J., Cieslik, C. J., Hooks, P., Clearman, D. R., Ray, L., Dunn, J. K., & Nader, P. R. (in press). Reliability and validity of self-report of aerobic activity: Family health project. *Research Quarterly for Exercise and Sport*.

Baranowski, T., Dworkin, R. J., Clearman, D. R., Dunn, J. K., Ray L., Vernon, S., & Nader, P. R. *Comparisons of dietary self-report methods: Family Health Project*. Unpublished manuscript, University of Texas Medical Branch, Galveston.

Baranowski, T., & Parcel, G. (in press). Social learning theory. In M. Kreuter & G. Christensen (Eds.), *Theories in health education*. Palto Alto, CA: Mayfield Press.

Baric, L. (1970). Conjugal roles as indicators of family influence of health-directed action. *International Journal of Health Education*, 13, 58–65.

Barrett-Connor, E., Suarez, L., & Criqui, M. H. (1982). A spouse concordance of plasma cholesterol and triglyceride. *Journal of Chronic Diseases*, 35, 333–340.

Becker, M. H., Drachman, R. H., & Kirscht, J. P. (1972). Predicting mothers' compliance with pediatric medical regimens. *Journal of Pediatrics*, 81, 843–854.

Becker, M. H., & Green, L. W. (1975). A family approach to compliance with medical treatment: A selective review of the literature. *International Journal of Health Education*, 18, 2–11.

Bentovim, A. (1976). Shame and other anxieties associated with breastfeeding: A systems theory and psychodynamic approach. In A Bentovim (Ed), *Breastfeeding and the mother* (p. 159). Ciba Foundation Symposium 45 (new series). New York: Elsevier, Excerpta Medica, North-Holland.

Berkman, L. A., & Breslow, L. (1983). *Health and ways of living: The Alameda County studies*. New York: Oxford University Press.

Biron, P., Mongeau, J. G., & Bertrand, D. (1975). Familial aggregation of blood pressure in adopted and natural children. In O. Paul (Ed.), *Epidemiology and control of hypertension* (pp. 387–395). New York: Grune & Stratton.

Block, G. (1982). A review of validations of dietary assessment methods. *American Journal of Epidemiology*, 115, 492–505.

Bogdan, R., Brown, M. A., & Foster, S. B. (1982). Be honest but not cruel: Staff/parent communication on a neonatal unit. *Human Organization*, 41, 6–16.

Borland, B. L., & Rudolph, J. P. (1975). Relative effects of low socio-economic status, parental smoking, and poor scholastic performance on smoking among high school students. *Social Science and Medicine*, 9, 27–30.

Brimblecomb, F. S. W., & Cullen, D. (1977). Influences on a mother's choice of method of infant feeding. *Public Health* (London), 91, 177–186.

Brittin, H. C., & Zinn, D. W. (1977). Meat-buying practices of Caucasians, Mexican-Americans, and Negroes. *Journal of the American Dietetic Association*, 71, 623–628.

Bryan, M. S., & Lowenberg, M. E. (1958). The fathers' influence on young children's food preferences. *Journal of the American Dietetic Association*, 34, 30–35.

Bryant, C. A. (1982). The impact of kin, friend and neighbor networks on infant feeding practices. *Social Science and Medicine*, 16, 1757–1765.

Bucher, K. D., Schrott, H. G., Clark, W. R., & Lauer, R. M. (1982). The Muscatine cholesterol family study: Familial aggregation of blood lipids and relationships of lipid levels to age, sex and hormone use. *Journal of Chronic Disease, 35,* 375–384.

Butcher, J. (1983). Socialization of adolescent girls into physical activity. *Addescence, 18,* 753–766.

Butensky, A., Faralli, B., Heebner, D., & Waldron, I. (1976). Elements of the coronary prone behavior patterns in children and teenagers. *Journal of Psychosomatic Research, 20,* 439–444.

Campbell, A. A., Kantner, J., Kincaid, H. V., Ridley, J. C., Taeuber, I. B., Valien, P., & Whitney, V. (Eds.). (1969). *The family in transition.* Bethesda, MD: National Institutes of Health, Fogarty International Center.

Charney, E., Bynum, R., Eldredge, D., Frank, D., MacWhinney, J. B., McNabb, N., Scheiner, A., Sumpter, E. A., & Iker, H. (1967). How well do patients take oral penicillin? A collaborative study in private practice *Pediatrics, 40,* 188–195.

Cooper, N. A., & Lynch, M. A. (1979). Lost to follow up. A study of nonattendance at a general pediatric outpatient clinic. *Archives of Disease in Childhood, 55,* 765–769.

Deutscher, S., Epstein, F. H., & Kjelsberg, M. O. (1966). Familial aggregation of factors associated with coronary heart disease. *Circulation, 33,* 911–924.

Diamond. E. L. (1982). The role of anger and hostility in essential hypertension and coronary heart disease. *Psychological Bulletin, 92,* 410–433.

Donabedian, A., & Rosenfeld, L. S. (1964). Follow up study of chronically ill patients discharged from hospital. *Journal of Chronic Diseases, 17,* 847–862.

Dowell, L. J. (1973). A study of physical and psychological variables related to attitudes toward physical activity. *International Journal of Sport Psychology, 4,* 39–47.

Eastham, E., Smith, D., Poole, D., & Neligan, G. (1976). Further decline of breastfeeding. *British Medical Journal, 1,* 305–307.

Ehmke, D. A., Stehbens, J. A., & Young, L. (1980). Two studies of compliance with daily prophylaxis in rheumatic fever patients in Iowa. *American Journal of Public Health, 70,* 1189–1193.

Elling, R. (1960). Patient participation in a pediatric program. *Journal of Health and Human Behavior, 1,* 183–189.

Eppright, E., Fox, H., Fryer, B., Lamkin, G., & Vivian, N. (1969). Eating behavior of preschool children. *Journal of Nutrition Education, 1,* 16–19.

Esler, M., Julius, S., Zweifler, A., Randall, O., Harburg, E., Gardiner, H., & DeQuattro, V. (1977). Mild high-renin essential hypertension, neurogenic human hypertension? *New England Journal of Medicine, 296,* 405–411.

Ewart, C. K., Burnett, K. F., & Taylor, C. B. (1983). Communication behaviors that affect blood pressure: An A–B–A–B analysis of marital interaction. *Behavior Modification, 7,* 331–344.

Ewart, C. K., Taylor, C. B., Kraemer, H. C., & Agras, W. S. (1983). *Reducing blood pressure reactivity during interpersonal conflict: Effects of marital communication training.* Unpublished manuscript.

Francis, V., Korsch, B. M., & Morris, M. J. (1969). Gaps in doctor-patient communication. Patients' response to medical advice. *New England Journal of Medicine, 280,* 535–540.

Freemon, B., Negrete, V. F., Davis, M., & Korsch, B. M. (1971). Gaps in doctor-patient communication: Doctor-patient interaction analysis. *Pediatric Research, 5,* 298–311.

Garn, S. M., Bailey, S. M., Solomon, M. A., & Hopkins, P. J. (1981). Effect of remaining family members on fatness prediction. *American Journal of Clinical Nutrition, 34,* 148–153.

Garn, S. M., Cole, P. E., & Bailey, S. M. (1976). Effect of parental fatness levels on the fatness of biological and adoptive children. *Ecology of Food and Nutrition, 6,* 1–3.

Gentry, W. D. (1976). Parents as modifiers of somatic disorders. In E. J. Mash, L. C. Handy & L. A. Hamerlynck (Eds.), *Behavior modification approaches to parenting* (pp. 221–230). New York: Brunner/Mazel.

Glueck, C. J., Laskarzewski, P. M., Rao, D. C., & Morrison, J. A. (in press). Familial aggregation of coronary risk factors. In W. Connor & D. Bristow (Eds.), *Complications in coronary heart disease.* Philadelphia: Lippincott.

Gordis, L., Markowitz, M., & Lilienfield, A. M. (1969). My patients don't follow medical advice: A study of children on long-term antistreptococcal prophylaxis. *Journal of Pediatrics, 75,* 957–968.

Gorton, T. A., Doerfler, D. L., Hulka, B. S., & Taylor, H. A. (1979). Intrafamilial patterns of illness reports and physician visits in a community sample. *Journal of Health and Social Behavior, 20,* 37–44.

Graham, H. (1980). Family influences in early years on the eating habits of children. In M. Turner (Ed.), *Nutrition and lifestyle.* London: Applied Science Publishers.

Griffiths, M., & Payne, P. R. (1976). Energy expenditure in small children of obese and non-obese parents. *Nature, 260,* 698–700.

Harburg, E., Erfurt, J. C., Schull, W. J., Schork, M. A., & Colman, R. (1977). Heredity, stress and blood pressure, a family set method. *Journal of Chronic Disease, 30,* 625–648.

Hartz, A., Giefer, E., & Rimm, A. A. (1977). Relative importance of the effect of family environment and heredity on obesity. *Annals of Human Genetics* (London), *41,* 185–193.

Hertzler, A. A. (1983). Children's food patterns—a review: II. Family and group behavior. *Journal of the American Dietetic Association, 83,* 555–560.

Hertzler, A. A., & Vaughan, C. E. (1979). The relationships of family structure and interaction to nutrition. *Journal of the American Dietetic Association, 74,* 23–27.

Jones, R. A. K., & Belsey, E. M. (1977). Breastfeeding in an inner London borough—A study of cultural factors. *Social Science and Medicine, 11,* 175–179.

Khoury, P., Morrison, J. A., Laskarzewski, P. M., & Glueck, C. J. (1983). Parent–offspring and sibling body mass index associations during and after sharing of common household environments: The Princeton School District Family Study. *Metabolism, 32,* 82–89.

Kintner, M. Boss, P. G., & Johnson, N. (1981). The relationship between dysfunctional family environments and family member food intake. *Journal of Marriage and the Family, 43,* 633–641.

Klein, B. E., Hennekens, C. H., Jesse, M. J., Gourley, J. E., & Blumenthal, S. (1974). Longitudinal studies of blood pressure in offspring of hypertensive mothers. In O. Paul (Ed.), *Epidemiology and control of hypertension* (pp. 387–395). New York: Grune & Stratton.

Klesges, R. C., Coates, T. J., Brown, G., Sturgeon-Tillisch, J., Moldenhauer, L. M., Holzer, B., Woolfrey, J., & Vollmer, J. (1983). Parental influences on children's eating behavior and relative weight. *Journal of Applied Behavioral Analysis, 16,* 371–378.

Klesges, R. C., Coates, T. J., Moldenhauer, L. M., Holzer, B., Gustavson, J., & Barnes, J. (in press). The FATS: An observational system for assessing physical activity in children and associated parent behavior. *Behavioral Assessment.*

Klesges, R. C., Malott, J. M., Boschee, P. F., & Weber, J. M. (in press). Parental influences on children's food intake, physical activity and relative weight: An extension and replication. *Journal of Behavioral Medicine.*

Korsch, B. M., Fine, R. N., & Negrete, V. F. (1978). Noncompliance in children with renal transplants. *Pediatrics, 61,* 872–876.

Korsch, B. M., Gozzi, E. K., & Francis, V. (1968). Gaps in doctor-patient communication. I. Doctor-patient interaction and patient satisfaction. *Pediatrics, 42,* 855–870.

Kramer, M. S., Barr, R. G., Leduc, D. G., Boisjoly, C., & Pless, I. B. (1983). Maternal psychological determinants of infant obesity. Development and testing of two new instruments. *Journal of Chronic Diseases, 36,* 329–335.

Langlie, J. K. (1979). Interrelationships among preventive health behaviors: A test of competing hypotheses. *Public Health Reports, 94,* 216–225.

Laskarzewski, P., Morrison, J. A., Khoury, P., Kelly, K., Glatfelter, L., Larsen, R., & Glueck, C. J. (1980). Parent-child nutrient intake interrelationships in schoolchildren ages 6 to 19: The Princeton School District Study. *American Journal of Clinical Nutrition, 33,* 2350–2355.

Lauer, R. M., & Shekelle, R. B. (Eds.). (1980). *Childhood prevention of atherosclerosis and hypertension.* New York: Raven Press.

Lawrence, R. (1980). *Breastfeeding, a guide for the medical profession.* St. Louis: Mosby.

Lecca, P. J., & McNeil, J. S. (1982). *Cultural factors affecting the compliance of older Mexican-Americans with hypertension regimens.* Paper presented at the annual meeting of the American Public Health Association, Montreal.

Linder-Pelz, S. (1982a). Social psychological determinants of patient satisfaction: A test of five hypotheses. *Social Science & Medicine, 16,* 583–589.

Linder-Pelz, S. (1982b). Toward a theory of patient satisfaction. *Social Science & Medicine, 16,* 577–582.

Livingood, A. B., Goldwater, C., & Kurz, R. B. (1981). Psychological aspects of sports participation in young children. *Advances in Behavioral Pediatrics, 2,* 141–169.

MacDonald, M. E., Hagberg, K. L., & Grossman, B. J. (1963). Social factors in relation to participation in follow-up care of rheumatic fever. *Journal of Pediatrics, 62,* 503–513.

Mackey, S., & Fried, P. A. (1981). Infant breast and bottle feeding practices: Some related factors and attitudes. *Canadian Journal of Public Health, 72,* 312–318.

Mechanic, D. (1964). The influence of mothers on their children's health attitudes and behavior. *Pediatrics, 30,* 444–453.

Mechanic, D. (1979). The stability of health and illness behavior: Results from a 16-year follow up. *American Journal of Public Health, 69,* 1142–1145.

Mohrer, J. (1979). Breast and bottle feeding in an inner-city community: An assessment of perceptions and practices. *Medical Anthropology, 3,* 125–145.

Moll, P. P., Harburg, E., Burns, T. L., Schork, M. A., & Ozgoren, F. (1983). Heredity, stress and blood pressure, a family set approach: The Detroit project revisited. *Journal of Chronic Diseases, 36,* 317–328.

Moll, P. P., Sing, C. F., Weidman, W. H., Gordon, H., Ellefson, R. D., Hodgson, P. A., & Kottke, B. A. (1983). Total cholesterol and lipoproteins in school children: Prediction of coronary heart disease in adult relatives. *Circulation, 67,* 127–134.

Moos, R. H., & Moos, B. S. (1981). *Family environment scale mannual.* Palo Alto, CA: Consulting Psychologists Press.

Nolte, A. E., Smith, B. J., & O'Rourke, T. (1983a). The relationshp between health risk attitudes and behaviors and parental presence. *Journal of School Health, 53,* 234–240.

Nolte, A. E., Smith, B. J., & O'Rourke, T. (1983b). The relative importance of parental attitudes and behavior upon youth smoking behavior. *Journal of School Health, 53,* 264–271.

Oakes, T. W., Ward, J. R., Gray, R. M., Klauber, M. R., & Moody, P. M. (1970). Family expectations and arthritis patient compliance to a hand resting splint regimen. *Journal of Chronic Diseases, 22,* 757–764.

O'Brien, M. E. (1980). Hemodialysis regimen compliance and social environment: A panel analyses. *Nursing Research, 29,* 250–255.

Oseid, B., Carter, J. P., Brown, J., Sullivan, J., Chang, C., & Gendel, P. (1982). *Characteristics and outcome of low-income urban women who choose to breastfeed.* Paper presented at the annual meeting of the Ambulatory Pediatric Association, Washington, DC.

Pantell, R. H., Stewart, T. J., Dias, J. K., Wells, P., & Ross, A. W. (1982). Physician communication with children and parents. *Pediatrics, 70,* 396–402.

Parcel, G., & Baranowski, T. (1981). Social learning theory and health education. *Health Education*, 12, 14–18.

Perrier Corp. (1979). *Fitness in America. The Perrier study*. Great Waters, NY.

Pratt, L. (1976). *Family structure and effective health behavior. The energized family*. Boston: Houghton-Mifflin.

Rantakallio, P. (1983). Family background to and personal characteristics underlying teenage smoking. *Scandinavian Journal of Social Medicine*, 11, 17–22.

Rassin, D., Richardson, J. D., Baranowski, T., Nader, P. R., Guenther, N., Bee, D., & Brown, J. (1984). Incidence of breastfeeding in a lower socioeconomic group of mothers in the United States. *Pediatrics*, 73, 132–137.

Robertson, T. S. (1979). Parental mediation of television advertising effects. *Journal of Communication*, 29, 12–25.

Rousseau, E. H., Lescop, J. N., Fontaine, S., Lambert, J., & Roy, C. C. (1982). Influence of cultural and environmental factors on breastfeeding. *Canadian Medical Association Journal*, 127, 701–704.

Schafer, L. C., Glasgow, R. E., McCaul, K. D., & Dreher, M. (1983). Adherence to IDDM regimens: Relationship to psychosocial variables and metabolic control. *Diabetes Care*, 6, 493–498.

Schwartz, R. M., & Gottman, J. M. (1976). Toward a task analysis of assertive behavior. *Journal of Consulting and Clinical Psychology*, 44, 910–920.

Sloper, K., McKean, L., & Baum, J. D. (1975). Factors influencing breastfeeding. *Archives of Diseases of Childhood*, 50, 165–170.

Smith, B. C. (1979). *Community health. An epidemiological approach*. New York: Mcmillan.

Snyder. E. E., & Purdy, D. A. (1982). Socialization into sport: Parent and child reverse and reciprocal effects. *Research Quarterly for Exercise and Sport*, 53, 263–266.

Spielberger, C. D., Jacobs, G. A., Crane, R. S., & Russell, S. F. (1983). On the relation between family smoking habits and the smoking behavior of college students. *International Review of Applied Psychology*, 32, 53–69.

Steele, J. L., & McBroom, W. H. (1972). Conceptual and empirical dimensions of health behavior. *Journal of Health and Social Behavior*, 13, 382–392.

Steidl, J. H., Finkelstein, F. O., Wexler, J. P., Feigenbaum, H., Kitsen, J., Kliger, A. S., & Quinlan, D. M. (1980). Medical condition, adherence to treatment regimens and family functioning. *Archives of General Psychiatry*, 37, 1025–1027.

Streltzer, J., Finkelstein, F., Feigenbaum, H., Kitsen, J., & Cohn, G. L. (1976). The spouse's role in home hemodialysis. *Archives of General Psychiatry*, 33, 55–58.

Tapp, J. T., & Goldenthal, P. (1982). A factor analytic study of health habits. *Preventive Medicine*, 11, 724–728.

Tennant, F. S., & Detels, R. (1976). Relationship of alcohol, cigarette and drug abuse in adulthood with alcohol, cigarette and coffee consumption in childhood. *Preventive Medicine*, 5, 70–71.

Ward, S., & Wackman, D. (1972). Television advertising and intra-family influences on children's purchase influence attempts and parental yielding. *Journal of Marketing Research*, 9, 316–319.

Waxman, M., & Stunkard, A. J. (1980). Calorie intake and expenditure of obese boys. *Journal of Pediatrics*, 96, 187–193.

Weinberger, M., Green, J. Y., & Mamlin, J. J. (1981). The impact of clinical encounter events on patient and physician satisfaction. *Social Science & Medicine*, 15E, 239–244.

Williams, A. F., & Wechsler, H. (1972). Interrelationship of preventive actions in health and other areas. *Public Health Reports*, 87, 969–976.

Windsor, R. A., Roseman, J., Gartseff, G., & Kirk, D. A. (1981). Qualitative issues in developing educational diagnostic instruments and assessment procedures for diabetic patients. *Diabetes Care, 4,* 468–475.

Windsor, R. A., Baranowski, T., Cutter, G., & Clark, N. (1984). *Evaluation of health promotion and education programs.* Palto Alto, CA: Mayfield Press.

Yeung, D. L., Pennell, M. D., Leung, M., & Hall, J. (1981). Breastfeeding: Prevalence and influencing factors. *Canadian Journal of Public Health, 72,* 323–330.

4

Family Involvement in Health Behavior Change Programs

Tom Baranowski

Philip R. Nader

The mechanical heart transplant story of Dr. Barney Clark received extensive national coverage. Every newspaper, newsmagazine, radio and television news program carried some coverage of his valiant struggle for life and the intelligence and concern of a team of medical professionals who created and tested the new mechanical heart. Extensive coverage was given to his wife, who supported him throughout the struggle, and his children and grandchildren who were concerned for his welfare and his

Support in part during the writing of this chapter is acknowledged by grants for "The Family Health Project" from the W. T. Grant Foundation (Nader & Baranowski), the W. L. Moody Foundation (Nader & Baranowski), and the Preventive Cardiology Division of the National Heart, Lung and Blood Institute of the National Institutes of Health (Baranowski).

dignity. This story received such extensive coverage because of the drama of the event: a good man with support from his loving family, fighting against the odds, helped by a team of medical superheroes.

Although Dr. Clark's medical problem was degenerative cardiomyopathy, which is not the result of the usual life style-related risk factors, many other patients with severe cardiovascular disease have in part been the victims of their own life styles. In most cases, heart failure is not an unanticipated random event. Heart failure instead is usually the final in a long chain of events. Most heart attack victims have spent their lives engaging in a variety of high-risk behaviors. These high-risk behaviors include overconsumption of calories, sodium, and saturated fats, underconsumption of potassium and polyunsaturated fats, inadequate participation in aerobic activity, smoking, exposure to high stress levels with poor coping skills, and an aggressive, anger-inducing, extremely time conscious (Type A) pattern for dealing with other people. One or more of these aspects of life style predispose an individual to develop heart disease. Heart failure is the culmination of a lifetime of such physically maladaptive behaviors.

There is also an extensive literature on compliance with medical regimens (Haynes, Taylor, & Sackett, 1979), which poses other problems for heart failure. Many heart disease patients do not take their medicines on a strictly followed time schedule, and do not strictly adhere to the dietary and other prescriptions of their physicians. Evidence is accumulating that major changes in the various life style factors may completely prevent or at least significantly delay the onset of disease (Nightingale, Cureton, Kalmar, & Trudeau, 1978). Adherence to medical prescriptions will prevent or at least postpone the development of complications from disease, at least from certain diseases (Haynes, Taylor, & Sackett, 1979). If individuals would implement these life style changes, and if heart disease patients would adhere more strictly to their medical regimens, the many future cases of heroic care for advanced heart disease may never make the evening television news. In fact, if the extensive time, expertise, and financial resources expended to help these advanced heart disease individuals had been expended to prevent heart disease, and prevent the complications of heart disease, many more lives might be affected.

Helping people make changes in their lives, however, has proven remarkably difficult (Foreyt, Goodrick, & Gotto, 1981). Although behavior change has often been obtained during the course of an intervention project, the behavior often reverts to baseline levels after discontinuation of the intervention. There has been some speculation that families have been key components in this backslide. The highly motivated patient comes home to an untrained and unmotivated family who resist the changes, or make the changes difficult to implement. The patient in turn decides it may be easier to do whatever the family is doing because the new behavior is considered aberrant from the family's point of view.

From this perspective, an intervention with the family poses several important possibilities. A family intervention has the potential for training and motivating all family members, attempting to minimize barriers posed by the family members, and training a variety of social supports in the family to enhance the behavior change process. Such training theoretically could lead to greater and broader scale behavior changes at the end of the project, and if the family habit patterns have changed, the new support mechanisms should maintain those changes over a longer period of time.

Let us review the literature to see whether these early hopes have been realized in the empirical literature.

FAMILY INVOLVEMENT IN HEALTH BEHAVIOR CHANGE PROGRAMS

The studies reported in the previous chapter were "naturalistic" in the sense that no attempt was made to promote change. The studies reported in this chapter will examine the efficacy of programs designed to change either health behaviors or regimen compliance. These studies have either systematically varied family involvement as a controlled experimental variable or have taken the family as the unit of intervention.

Preventive Health Behavior Change Trials

Families have been involved in programs to promote weight reduction (among spouses and among parent–child pairs) and other components of cardiovascular risk reduction. We report each separately.

Couples Training for Weight Loss.   The first report of spouse involvement in weight loss was casually made by Stuart and Davis (1972). They reported that in two of their case studies the spouse of the weight loss program participant acted against the goals of the program in that he nagged, criticized, or enticed the participant with the wrong foods. Mahoney and Mahoney (1976) developed an index of social support for weight loss based on family attendance during a ten-week program and family reports of the "cooperation and encouragement they received from family and friends" (p. 35). They reported correlations of .92 between this index and weight loss at the end of the program and of .63 two years after the program ended. Although both samples were exceedingly small, these two studies led to ensuing research in the behavior modification literature to further validate and explicate these results.

In the first experimental study of married obese women in behavior therapy for weight loss, Wilson and Brownell (1978) reported no effect on weight loss when involving versus not involving the husbands. Husband involvement meant that husbands attended all eight training sessions, in which they were taught the philosophy of behavior modification, were instructed to cease criticizing their partners' weight and eating behaviors, were trained to provide positive reinforcement as appropriate, and find ways to help the obese wife rearrange the conditions and consequences of eating at home. No measures were obtained, however, of whether these trained support behaviors were successfully employed by the spouses.

Apparently not satisfied with the results of the first experimental study, Brownell, Heckerman, Westlake, Hayes, and Monti (1978) assigned 29 obese men and women to two conditions—couples training or subjects alone—and created a third category, noncooperative spouses, in which individuals whose spouses refused to participate were assigned. As far as can be gleaned from the published reports, spouse training in this study was similar to that in Wilson and Brownell (1978). (Colletti and Brownell, 1982, however, report more active involvement of the spouse in the later study.) Although no statistically significant differences were evident across the three groups immediately after the ten intervention sessions, the couples-training group had lower weights than the other two groups. Statistically significant differences did appear at the three- and six-month follow-ups for the couples-training group versus the other groups. The mean weight loss for the couples-training group at three months and six months was about 30 lb, which is more than double the 11 to 12 lb weight losses at the end of the program that is commonly reported in the literature (Foreyt, Goodrick, & Gotto, 1981). Heckerman and Zitter (1979) reported that at three years after the ten-session training program, the couples training had maintained a 31.5 lb weight loss, whereas the subjects alone and the noncooperative spouse groups maintained 10.1 lb and 11.8 lb, respectively. Although the latter figures were based on an incomplete sample, and were not statistically significantly different, they have been pointed to as dramatic evidence for the potential of couples training for weight loss. Brownell et al. (1978) therefore provided a benchmark against which subsequent studies have measured themselves. Brownell, however, was not able to replicate his own findings (Brownell & Stunkard, 1981), which means that no one can be sure what the crucial ingredients were for the success in the Brownell et al. (1978) intervention.

A flurry of related articles have appeared. Saccone and Israel (1978) obtained no statistically significant difference between a group in which a significant other (it is not clear if this group included spouses only or others) provided a reward either for weight loss or for dietary behavior changes. Israel and Saccone (1979) reported on the three and 12 months follow-up data from this study and showed that the group with reinforcement provided by a significant other for eating behavior changes produced the most persistent weight loss. The magnitude of weight loss for this group at one year was only 10 lb. This study appears to have shown that a primary component in couples training is the spouse's provision of reinforcement contingent on dietary behavior change.

The level of spouse involvement was the next aspect to be varied. Rosenthal, Allen, and Winter (1980) conducted a study of obese women randomly assigned to full spouse involvement, partial spouse involvement, and no spouse involvement conditions. All three conditions included training in positive and negative reinforcement, shaping, extinction, and contracting during the first four sessions. Spouses attended four additional sessions in the full spouse involvement condition in which discussions took place of the "couples" specific situations and needs, and refinement of techniques to meet these needs" (p. 167). The analyses revealed no statistically significant differences at posttreatment, but showed significant differences between both spouse involvement and no spouse involvement conditions at the six week follow-up. This study indicates no additional value is gained from problem solving with couples adapting the behavior modification tools to meet the specific needs. Consistent with this, Pearce, LeBow, and Orchard (1981) reported that best results in both weight loss and loss maintenance were obtained in a nonparticipating spouse condition in which the spouse was asked not to nag or otherwise give the spouse a hard time in regard to weight loss. This indicates that removing the spouse as a detriment to change may be just as important as training the spouse to be helpful.

Several additional studies showed no additional effect on weight loss from spouse involvement (Dubbert & Wilson, in press, Zitter & Fremouw, 1978, O'Neil et al., 1979, Weisz & Bucher, 1980). In contrast Murphy et al. (1982) reported that couple training with two-party contracting maintained greater weight loss at two years posttreatment. Although Weisz and Bucher (1980) reported no weight loss at the end of treatment, they did find that their trained couples reported fewer depressive symptoms and better marital adjustment at posttreatment and follow-up, thus demonstrating a positive, but unintended, outcome from family intervention. Alternatively, Dubbert and Wilson (in press) found no marital adjustment effects from the couples treatment, but did find that higher marital adjustment scores correlated with more weight loss.

Conclusions are not as clear as they might be and interpreting this literature is not straightforward. The participants have varied on a variety of characteristics. Some studies have used obese women alone, whereas others have used men and women. This may be unfortunate because Burke and Weir (1974) have reported that wives are generally supportive of husbands but not vice-versa. Although a broad range of ages has been reported in several of these studies, no statement has been made on the social class, ethnicity/race, employment status, and other potentially relevant demographic characteristics of these participants. This is a serious shortcoming because the most important source of support for other behavior has been shown to vary by ethnicity (Bryant, 1982; Baranowski, Bee et al., 1983) and may vary by other characteristics.

There seems to be little comparability in treatment as well. The number of sessions varied from six to 18. We know little about the duration (e.g., one hour) or timing (e.g., during Christmas break) of these sessions, which may also account for differences across studies. The content of the intervention appears to vary greatly. There seems to be an assumption of commonality of interventions across studies when describing a particular intervention component. When an article, however, states "trained in contracting," what is meant by contracting? And how extensive was the training? Training could vary from distributing the forms with a minor explanation to intensive step-by-step explanation with practice, problem identification, and problem solving at each step. Because the interventions are most often described in one or two sentences, it is impossible to determine whether two authors are using equivalent techniques or simply using the same word. Such lack of consistency in program structure across studies would be valuable if positive results were obtained, because it would document the robustness of the treatment. When positive results are hard to demonstrate, however, the lack of consistency makes the job of comparison and interpretation difficult, if not impossible. A major contribution to this literature would be the delineation of a standard treatment protocol for each type of intervention. An alternative would be to describe two or three alternative kinds of complexity in standard treatment protocol for the same type of intervention. An investigator could then select and identify the level of treatment most appropriate to his or her population, thereby introducing some commonality and resulting in some comparability across studies.

A variety of research designs have been employed. Some studies have randomized participants to conditions, and others have not. The most dramatic success was a report in which cases with refusing spouses were placed in a separate control group. Although this research design can be appreciated from the viewpoint of wishing to obtain an assessment of the intervention's true effect, it is also likely that a high proportion of couples with marital conflict was deleted from the intervention groups, thereby eliminating the couples for whom a family intervention is least likely to work.

It may be that the positive results obtained to date have been a function of some experimenter-expectancy effect (Kazdin, 1979). No studies have controlled for this possibility by using multiple intervenors and systematically varying the assignment of couples to intervenors. The only two authors to attempt a couples-training program more than once (Wilson & Brownell, 1978; Brownell et al., 1978; Brownell & Stunkard, 1981; Dubbert & Wilson, in press) have failed to obtain an effect in three of the four studies.

The method of recruitment has gone virtually unreported (Hooks, Baranowski, Vanderpool, & Nader, 1983). Participants who have been intensively recruited are likely to be less responsive to a program than those who come seeking assistance. The sample sizes have also been exceedingly small. There is no evidence that sample sizes have been estimated prior to the studies to be sure of having the opportunity to detect some likely or acceptable differences in weights. This has been a particular problem for comparisons at follow-up points because the inevitable attrition has reduced samples in some cases to less than half. Future work must use the variances obtained in the published work—the obtained differences in mean weight loss and the obtained sample attrition to estimate the number of subjects necessary to obtain those differences at a prespecified follow-up point. Although the samples in some of the studies were obviously large enough to detect some differences, they have not been large enough to conduct extensive within-group analyses of mediating variables.

This brings us to the last point. The couples research has ignored existing family theory. Investigators have involved spouses or significant other in an ad hoc fashion. The basic premise seems to have been that the significant other could participate in the operant control of the desired behaviors. Because the results from this simple conceptualization have not resulted in extensive weight loss, other theoretical formulations should be explored (e.g., family systems theory, see Turk & Kerns, Chapter 1, this volume).

Process Studies of Weight Loss. Preliminary research has been conducted that begins to explicate the problems in couples treatment for weight loss. Using instruments similar to those reported by Baranowski, Chapin, and Evans (1982b), Schafer, Glasgow, McCaul, and Dreher (1982), Mahoney and Mahoney (1976), and Mermelstein, Lichtenstein, and McIntyre (1983), Dubbert et al. (1981) employed a checklist of the frequency of spouse behaviors that were possibly supportive or nonsupportive of weight loss. Although spouse involvement in their intervention did not increase significantly the frequency of performance (or reporting) of these behaviors, and the scores did not predict weight loss at the immediate posttreatment assessment, the scores were correlated with weight loss three months after treatment. Of equal interest, the Locke-Wallace Marital Adjustment Scale also correlated with three-month posttreatment weight loss. Dubbert and Wilson (in press), however, reported that these relationships did not hold at the three-year posttreatment follow-up. Dubbert (private communication, 1983) also reported "many of our involved spouses (mostly males) were very reluctant to engage in discussions of supportive behaviors and simply refused to make written contracts to perform specified supportive behaviors." The delayed effect of social support, noted in these studies, may indicate that the support provided by the therapist is sufficient in all cases during therapy, and support from the spouse is most important once contact with, and thereby the support from, the therapist declines. This spouse support, however, either declines in frequency or wanes in effectiveness as time passes.

In a study of the weight loss process, Streja, Boyko, and Rabkin (1982) found a positive relationship between perceived support on the part of the spouse and weight loss. The nature of this support, however, was not defined. Gierszewski (1983), on the other hand, found no relationship between social support and weight loss across all participants. This was despite the fact that the highest levels of reported support for weight loss came from the spouse. Subanalyses revealed, however, that social support for weight loss was negatively correlated ($r = -.64$) with weight loss among individuals with an internal locus of control. No subanalyses were reported by the ten individual sources of support assessed. These data suggest an interactional effect between social and personality variables in inhibiting weight loss.

Saltzer (1980) explored the process of weight loss within the framework of a Fishbein value-expectancy model. She demonstrated that the perceived social norms were more important than the perceived consequences for weight loss in predicting both the behavioral intentions for and the actual weight loss. Within the social norm component, Saltzer reported that the expectations of close friends for weight loss were most strongly related to actual weight loss, whereas those of the spouse were not related. Spouses had the highest mean perceived preference for weight loss and the lack of correlation may have been the reflection of a ceiling effect.

Marshall and Neill (1977) conducted intensive interviews with couples in which one partner had undergone intestinal bypass surgery for extreme obesity. Although the sample was small and the data nonquantitative, these authors described marital relationships in which the obesity served important functions. For the husbands of the obese person, "the obesity of their wives protected them from excessive sexual demands, competition with other males, and the possibility of abandonment and allowed them to adopt a passive-dependent role" (P. 179). The wives in turn appreciated their husbands not being critical of their obesity and thus accepted the dependency of the spouse. The loss of weight disrupted this equilibrium, providing the formerly obese person with newfound freedom and attractiveness that threatened the relationship the spouses had developed. This research indicates that the prior marital relationship may be important in determining the effect of a weight loss program. If these findings are supported by subsequent research, a successful intervention for weight loss may require some marital therapy as a component. Rand, Kuldau, and Robbins (1982), however, reported data that found no such dependency relationships nor their alleviation after surgery.

An alternative approach to unraveling the complex strands of intervening with couples for weight loss is A–B–A-type single-case interventive designs. Heckerman and Zitter (1979) reported an intensive analysis of a single case in which spouse reinforcement was far superior to spouse-monitoring or self-monitoring for weight loss. Although generalizations from such studies must be retested with larger and representative samples, these designs provide an opportunity to systematically vary components of an intervention and develop a detailed understanding of the relationship of interventive techniques to the processes of weight loss.

These studies provide hypotheses for ensuing more generalizable and defensible research.

Studies on the process of weight loss are sparse and the findings are inconsistent. In some cases social support from spouse was important and in others it was not. In one case preexisting marital dependency among obese couples vitiated the long-term effects of intervention (Marshall & Neill, 1977), whereas in another no such evidence was found (Rand, Kuldau, & Robbins, 1982). In part, these differences may be due to differences in the sources or the composition of the sample. It is hard to believe that in the extensive amount of research on weight loss we do not know to whom to generalize the results because the participants were not selected from some known population. All this research has relied on volunteers of unknown origin.

Including more process measures in conducting intervention studies would enable us to answer several theoretical and practical questions. Which family member has been involved? Does effectiveness differ by family member? Does effectiveness differ by preexisting family functioning? Do family members actually perform the behaviors at home that are encouraged during the sessions? Does the higher performance of these behaviors lead to greater weight loss? What procedures can be used to promote the higher frequency performance of these behaviors at home? What impact does the intervention and compliance with the regimen have on family functioning and family diet and exercise patterns?

The problem with obtaining measures for process analysis is that larger sample sizes are needed to conduct the correlational analyses. This means larger staffs are needed and higher costs incurred to conduct the interventions and collect the measures. It is not until process measures are collected, however, that we can have some confidence that our interventions are working in the way we theorize they are, and that we can identify the additional problems that our interventions were not originally designed to handle.

Parent–Child Intervention for Weight Loss.   The role of the family in pediatric obesity was clearly documented in the previous chapter. Children had a 27.5% or 24.1% chance of being obese if both their parents were obese (Garn, Bailey, Solomon & Hopkins, 1981). Mothers gave larger portions to obese children as opposed to nonobese children (Waxman & Stunkard, 1980). Parents of obese children gave a higher frequency of encouragements to eat and more food prompts to eat (Klesges, Coates, Brown et al., 1983, Klesges, Malott, Boschee, & Weber, in press). The children of obese parents participated in exercise less frequently than children of nonobese parents (Griffiths & Payne, 1976), and parents encouraged obese children to exercise less often than nonobese children (Waxman & Stunkard, 1980; Klesges, Coates, Moldenhauer et al., in press; Klesges, Malott, Boschee, & Weber, in press). Because parents are such an integral aspect of a child's eating behavior, an intervention for controlling pediatric obesity would most likely involve modifying the parents' behavior as well as the child's. For example, Huse et al. (1982) reported a five-stage childhood obesity problem-solving sequence in which the importance of family and other social actors has been identified. The problems posed by family, for example, offering food at nonmeal times (rather than family strengths), were emphasized in this model.

The family intervention for childhood obesity literature began with a young target group—5- to 10-year-old children. Aragona, Cassaday, and Drabman (1975) compared two forms of parent training for weight loss with a no-treatment control group. Both parent training groups involved a structured exercise program, nutrition, and stimulus control information. In addition, one of the groups included daily self-monitoring and graphing of dietary calorie intake and weight, instructions in reinforcement procedures and response-cost contracting for attendance, graph completion, and child weight loss. Although the children in both parent groups lost more weight than children in the control, there were no differences between the parent groups. The authors concluded that parent training would be a successful approach to weight loss, even without the trappings of a sophisticated behavior management program. Their sample, however, was exceedingly small.

Wheeler and Hess (1976) explored parent training for weight loss for children from two to 11 years old. Parents in the experimental groups received training in situational analysis of the eating behavior of their children, problem solving for identified eating contingencies, and record keeping on eating behavior. The results revealed that the experimental group (even including the dropouts) significantly outperformed the control. The treatment completors reduced their average percent overweight from 40.4 to 34.9, whereas the controls increased from 38.9 to 44.4. Another study thus showed reason to believe in the effectiveness of parent training for juvenile obesity.

Kingsley and Shapiro (1977) focused on a slightly older age group, that is 10- and 11-year-olds, and compared family involved with no family involved interventions. They systematically varied child involvement and parent involvement in a factorial design. In all conditions except the control, the interventions involved maintaining a daily calorie consumption record, and parents being encouraged to institute a token economy for appropriate dietary behavior changes. In addition, in the mother only group, emphasis was placed on "having the mothers help the children to overcome their weight problems by teaching them the necessary behavioral techniques." (This intervention was not further defined or clarified.) At immediate posttreatment, the children in the three interventive groups had lost roughly equal amounts of weight (about 3.5 lb) with no significant differences between groups, but all different from the control. At six weeks posttreatment and 20 weeks posttreatment, there were no statistically significant differences among the intervention groups. These findings tend to question the added effectiveness of parental involvement in weight loss therapy, thus suggesting that any therapy is better than none for children weight loss. Child-alone intervention, however, may not be possible for children younger than ten years old.

Kingsley and Shapiro also analyzed weight loss among mothers in their child weight loss program. At immediate posttreatment, the mothers in the mother-only condition lost 6.25 lb, significantly more than any of the other groups. This effect was maintained for the first follow-up assessment but not for the second follow-up assessment. These data reveal an unintended transference of learning from modifying a child's eating habits to modifying the mother's.

Epstein, Wing, Steranchak, Dickson, and Michelson (1980) compared behavior modification with nutrition education techniques in promoting weight loss in mother–preadolescent child pairs. Among other components, the behavior modification treatment involved training parents and children to praise one another for desired dietary and exercise changes, and to act as models for one another. According to the authors, not only did the behavior modification group outperform the other in percent overweight loss, but a correlation of .75 was obtained in this group between parent and child in their percent overweight losses. This finding supported their intent that parents and children lose weight in pairs. The corresponding correlation for the nutrition education group was − .26 (n.s.). Lavigne and Daruna (1982), however, challenged the data analyses and interpretations of Epstein, Wing, Steranchak, Dickson, and Michelson (1980), inferring that the study did not establish the greater effectiveness of behavioral over nutrition education treatment for childhood obesity, but only that mothers were more likely to lose weight in the behavioral treatment condition. Their criticisms did not concern the correlations between parent and child.

Epstein, Wing, Koeske, Andrasik, and Ossip (1981) replicated parts of the design of Kingsley and Shapiro (1977) by studying parent and child weight loss in three conditions: (1) parent and child as focus of behavior modification program; (2) child alone as focus; and (3) unspecified focus. The intervention program included common behavioral techniques. In addition, the first two groups were taught to act as positive models for eating and to praise family members for positive eating and exercise behaviors— much as in Epstein and his colleagues (1980). No significant differences were obtained across conditions by time periods for children. The adults in the parent and child focus condition, however, were significantly lower at the eight month follow-up, but were equal with the other groups at the 21 month follow-up. (This was in contrast to Kingsley and Shapiro (1977), in which the mother-only condition maintained the greatest weight loss.) Child and parent weight losses were correlated at eight months, but not 21 months. In using a different approach to the analysis of weight loss maintenance, 100% of the children in the parent and child focus group who were nonobese (under 20% overweight) at the eight-month follow-up were also noneobese at 21 months. The corresponding proportions for the children in the child and unspecified focus groups were 30 and 33%, respectively. These results indicate a delayed and modest effect of parent–child training for adults, but a potential enduring effect for children who were able to get under 20% overweight during the initial training.

Shifting the focus to adolescents, Coates and Thoresen (1981) compared three single-subject interventions, two of which involved family participation. Among a variety of other aspects of the intervention, the families were trained in food storage, buying and preparation patterns, and in ways that related to one another in regard to food. The two experimental participants demonstrated weight losses, whereas the control participant gained. Coates, Killen, and Slinkard (1982) pursued this lead and compared parent participation with a no-parent participation group. The intervention in both adolescent groups consisted of 20 weekly sessions in which calorie estimation, exercise, reinforcement, problem solving, imagery, and goal setting skills were trained. The parents in the parent participation condition received similar training in separate sessions, with an emphasis on how to be supportive of their child's weight loss efforts. Both groups lost weight with no statistically signficant differences between groups. There were also no differences between groups in other aspects of a healthy diet (e.g., calories, cholesterol intake, and saturated fats), or lipid status. These results support the notion that the behavioral techniques and not the family involvement were responsible for the weight loss. These techniques were similar to those in Coates and Thoreson (1981) and therefore serve to emphasize caution for interpreting single case study designs.

Brownell, Kelman, and Stunkard (1983) varied the type of parent–child involvement with adolescents. These authors had parent–child trained together, parent–child trained separately, and child–alone groups. The training involved 16 sessions in which a series of behavioral and cognitive-behavioral techniques was taught. One session was devoted to social support. No more in-depth statement of the social support treatment was provided in that paper. The parent–child-trained separately group achieved the greatest posttreatment weight loss, and was the only group to maintain weight loss at one year follow-up. In contrast to the previous work no differences occurred in weight across the groups on the part of the involved parents (they were not asked to lose weight), and no significant correlation appeared between parent and child weight losses. Brownell et al. interpreted the differences in child weight loss across groups to reflect a moderate level of parent involvement between extremes of disengagement with excessive freedom for the child and overinvolvement with an exacerbation of usual adolescent–parent dependency conflicts. They interpreted this moderate level of parental involvement as providing training to the parent, allowing the parent and child to openly discuss problems of dealing with the other, and encouraging the child to take personal control for the obesity and weight loss. These conclusions, however, remain speculative. It may be that the parent–child separate group did best because the mothers in this group alone were counseled and trained by Brownell himself, who has more experience—and perhaps more dynamism or charisma—than the primary counselor/trainer for the other groups.

Across all the studies the findings in this area are confusing, once again. Several authors found an effect for parent involvement (Argona, Cassady, & Drabman, 1975; Wheeler & Hess, 1976) and others did not (Kingsley & Shapiro, 1977). Some found an effect for training the parent and the child together (Aragona et al., 1975); others found an effect for training the parent and child separately but not together (Brownell, et al., 1983); and still others found an effect for training separately but no additional effect over individual treatment (Coates, Killen, & Slinkard, 1982). Some found an effect from parent involvement on the parents' weight (Kingsley & Shapiro, 1977; Epstein et al., 1980), whereas others found an isolated fleeting difference (Epstein et al., 1981). At least one report questioned the value of including training in the sophisticated and time-consuming behavior management procedures (Aragona et al., 1975). Despite the evidence presented in the previous chapter for family influence on dietary patterns, only one study (Brownell, Kelman, & Stunkard, 1983) provided evidence for an enhanced effect of parent involvement beyond that from training the child alone, and this study trained parents and children separately. Of course, child-alone training does not make sense for children under ten years of age, and combined parent and child training has been shown to work in that age group. It is too early in this research to resolve these inconsistencies, or to determine with confidence whether family involvement or what form of family involvement in pediatric weight loss is effective; and if effective, effective for what outcome—child weight loss, parent weight loss, family harmony?

Although the parent–child intervention literature is not as extensive as that for couples training, most of the same problems exist. Samples are small. The interventions are inconsistent and noncomparable. The measures differ across studies. No family theory is employed for identifying the best means for involving the family. At a minimum we need to know more about how families can be supportive of a child's dietary changes, so that training for these behaviors can be incorporated into the weight loss programs. Given that the major task of adolescence is establishing independence from the parents, modes of parental support may be particularly difficult to determine. Furthermore, the identification of supportive behaviors is not independent of the relationship within which they are provided. What behaviors may be considered as supportive in one relationship may be interpreted as nonsupportive in another. There appear to be some parent–child relationships in which emotions are not easily expressed and supportive behaviors are not easily performed. We need to know more about these relationships and behaviors before we can determine the design that is likely to be effective parent–child interventions.

Cardiovascular Disease Risk—Related Behavior Changes.   Health behavior changes have been attempted for other cardiovascular risks as well. School age children have often been the target of these programs because the school provides both an institution for promoting change through school-based health education and a setting for evaluating easily the impact of such a program. Several of these programs have attempted to involve the family on the assumption that both family involvement will facilitate greater child change and children can affect parental behavior throughout the life cycle (Rapoport, Rapoport, & Strelitz, 1977) and particularly in adolescence (Baranowski, 1978).

One such approach was designed for fifth- and sixth-grade students (Coates, Jeffery, & Slinkard, 1981) to assist them to increase their consumption of complex carbohydrates, decrease their consumption of saturated fats, cholesterol, sodium, and sugar, increase their level of habitual physical activity, and generalize these changes to other family members. The program's 12 class sessions used participative activities, personal goal setting, handouts of information for parents, feedback, and reinforcement for behavior change. For example, children were intermittently reinforced (given stickers with red hearts) at lunch for bringing predominately heart-healthy lunches prepared at home. The authors expected that this strategy would stimulate parents to change food purchasing and eating patterns in directions encouraged by the program. Evaluation of the impact of this program used direct observation of the children's eating and physical activity at school as well as questionnaires at the end of the academic year. Results indicated substantial changes in eating behavior at school, knowledge about heart health, food preferences, and family eating patterns, as reported by parents. No effect was obtained in exercise when observed at the beginning of the ensuing academic year. A subsequent replication of the experiment and component analyses revealed that only those students and their families receiving the full program (containing both instructional and motivational behavior components) showed positive and sustained changes in behavior at four months (Coates, Slinkard, & Perry, 1983). Thus family involvement may have been a key element in a successful school-based cardiovascular risk behavior change program.

In a study of a high school-based education program designed to increase family awareness of an ongoing community cardiovascular-risk reduction program (Nader et al., 1982), only one third of tenth-grade students expressed a high level of confidence in their ability to help a parent change dietary or exercise behaviors. Both boys and girls expressed less confidence that they could help their fathers make changes than help their mothers. A simple two class intervention did result in more family members of those students viewing a communitywide media event broadcast ten days following the class sessions (Nader et al., 1982). However, no effects on parental health knowledge, attitudes, or behaviors were detected.

Another study conducted over a three-year period explored the feasibility of a family educational intervention for the purpose of reducing the risk factors of coronary heart disease (Hopp & Zimmerman, 1982). Although no change in risk factors was statistically significant, behavior change did occur and was maintained over a year's period. Any changes in behaviors and risk factors that did occur were in a positive direction.

The Chicago Heart Health Curriculum Program (Sunseri et al., 1983) focused on the impact of their curriculum on smoking attitudes and behaviors among predominantly preadolescent children. Their approach to family involvement was to send home educational materials specifically designed to involve the parents in the program. Sunseri et al. (1983) reported statistically significant, but only slightly, higher knowledge and attitudes for the parent involved group. Children in the family-involved condition were less likely to "purchase" cigarettes in a simulated test situation, but no less likely to actually smoke. The predominant variable in their study was reading level that was significantly related to every outcome variable. It is not clear how to interpret the relationship with this reading variable. If treated as a measure of social class, it may indicate that upper class, upwardly mobile children were somehow immune to the pressures to smoke. Alternatively, as a measure of cognitive ability, it may indicate that children who had difficulty reading could not understand the program materials.

In a study to assess the effects of modifying sodium intake, 80 schoolchildren from the Minneapolis Children's Blood Pressure Study who had blood pressures above the 95th percentile for age and sex, but below 130/90 mmHg at school screening, were randomized to a family intervention program or a control group (Gillum, Prineas, & Surbey, 1981). Intervention group meetings, attended by both children and parents, included four biweekly intensive 90-minute lecture demonstration sessions followed by 90-minute maintenance sessions at approximately bimonthly intervals over the remainder of the year. At each session, families were separated into children and parent groups for a 60-minute educational session and then reunited for a low sodium refreshment period with discussion. Parents were given dietary guidelines of 70 mmol sodium per day for each family member. Other topics included blood pressure and sodium, dietary sources of sodium, salt point (one salt point = 3 mmol sodium) counting, cooking without salt, and avoiding salt when eating out. Children learned by means of crafts and games, food preparation, and taste activities. Adherence was examined by three-day food records and overnight urine collections for urinary sodium excretion. Sodium intake was significantly lower in the intervention group active participants as compared to the control group or those who dropped out of the intervention (87 versus 130 versus 133 mmol per 24 hours). The authors also measured and found no detrimental effects of the intervention on family environment and children's personality measures.

Direct programmatic interventions have also been developed with and for families. Witschi, Singer, Wu-Lee, and Stone (1978) examined family cooperativeness in a four-week baseline and three-week diet change period. In this short term, family-centered study in which dietary cholesterol and saturated fat sources were decreased and sunflower oil and margarine were added as the major sources of polyunsaturated fat, an average reduction in serum cholesterol approximating 10% was achieved within ten days and maintained throughout a three-week period. Witschi et al. stated: "A high correlation of decreasing cholesterol levels among family members, particularly adults, strengthens the hypothesis that dietary manipulation is best achieved as a family activity." (p. 388)

A recent pilot project involving 24 families with children in the third to sixth grades from three ethnic groups (Anglo, Black, and Hispanic) combined behavior change efforts for diet and exercise (Nader et al., 1983). The intervention was based on principles of both cognitive social learning theory (Bandura, 1977; Parcel & Baranowski, 1981) and family social support (Baranowski, Nader, Dunn, & Vanderpool, 1981). The families, randomly assigned within ethnic groups to treatment or control groups, attended eight weekly 90-minute sessions designed to initiate a process of behavior change. The sessions began with a period of enjoyable physical activity to introduce the families to types of activity in which they could participate together later. This was followed by a nutritious low sodium, low saturated fat snack and beverage—initially provided by the project staff and later brought by participant families. An educational session followed in which adults and children met separately and engaged in adult discussion and child games and role-playing activities. Finally, families were reunited into family groups for behavior management activities and to discuss ways each family member was going to support each other's attempts at behavior change in the ensuing week.

Each participant monitored the daily frequency of their consumption of foods high in sodium and saturated fats, and used this record as a basis of selecting food items to target (decrease or substitute) and as the record for reinforcement. Physical activity was also monitored on a daily basis. Statistically significant differences in reported consumption of high sodium and high saturated fat foods were obtained between the treatment and the control groups at the posttreatment assessment. Participants in the treatment group also gained significantly more knowledge of factors influencing cardiovascular risk, even though the intervention did not emphasize a cognitive approach. The Mexican-American adults evidenced the greatest dietary changes. This pilot experience suggests that the method of health promotion including families, support, and skill enhancing behavioral strategies deserves more extensive investigation.

A range of other studies refers to family involvement in health behavior change programs for the general population and for high-risk populations. In the North Karelia project (Puska et al., 1982), an intervention that was aimed at schoolchildren focused on diet, exercise, and nonsmoking. The approach was comprehensive, involving the children in school, their teachers, the parents, and even the school lunch service. Statistically significant effects were noted in lowered smoking rates, decreased sodium use, increased use of polyunsaturated fats, and switches to low fat milk from whole milk. Because of the comprehensiveness of the approach, it was impossible to separate the relative contributions of the school, peers, the family, or general community awareness. Other complex studies have mentioned the involvement of families as well. Although not explicitly described, nor controlled for, workers responsible for carrying out the multifactor intervention program in the Multiple Risk Factor Intervention Trial (MR FIT, 1982) with 12,886 high-risk men aged 35–57 years reported involvement of spouse and significant others in the health-counseling procedures.

The mechanisms by which families may be helpful to one another in these health behavior change programs have not been the subject of extensive research. In a study examining how possibly socially supportive behaviors (Baranowski, Nader et al., 1982) related to diet and exercise behavior change, generally low levels of the frequency of performance of these behaviors were identified at the beginning of a program (Nader, Baranowski, Vanderpool, Dworkin, & Dunn, 1983), with greater increases in the experimental than in the control groups at the end of the program. It may be that families in which more generally supportive behaviors are performed, for example, making positive comments contingent on the performance of desired behavior, is a key to assisting people to change health behavior. It also seems clear that the behaviors in which one family member engages to be supportive of a particular change may not be construed as positively supportive by the receiver. In fact, some of these behaviors may be interpreted as negatively influencing the adoption and maintenance of health behaviors (Baranowski, Nader, Dunn, & Vanderpool, 1982).

Mermelstein, Lichenstein, and McIntyre (1983) reported a similar set of analyses of socially supportive behaviors in the area of smoking cessation. Program participants rated both the frequency and the helpfulness of a set of 76 behaviors performed by a partner at each of three points (one month, three months, and six months) postprogram. The authors reported increasing differences in mean support over time between three groups: (1) those who never quit, (2) those who quit but relapsed; and (3) continued abstainers, with continued abstainers consistently reporting most support. The pattern of correlations indicated that positive support was more important in maintaining the behavior changes than negative support was in inhibiting the behavior changes.

The value of involving families in cardiovascular-risk behavior change as enhancing effectiveness has not been adequately tested. It is still not clear that we know how to meaningfully involve the family in the school-based programs. The direct family intervention studies have not systematically varied family involvement sufficiently to asssess the effectiveness of such a therapeutic modality.

Alternatively, much of this literature, has assumed that involvement of the family was important in itself. We know from other work that families influence the health behaviors of all members, and that families having one member with an unhealthy behavior probably have other members with that unhealthy behavior. The children and the parents, the husbands and the wives can benefit from these health-promoting behaviors. Perhaps what we should try to learn from this literature is not whether a family-based intervention is more effective than an individual-based intervention but rather how we can best work with families to promote familywide health behavior changes.

If we take the perspective that the whole family should be the unit of concern in promoting healthy behaviors, then the school-based programs do not seem to have a handle on how to meaningfully involve the family. The more direct approach to the family has to be further developed to assess our ability to change health behaviors over the long term. All the criticisms leveled at the family and weight loss studies, (e.g., poorly specified interventions, little documentation of demographic characteristics, no theoretical foundation for involving the family) can also be leveled at most of the cardiovascular-risk reduction literature.

Regimen Compliance Trials

We found no literature in which an intervention for promoting regimen compliance by involving families was evaluated with a pediatric population. This review is thereby limited to interventions involving families with adult patients. One of the earliest approaches to the systematic involvement of family in regimen compliance comes from the family therapy literature, emphasizing family systems and "paradoxical" interventions. Jacob and Moore (in press) have defined paradoxical techniques as those "involving instruction to deliberately increase a symptom, to continue a symptom at its present level, or (at least) not to improve too quickly." On the face of it, these interventions promote change by maintaining or exacerbating the symptoms that we desire removed (i.e., a paradox). In the vernacular, these techniques have sometimes been called "reverse psychology."

Hoebel (1976) reported the effects of a paradoxical intervention with cardiac patients concerning their change of risk-related behaviors (e.g., smoking, weight loss). The study was conducted with nine males who had been referred as being particularly resistant to changing their risk behaviors. In the single case described, the authors used five one-hour sessions (held at one- to three-week intervals) to have the wife *stop* encouraging dietary change and just develop a closer relationship with the patient. In this case, the patient initiated dietary change for weight loss completely on his own after removal of wife influence, and went on to lose a significant, but unreported, amount of weight. Hoebel suggested that parallel processes occurred in the other eight cases and provided an indication of changes in each case. He interpreted his intervention as relieving the maladaptive behavior-maintaining forces in the family, thereby in a sense freeing the patient to comply.

A more traditional, nonparadoxical family approach to regimen compliance was reported by Levine et al. (1979) for hypertensive patients attending inner city university-affiliated clinics. In a baseline survey of these hypertensive patients, these authors found that 70% of the patients expressed a desire for a family member to learn something about the disease, whereas 30% reported no social support. In response to these documented needs, Levine and his colleagues designed a three-part intervention, applying the parts in a factorial design to eight groups with 50 participants per group. One part consisted of a home visit by a trained community interviewer with no background in health care. An adult, usually the spouse, was identified as the target of training for the home visit. The goal of the training was to find ways in which the spouse could assist the patient in complying with the regimen, to explain the need for compliance even when the patient was feeling well, and to obtain a commitment from the spouse to help the patient take medications and keep appointments.

Results revealed that the family support home visit by itself produced an 11% increase over baseline in percentage of patients under hypertension control. This was better than the control group and one of the other intervention components by itself, but not quite as effective as participation in three one-hour group sessions. On the average, all groups with single and combined double interventions achieved roughly a 12% increase in percentage of patients under control. The group with the combined three interventions, however, achieved a 28% increase in percentage under control. The family support training therefore was effective by itself in producing an increase in the percent of patients under control, and was particularly valuable as a component in a more comprehensive program. The authors noted that the family support home visit was significantly more effective with male patients, which is consistent with the data on supportiveness of wives but nonsupportiveness of husbands (Burke & Weir, 1974).

Five-year follow-up data from this study were reported by Morisky et al. (1983). They found an increased likelihood of keeping appointments at five years by the groups receiving the family support home visit. The family support visit, however, did not have an effect on weight loss or blood pressure control. These authors documented a 53% decrease in the five-year mortality rate among all the combined intervention groups as compared to the control group. This is the first study to document a five-year decrease in mortality from any health education intervention. Knowing how difficult it is to change compliance behaviors, and the modest correlation between compliance and disease control, it is hard to believe that a single home visit even in conjunction with other interventions had such an extensive impact on hypertension regimen-compliance behaviors and the resulting disease process as to affect the mortality rate.

A rural community hypertension control project was conducted from a rural primary care clinic in West Virginia (Baranowski, Chapin, Evans, Wagner, & Warren, 1980). A part of this demonstration project was an experiment to promote hypertension care utilization and regimen compliance with family involvement as one factor in a factorial design. The patients in the two family involvement conditions had their spouses or significant others attend the hypertension-related clinic visits; they were trained in all aspects of regimen compliance (as was the patient), encouraged to help the patients in all facets of compliance, and included the spouse/significant other in all facets of a verbal regimen compliance contracting process. (Formal written contracting was not readily accepted in this population and had to be dropped.) Ways for the spouse to promote compliance were discussed at each clinic visit. Another factor in the design was daily home self-monitoring of blood pressure. All patients in these four groups received medication self-monitoring, phone call reminders for appointments, and care from a specially trained nurse hypertension counselor. To control for these factors, a fifth other-provider control group was added. Participants were randomly assigned to the five groups.

After one year of functioning, the data revealed that the blood pressures in all conditions were reduced and that significantly more patients in the neither groups and in the other provider-care control groups had their blood pressures under control (≤ 90 mm Hg). A significant interaction effect was detected with those patients who received both the family involvement and self-blood pressure monitoring, and those receiving neither, had the lowest mean diastolic blood pressures. Although randomization was conducted, there were significant prior differences across groups in education. The effects of education could not be covaried from the impact of the program on blood pressure because nonparallel slopes were obtained between education and blood pressure across the groups. These data thereby revealed a possible effect of family involvement in this rural Appalachian population if pursued in conjunction with daily self-blood pressure monitoring. This conclusion must be drawn with caution because of the three-month long coal miners strike in the first year of the project that confounded utilization of clinical care. An attempt to evaluate the impact of this program two-and-a half years after its initiation (Baranowski, Chapin, & Evans, 1982a) was confounded by a severe economic recession in the mining industry that caused half the miners to move out of this area, and others not to seek care for hypertension because no money was available. Of those remaining in the program after two-and-a half years, no differences were found across groups in compliance, utilization of clinical care, or blood pressures.

An effort was made to detect differences in the way families related to the hypertensive patients in the above study (Baranowski, Chapin, & Evans, 1982b). Within the framework provided by Caplan, Robinson, French, Caldwell, and Shinn (1976), Baranowski et al. (1982b) developed 22 behaviors potentially performed by family and significant others that could be interpreted to be materially (instrumentally), informationally (cognitively), or social-emotionally (affectively) supportive of hypertensive regimen compliance. Their results revealed that in two groups of hypertensive patients (those participating in the experiment versus those not), the median and the modal response on the frequency of performance of each item was "never." This indicated that there was little naturally occurring social support for hypertension regimen compliance in this population. In a factor analysis, the items factored along components of the regimen (e.g., salt consumption, medication ingestion) rather than types of suppport (e.g., informational, material, or emotional), and the factors included both positively and negatively supportive behaviors. The authors inferred that training families in supportive behaviors had the effect of the family selecting the particular component of the regimen and the particular approach to support that he or she found most comfortable. These are obviously tentative and preliminary results.

The value of family involvement in regimen compliance was questioned by Earp, Strogatz, and Ory (1982). These authors introduced two forms of social support in comparison with a usual care control group. The first form of support involved home visits by public health nurses or pharmacists over an 18-month period. The second group received the same home visits, and in addition had a family member or some significant other participate in these home visits and participate in daily self-monitoring of blood pressure. (Fifty percent of the patients chose a spouse, 25% a son or daughter, and only 7% a nonrelative.) Their results revealed no differences in blood pressure control between the two support groups at one or two years after the introduction of the program, although there were marked reductions in the percent of patients above the level of diastolic blood pressure control at year one and continued improvement at the end of two years. The two experimental groups were better than the control group only at the two-year assessment. These results only question the value of family support as an addition to that provided by professionals.

Earp, Strogatz, and Ory (1981) showed with the same group of patients at the two-year assessment that providing social support from family and friends moderated the impact of stress on utilization noncompliance, and showed that highly supported individuals had significantly more medication compliance than the low support group, regardless of level of stress. Family support as measured by process variables thereby was shown to be significantly related to utilization and medication compliance. Two inferences can be drawn. The family involvement intervention was not strong enough to increase support by the family members. Some families in the control groups had existing high levels of support.

A different type of family involvement was tested with dietary compliance among hemodialysis patients. Cummings, Becker, Kirscht, and Levin (1981) compared three approaches to intervention (behavioral contract, behavioral contract with a family member or friend, or weekly telephone contact) with a control group. The family involvement in the contracting group involved three-participant contracting in which specific self-care behaviors and contingencies for the patient were also identified. The results revealed that the effect of family involvement in contracting varied by area of compliance. Immediately, posttreatment, the behavioral contract with a family member or friend group, displayed the least effect on mean serum potassium level and was worse than the control group at three months postintervention. On the other hand, this group had the lowest mean weight gain at both assessment points.

The value of family involvement in a structured program for regimen compliance is no more clear than it was for health behavior changes. One study showed the value of a singlefamily home visit, the other questioned involving the family over multiple home visits. One reported an interactive effect with self-blood pressure monitoring, which, however, was no more effective than a program without either of these components. The last study showed positive effects from family involvement in one outcome area, but not others.

A strong conceptual case can be made for continued exploration of family involvement in regimen compliance. Many regimen tasks require the assistance of family members in their support. For instance, some tasks (e.g., dietary changes) would be facilitated by entire family changes rather than changes on the part of the patient alone. The manner in which families participate in regimen task performance may vary in effectiveness. Future research in this area, however, must take a more sophisticated approach. Diseases must be differentiated into groups that vary by the demands made on the family; practical ways for families to be supportive without nagging must be identified; methods must be developed for training family members in the performance of these support behaviors and for increasing the frequency of their performances; steps must also be taken to evaluate the credibility and integrity of interventions; and preexisting family relationship and interaction patterns must be assessed and factored into the intervention program. The literature thus shows that good intentions for involving the family are not enough. More sophisticated interventions for behavior change must be devised and tested. A potential contribution can come from integrating the behavior change techniques with what we know about family functioning and from the descriptive literature on family aspects of health behaviors and compliance.

CONCLUSION

Studies designed to deliberately change health-related behavior by involving families were described. Future intervention research must capitalize more on what is known about families in order to design more effective interventions. More standardization must be introduced into the intervention components so that it is possible to compare the results of intervention attempts across studies. Many other methodological shortcomings have been identified in this review and deserve attention in the future.

REFERENCES

Aragona, J., Cassady, J., & Drabman, R. S. (1975). Treating overweight children through parental training and contingency contracting. *Journal of Applied Behavior Analysis, 8,* 269–278.

Bandura, A. (1977). *Social learning theory.* Englewood Cliffs, NJ: Prentice-Hall.

Baranowski, M. (1978). Adolescents attempted influence on parental behaviors. *Adolescence 13,* 585–604.

Baranowski, T., Bee, D., Rassin, D., Richardson, C. J., Brown, J., Guenther, N., & Nader, P. R. (1983). Social support, social influence, ethnicity, and the breastfeeding decision. *Social Science & Medicine, 17:* A, 1599–1611.

Baranowski, T., Chapin, J. & Evans, M. (1982a). *Hypertension regimen compliance at Cabin Creek: Analyses of final survey data.* Galveston: University of Texas Medical Branch.

Baranowski, T., Chapin, J., & Evans, M. (1982b). *Dimensions of social support for hypertension regimen compliance.* Galveston: University of Texas Medical Branch.

Baranowski, T., Chapin, J., Evans, M., Wagner, G., & Warren, S. G. (1980). Utilization and medication compliance for high blood pressure: An experiment with family involvement and self blood pressure monitoring in a rural population. *American Journal of Rural Health, 6,* 51–67.

Baranowski, T., Dworkin, R. J., Clearmen, D. R., Dunn, J. K., Ray, L., Vernon, S. & Nader, P. R. (1983). *Comparisons of dietary self-report methods: Family Health Project.* Unpublished manuscript. Galveston: University of Texas Medical Branch.

Baranowski, T., Nader, P., Dunn, J. K., & Vanderpool, N. A. (1982). Family self-help: Promoting changes in health behavior. *Journal of Communication, 32,* 161–172.

Baranowski, T., & Parcel, G. (in press). Social learning theory. In M. Kreuter & G. Christensen (Eds.), *Theories in health education.* Palto Alto, CA: Mayfield Press.

Brownell, K. D., Heckerman, C. L., Westlake, R. J., Hayes, S. C., & Monti, P. M. (1978). The effect of couples training and partner co-operativeness in the behavioral treatment of obesity. *Behavior Research and Therapy, 16,* 323–333.

Brownell, K. D., Kelman, J. H., & Stunkard, A. J. (1983). Treatment of obese children with and without their mothers: Changes in weight and blood pressure. *Pediatrics, 71,* 515–523.

Brownell, K. D., & Stunkard, A. J. (1981). Couples training, pharmacotherapy, and behavior therapy in the treatment of obesity. *Archives of General Psychiatry, 38,* 1224–1229.

Bryant, C. A. (1982). The impact of kin, friend and neighbor networks on infant feeding practices. *Social Science and Medicine, 16,* 1757–1765.

Burke, R. J., & Weir, T. (1974). Husband-wife helping-relationships: The "mental hygiene" function in marriages. *Psychological Reports, 40,* 911–925.

Caplan, R. D., Harrison, R. V., Weltons, R. V., & French, J. R. P., Jr. (1980). *Social Support and patient adherence: Experimental and survey findings.* Ann Arbor: University of Michigan.

Caplan, R. D., Robinson, E. A. R., French, J. R. P., Jr., Caldwell, J. R., & Shinn, M. (1976). *Adhering to medical regimens.* Ann Arbor: University of Michigan.

Coates, T. J., Jeffery, R. W., & Slinkard, S. A. (1981). Heart healthy eating and exercise: Introducing and maintaining changes in health behaviors. *American Journal of Public Health, 71,* 15–23.

Coates, T. J., Killen, J. D., & Slinkard, L. A. (1982). Parent participation in a treatment program for overweight adolescents. *International Journal of Eating Disorders, 1,* 37–48.

Coates, T. J., Slinkard, L. A., & Perry, C. (1983). *Heart healthy eating and exercise: A replication and component analysis.* Unpublished manuscript, University of California, San Francisco.

Coates, T. J., & Thoresen, C. E. (1981). Behavior and weight changes in three obese adolescents. *Behavior Therapy, 12,* 383–399.

Colletti, G., & Brownell, K. D. (1982). The physical and emotional benefits of social support: Application to obesity, smoking, and alcoholism. *Progress in Behavior Modification, 1,* 383–399.

Cummings, K. M., Becker, M. H., Kirscht, J. P., & Levin, N. W. (1981). Intervention strategies to improve compliance with medical regimens by ambulatory hemodialysis patients. *Journal of Behavioral Medicine, 4,* 111–128.

Dubbert, P. M., & Wilson, G. T. (in press). Goal setting and spouse involvement in the treatment of obesity. *Behavior Research and Therapy.*

Dubbert, P. M., Wilson, G. T., Augusto, F., Longenbucher, J. McGee, D. H., & Allen, C. (1981, November). *Cooperative behavior of involved and noninvolved spouses of weight control program participants.* Paper presented at the annual meeting of the Association for the Advancement of Behavior Therapy, Toronto.

Earp, J. A. L., Ory, M. G., & Strogatz, D. S. (1982). The effects of family involvement and practitioner home visits on the control of hypertension. *American Journal of Public Health, 72,* 1146–1154.

Earp, J. A. L., Strogatz, D. S., & Ory, M. G. (1981). *The relationship between stressful life events, social support, and high blood pressure control.* Paper presented at the National Conference on High Blood Pressure Control, New York.

Epstein, L. H., Wing, R. R., Koeske, R., Andrasik, F., & Ossip, D. J. (1981). Child and parent weight loss in family-based behavior modification programs. *Journal of Consulting and Clinical Psychology, 49,* 674–685.

Epstein, L. H., Wing, R. R., Steranchak, L., Dickson, B., & Michelson, J. (1980). Comparison of family-based behavior modification and nutrition education for childhood obesity. *Journal of Pediatric Psychology, 5,* 25–36.

Foreyt, J. P., Goodrick, G. K., & Gotto, A. M. (1981). Limitation of behavioral treatment of obesity: Review and analysis. *Behavioral Medicine, 4,* 159–174.

Garn, S. M., Bailey, S. M., Solomon, M. A., & Hopkins, P. J. (1981). Effect of remaining family members on fatness prediction. *American Journal of Clinical Nutrition, 34,* 148–153.

Gierszewski, S. A. (1983). The relationship of weight loss, locus of control, and social support. *Nursing Research, 32,* 43–47.

Gillum, R. F., Elmer, P. J., Prineas, R. J., & Surbey, D. (1981). Changing sodium intake in children. The Minneapolis Children's Blood Pressure Study. *Hypertension 3*, 698–703.

Griffiths, M., & Payne, P. R. (1976). Energy expenditure in small children of obese and non-obese parents. *Nature, 260*, 698–700.

Haynes, R. B., Taylor, D. W., & Sackett, D. L. (1979). *Compliance in health care*. Baltimore: Johns Hopkins University Press.

Heckerman, C. L., & Zitter, R. E. (1979). *Spouse monitoring and reinforcement in the treatment of obesity*. Paper presented at the annual meeting of the Association for the Advancement of Behavior Therapy, San Francisco.

Hoebel, F. C. (1976). Brief family-interactional therapy in the management of cardiac-related high-risk behaviors. *Journal of Family Practice, 3*, 613–618.

Hoebel, F. C. (1977). Coronary artery disease and family interaction: A study of risk factor modification. In P. Watzlawick & J. H. Weakland (Eds.), *The interactional view* (pp. 363–374). New York: Norton.

Hooks, P., Baranowski, T., Vanderpool, N., & Nader, P. R. (1983) *Issues in recruiting families for community based cardiovascular disease prevention research*. Unpublished manuscript, Galveston: University of Texas Medical Branch.

Hopp, J., & Zimmerman, G. (1982). Family intervention for the reduction of coronary heart disease risk factors: A community case study. In Carlow R. W. (Ed.), *Perspectives in community health education*, Oakland, CA: Third Party Publishing.

Huse, D. M., Branes, L. A., Colligan, R. C., Nelson, R. A., & Palumbo, P. J. (1982). The challenge of obesity in childhood. I. Incidence, prevalence, and staging. *Mayo Clinic Proceedings. 57*, 279–284.

Israel, A. C., & Saccone, A. J. (1979). Follow-up of effects of choice of mediator and target of reinforcement on weight loss. *Behavior Therapy, 10*, 260–265.

Jacob, R. G., & Moore, D. J. (In press). Paradoxical interventions in behavioral medicine. *Journal of Behavior Therapy and Experimental Psychiatry*.

Kazdin, A. E. (1979). Therapy outcome requiring control of credibility and treatment-generated expectancies. *Behavior Therapy, 10*, 81–93.

Kingsley, R. G., & Shapiro, J. (1977). A comparison of three behavioral programs for the control of obesity in children. *Behavior Therapy, 8*, 30–36.

Klesges, R. C., Coates, T. J., Brown, G., Sturgeon-Tillisch, J., Moldenhauer, L. M., Holzer, B., Woolfrey, J., & Vollmer, J. (1983). Parental influences on children's eating behavior and relative weight. *Journal of Applied Behavioral Analysis, 16*, 371–378.

Klesges, R. C., Coates, T. J., Moldenhauer, L. M., Holzer, B., Gustavson, J., & Barnes, J. (in press). The FATS: An observational system for assessing physical activity in children and associated parent behavior. *Behavioral Assessment*.

Klesges, R. C., Malott, J. M., Boschee, P. F., & Weber, J. M. (in press). Parental influences on children's food intake, physical activity and relative weight: An extension and replication. *Journal of Behavioral Medicine*.

Lavigne, J. V., & Daruna, J. H. (1982). A comment on Epstein et al.'s "Comparison of family-based behavior modification and nutrition education for childhood obesity." *Journal of Pediatric Psychology, 7*, 95–98.

Levine, D. M., Green, L. W., Deeds, S. G., Chwalow, J., Russell, R. P., & Finlay, J. (1979). Health education for hypertensive patients. *Journal of the American Medical Association, 241*, 1700–1703.

Mahoney, M. J., & Mahoney, K. (1976). Treatment of obesity: A clinical exploration. In B. J. Williams, S. Martin, & J. P. Foreyt (Eds.), *Obesity, behavioral approaches to dietary management* (pp.   ). New York: Brunner/Mazel.

Marshall, J. R., & Neill, J. (1977). The removal of a psychosomatic symptom: Effects on the marriage. *Family Process, 16,* 273–280.

Mermelstein, R., Lichtenstein, E., & McIntyre, K. (1983). Partner support and relapse in smoking-cessation programs. *Journal of Consulting and Clinical Psychology, 51,* 465–466.

Morisky, D. E., Levine, D. M., Green, L. W., Shapiro, S., Russell, R. P., & Smith, C. R. (1983). Five-year blood pressure control and mortality following health education for hypertensive patients. *American Journal of Public Health, 73,* 153–162.

Multiple Risk Factor Intervention Trial Research Group. (1982). Multiple risk factor intervention trial. *Journal of the American Medical Association, 248,* 1465–1477.

Murphy, J. K., Williamson, D. A., Buxton, A. E., Moody, S. C., Absher, N., & Warner, M. (1982). The long-term effects of spouse involvement upon weight loss and maintenance. *Behavior Therapy, 13,* 681–693.

Nader, P. R., Baranowski, T., Vanderpool, N., Dworkin, R. J., & Dunn, K. (1983). The Family Health Project: Cardiovascular risk reduction education for children and parents. *Developmental and Behavioral Pediatrics, 4,* 3–10.

Nader, P. R., Perry, C., Maccoby, N., Solomon, D., Killen, J., Telch, M., & Alexander, J. K. (1982). Adolescent perceptions of family health behavior: A tenth grade educational activity to increase family awareness of a community cardiovascular risk reduction program. *Journal of School Health, 52,* 372–377.

Nightingale, E. D., Cureton, M., Kalmar, V., & Trudeau, M. B. (1978). *Perspectives on health promotion and disease prevention in the United States.* Washington, D.C.: National Academy of Sciences, Institute of Medicine.

O'Neil, P. M., Curey, H. S., Hirsch, A. A., Riddle, F. E., Taylor, C. I., Malcolm, R. J., & Sexauer, J. D. (1979). Effects of sex of subject and spouse involvement on weight loss in a behavioral treatment program: A retrospective investigation. *Addictive Behaviors, 4,* 167–177.

Parcel, G., & Baranowski, T. (1981). Social learning theory and health education. *Health Education, 12,* 14–18.

Pearce, J. W., LeBow, M. D., & Orchard, J. (1981). Role of spouse involvement in the behavioral treatment of overweight women. *Journal of Consulting and Clinical Psychology, 49,* 236–244.

Puska, P., Vartiainen, E., Pallonen, U., Salonen, J. T., Poyhia, P., Koskela, K., & McAlister, A. (1982). The North Karelia Youth Project: Evaluation of two years of intervention on health behavior and cardiovascular risk factors among 13 to 15 year old children. *Preventive Medicine, 11,* 550–570.

Rand, C. S. W., Kuldau, J. M., & Robbins, L. (1982). Surgery for obesity and marriage quality. *Journal of the American Medical Association, 247,* 1419–1422.

Rapoport, R., Rapoport, R., & Strelitz, Z. (1977). *Fathers, mothers and society: Towards new alliances.* New York: Basic Books.

Rosenthal, B., Allen, G. J., & Winter, C. (1980). Husband involvement in the behavioral treatment of overweight women: Initial effects and long-term follow-up. *International Journal of Obesity, 1,* 165–173.

Saccone, A. J., & Israel, A. C. (1978). Effects of experimenter versus significant other-controlled reinforcement and choice of target behavior on weight loss. *Behavior Therapy, 9,* 271–278.

Saltzer, E. B., (1980). Social determinants of successful weight loss: An analysis of behavioral intentions and actual behavior. *Basic and Applied Social Psychology, 1,* 329–341.

Schafer, L. C., Glasgow, R. E., McCaul, K. D., & Dreher, M. (1983). Adherence to IDDM regimens: Relationship to psychosocial variables and metabolic control. *Diabetes Care, 6,* 493–498.

Streja, D. A., Boyko, E., & Rabkin, S. W. (1982). Predictors of outcome in a risk factor intervention trial using behavior modification. *Preventive Medicine, 11,* 291–303.

Stuart, R. B., & Davis, B. (1972). *Slim chance in a fat world: Behavioral control of obesity.* Champaign, IL: Research Press.

Sunseri, A. J., Alberti, J. M., Kent, N. D., Schoenberger, J. A., Sunseri, J. K., Amuwo, S., & Vickers, P. (1983). Reading, demographic, social and psychological factors related to preadolescent smoking and non-smoking behaviors and attitudes. *Journal of School Health, 53,* 257–263.

Waxman, M., & Stunkard, A. J., (1980). Calorie intake and expenditure of obese boys. *Journal of Pediatrics, 96,* 187–193.

Weisz, G., & Bucher, B. (1980). Involving husbands in treatment of obesity-effects on weight loss, depression, and marital satisfaction. *Behavior Therapy, 11,* 643–650.

Wheeler, M. E., & Hess, K. W. (1976). Treatment of juvenile obesity by successive approximation control of eating. *Journal of Behavior Therapy and Experimental Psychiatry, 7,* 235–241.

Wilson, G. T., & Brownell, K. (1978). Behavior therapy for obesity: Including family members in the treatment process. *Behavior Therapy, 9,* 943–945.

Windsor, R. A., Baranowski, T., Cutter, G., & Clark, N. (1984). *Evaluation of health promotion disease prevention programs.* Palto Alto, CA: Mayfield Press.

Windsor, R. A., Roseman, J., Gartseff, G., & Kirk, D. A. (1981). Qualitative issues in developing educational diagnostic instruments and assessment procedures for diabetic patients. *Diabetes Care, 4,* 468–475.

Witschi, J. C., Singer, M., Wu Lee, M., & Store, F. (1978). Family cooperation and effectiveness in a cholesterol-lowering diet. *Journal of the American Dietetic Association, 72,* 384–389.

Zitter, R. E., & Fremouw, W. J., (1978). Individual versus partner consequation for weight loss. *Behavior Therapy, 9,* 808–813.

Zitter, R. E., & Heckerman, C. L. (in press). Long term follow-up of couples treatment of obesity. In D. Upper & S. Ross (Eds.), *Annual review of behavioral group therapy.*

5

Reactions of Families to Illness: Theoretical Models and Perspectives

Howard Leventhal

Elaine A. Leventhal

Tri Van Nguyen

The occurrence of chronic illness in an adult member of a family introduces a host of pressures that may lead to changes ranging from the dissolution of the family unit to an increase in its cohesiveness and in a sense of well-being of its members (Boss, in press). What is responsible for these varied outcomes? Are they produced by the specific features of the illness in interaction with the family and its ways of coping with stress? Do factors such as cohesiveness, dissolution, or well-being of the family and its members adequately define the set of dependent variables for evaluating response to chronic illness, or must we include other factors such as role conflict, role definition, and communication in our set of end points? Are these end points dependent upon the social context in which the family resides? Does illness in an adult member merely bring out or hasten the appearance of strains and strengths existent in the family unit? Do these outcomes depend upon the point in the life cycle of the individual or the life course of the family at which illness strikes?

It would take a substantial body of research to answer these questions or to determine whether they are the most appropriate questions to ask. Unfortunately, such data do not exist and in their absence we cannot select the most plausible theory and use it either to suggest future research or to recommend solutions to the practical problems of identifying and assisting families that are at high risk when illness strikes an adult member. Our more modest, yet perhaps still too ambitious, goal is to propose a systems framework in which we can generate questions and develop methods for the study of families responding to chronic illness in an adult member (e.g., Arbib, 1972; Carver & Scheier, 1982; Leventhal & Nerenz, 1982; Powers, 1973; Schwartz, 1979). This framework can be helpful in two quite different ways. First, it can serve as a structure within which to describe the relationships between quite different levels of data, for example, data from the social system, the family system, the individual's psychological and biological systems, and the disease system. Second, it can be used to describe the content, organization, and operation of the components at each level of description.

Our second major goal is to provide a temporal perspective for looking at the social, family, individual, and illness systems. We are looking at systems within a life-course perspective, that is, as processes that can change and become more or less elaborate over time. The family exists at a particular point in the history of its culture, and the culture establishes values, resources, and behavioral rules respecting social relationships both within and without the family for age- and sex-related role behaviors (Caplow, Bahr, Chadwick, Hill, & Williamson, 1982) and for the perception and response to illness. These varied effects, with some related to cohort and others to individual and family development, are difficult to study (see Baltes & Nesselroade, 1973; Boss, in press; McCubbin et al., 1983; McCubbin & Patterson, 1981), but are critical for understanding the way a family responds to illness in one of its adult members. Within this complex structure we can search for pattern, for different types or modes of adjustment as a function of where the individual and family may be with respect to their life course. The individual and the nuclear family are born, differentiate and mature, pass through one or more periods of stable productivity, retire in some respects from active participation in the marketplace, and face dissolution or death. The extended and cross-generational family, however, has greater psychological longevity.

Finally, chronic illnesses vary in duration and outcome, and each type of illness has its natural history. Moreover, the history of the illness in any particular family is a function of when the illness occurs in both the family and in the individual life history and how it changes the individual and family system. Illness alters the relationship of family members to the ill person and of well persons to one another. The changes in relationship can occur in problem-focused actions, for example, in work, household tasks, and economics, and especially in emotional responses both in problem areas and in interpersonal areas rich in emotional meaning, such as, solidarity or belonging and sexuality and love. Such changes can be stimulated by the action of a specific person or brought about by collective changes, either consciously thought out and considered by the individual and the family or generated automatically in thoughtless, affective reactions by (or toward) the ill person or by well persons toward one another. The family system also has an impact on the illness system and can influence whether an illness is controlled or claims its target. Finally, many of the changes created by illness can accelerate the aging of the family and its members, and these changes may be resisted and intensely resented.

Because our topic includes so many systems and system interactions and a large number of chronic diseases, we must narrow our focus. First, we will draw the most heavily from studies of families coping with cancer, but we also will use data from studies of other chronic diseases to develop our topic. Second, we will focus primarily upon intrafamily relationships, even though we appreciate that extrafamily factors ranging from economic to social support can alter and sometimes reverse interaction patterns and outcomes that may seem "inevitable" when examined from within the family's perspective. And third, we will focus on the interrelationships between the family system and the illness system.

THE SYSTEMS FRAMEWORK

There are a number of important implications of the decision to conceptualize the family, the individual, and the illness in a systems framework. Two are of special importance: (a) systems have components and structure and (b) systems operate and change over time.

Systems Organization: Goals, Actions, Appraisals

The structure of a system is defined by the organization of variables in stages or components and by a specifiable pattern of relationships between these components. Some variables will function as target values or goals that the system attempts to reach or maintain (Miller, Gallanter, & Pribram, 1960; Powers, 1973). Target values at the biological level are often referred to as set points, for example, the weight that the body attempts to maintain; the level of oxygen and sugar in the blood. Set points may vary over the day in association with circadian rhythms (Aschoff, 1965), over the year (Brown, 1972; Pengelley & Asmundson, 1971), and over the life span (Tanner, 1973). Reference values at the psychological level are typically referred to as goals or incentives, and at the social level as role demands or role requirements. Role definitions, such as the tasks of parenting and the status and tasks of the aged, are culturally defined and may vary by cohorts (Featherman, 1984). The set of goals defined by illness (or by any specific problem) is defined as the representation of the illness.

Systems also contain mechanisms for reaching and maintaining reference values. At the biological level there are a variety of mechanisms useful for homeostatic adjustments. At the psychological level there are a variety of coping mechanisms for goal attainment; and at the social level there are a variety of groups and group processes to help with goal attainment. The mechanisms for adjusting to illness will include adaptations from all of the above domains.

Finally, systems contain mechanisms for detecting and appraising the consequences of adjustive actions. Thus biological, individual psychological, and social systems can detect the consequences of adjustive actions and determine whether those actions are closing or failing to close the gap between an immediately preceding state and a reference value. These appraisal mechanisms may be simple or complex. A simple mechanism may only appraise movement toward a goal. A complex mechanism will also appraise the efficiency of movement, the adequacy of the representation of the goal itself (Is the goal accurately defined?), and the adequacy of the appraisal rules (Are the appraisal expectations reasonable?).

Parallel and Hierarchical Organization

The systems we are dealing with—social, psychological, and biological—are yet more complex because they are both parallel and hierarchical in organization (Leventhal, 1982; Powers, 1973). They are parallel in that several operate simultaneously and their simultaneous operations may only be loosely interconnected. For example, at the biological level chemical exchanges are taking place in the cells of the liver, kidneys, and skin, and barring cataclysm, these exchanges proceed in relative independence of one another. These exchanges are also organized hierarchically; cellular exchanges, for instance, are affected by levels of hormones such as the bursts of epinephrine that occur during demands for intense work. Similar complexity exists at the psychological level. We process various types of information simultaneously, for example, data relevant for writing or reading this chapter along with data relevant for maintaining our upright posture while doing so. Each of these parallel processes involves a hierarchy of automatic mechanisms ranging from lower-level or automatic processes to decisional and integrative processes, such as formulating one's current research activities in a systems framework.

Construction of New Goals

Both social theorists (Buckley, 1967; Deutsch, 1948–1949) and family theorists (Speer, 1970) hypothesize that any operating system can create or generate new goals and new skills, that is, new social roles or new ways of perceiving and coping with situations. This constructive aspect of systems is readily apparent in disease. Diseases such as cancer create a novel biological system that may overwhelm the organism's natural defenses and eventually destroy it (Frei, 1978). At the psychological level, cancer creates new perceptions of the self and life, that is, new structures, new roles, and definitions of self within the family. Indeed, these psychologically and socially generated structures define the illness as a psychosocial syndrome distinct from the biomedical definition of disease (Engel, 1977; Fabrega, 1973, 1975; Nerenz & Leventhal, 1983).

Illness and Nonillness Systems.   Family and individual interactions that are disease- or illness-related need to be distinguished from those that are perceived as nonillness-related. The degree to which the two are segregated, that is, reacted to as separate or distinct, or integrated, that is, where illness beliefs and perceptions affect nonillness-related functions, is critical to an understanding of the extent to which the family and its members are dominated by the illness or by needs to satisfy other goals (Nerenz & Leventhal, 1983). Adaptation to chronic disease poses important questions with respect to the overlap or separation of systems. A disease such as cancer is biomedically chronic, that is, if Mr. Smith has cancer, he "has it all of the time," but his behaviors directed toward the disease can be episodic. Patients typically strive to act as noncancer or "normal" cases when outside the treatment setting, thus restricting the sick role to treatment episodes. This separation may be disrupted and replaced by hypervigilance or depression as a disease makes permanent, visible changes in the individual's physical self or reduces his physical, mental, or emotional competency (Janis, 1958, 1962). Even in the case of severe physical dysfunction, however, individuals encapsulate or segregate episodes of disease from episodes of wellness and act to expand and obtain pleasure in the nondisease domains (Nerenz & Leventhal, 1983). How and when this happens will have critical effects on the family and be critically influenced by it.

BIOLOGICAL, PSYCHOLOGICAL, AND FAMILY SYSTEMS

Our basic goal—to understand how illness in an adult member affects the family—requires that we attend to three types of systems simultaneously: (a) the biological or pathophysiological process of the disease and its natural history; (b) the psychological, or the individual's, representations and efforts to cope with the disease; and (c) the social, or the family's, response to the disease. It is important therefore to be clear about the terms we will use to describe each of these systems before attempting to discuss their interaction.

Biological System: Disease and Its Treatment

Practitioners and investigators have found it useful to adopt stage models to describe both the natural history of specific illnesses and the patient's and family's experience of them. Most of these "systems" divide the history into prediagnostic, diagnostic and pretreatment, treatment, and rehabilitation or resolution phases. Biologically, the prediagnostic phase of illness includes a set of processes that occur in sequence at the cellular and systemic levels before the disease state is manifested or symptomatic. This "predisease" phase can exist for many years without assayable clues. Cancer is a prototypic example of multistage disease development, in which a normal cell becomes malignant and grows uncontrollably at the expense of surrounding normal cells and eventually of the organism itself.

The two major events in the development of a cancer are initiation and promotion (Scott, Wille, & Wier, 1984; Pitot, 1981). In initiation, the genetic information of the normal cell is altered; the cell can be derepressed or two or more oncogenes can be introduced into the genome, so that it is primed or receptive for the events that promote or trigger the actual malignant transformation. Promotion can be effected by environmental pollutants, chemicals, or viruses (Scott, Wille, & Wier, 1984; Pitot, 1981; Todaro, 1977). Neither initiation nor promotion alone is sufficient to produce malignancy; only an initiated cell can be promoted to become cancerous, and these processes may be separated temporally by years.

Other chronic illnesses also occur only after a variety of defined events occur in sequence. Type II diabetes mellitus is the end result of an interaction between a specific genome present since birth and a defined set of biological factors including exogenous obesity, decreased energy demands secondary to decreased activity, and age-related losses of the small beta cells in the pancreatic islets (Raskin, 1982). Parkinsonism (Calne & Langston, 1983) also reflects encephalopathic virus-induced loss of neurons in the basal ganglia, and substantia nigra superimposed on "normal" age-related nerve cell loss in the extrapyramidal system, thus accelerating the degenerative process and producing the signs and symptoms of this neurological motor disorder.

Biological phenomena such as the above generate the characteristic signs and symptoms of specific diseases and influence the psychological events that comprise the prediagnostic phase of illness: the awareness or appraisal (hypothesis-testing) stage, where the individual recognizes vague sensations that suggest the possibility of illness and thus gathers information (reads, engages in social comparison) to decide if expert help is needed; the illness stage in which the individual is certain something is wrong; and the utilization stage in which the individual makes efforts to seek expert help (Matthews, Siegel, Kuller, Thompson, & Varat, 1983; Safer, Tharps, Jackson, & Leventhal, 1979; Suchman, 1965). Each step may involve the sharing of different types of information, different expressions of emotional solidarity, and different role adjustments. The appraisal or hypothesis-testing stage may be brief or drawn out. With many types of cancer, initial contact with practitioners results in alternative questions about the nature of the problem and in the need for additional tests to reject or confirm specific hypotheses. To the family certain that the patient has cancer, these steps may appear as unnecessary delays, and there are occasions when the patient and family are correct (Hackett & Cassem, 1969). Treatment, recovery, and rehabilitation or resolution phases differ widely between different diseases, but there are many features shared by most chronic conditions. One of the most important is the possibility of recurrence! The patient (and family) who has experienced, been treated for, and seemingly recovered from cancer or a heart attack continue to be emotionally and defensively tuned or readied for the threat of recurrence (Wikler, 1981). Recurrence is particularly threatening because subsequent episodes are likely to be more severe and to signal probable mortality.

Psychological Models of Illness

There is a growing literature examining illness from the perspective of the sick individual (see Hayes-Bautista, 1976; Kleinman, 1980; Leventhal, Meyer, & Nerenz, 1980; Leventhal & Nerenz, 1982; Nerenz & Leventhal, 1983). These studies have begun to define the variables involved in the representation of illness, coping with illness, and the appraisal of outcomes (Lazarus, 1966). It will help to describe briefly these components, for they form the substance of the social psychology of illness.

Representation of Illness. Four attributes seem to be important in setting goals and subgoals of the illness problem and become a focus for sharing information and developing coping strategies: (1) the *identity* of the illness; (2) its *causes*; (3) its *consequences*; and (4) its *duration* or time line. Each of the four can be represented hierarchically, that is, both concretely and abstractly (see Leventhal, Nerenz, & Steele, 1984). Thus an illness can be identified by its signs and symptoms (pain, rash, tiredness, cough), some but not all of which will be public, and by its abstract label (viral pneumonia, cancer, etc.). Causes can also be construed concretely—for example, the cancer was caused by a blow—or abstractly—for example, my cancer was caused by a breakdown in control of cell division because I am aging. Many diseases are perceived to be caused by external agents (such as, infections or environmental poisons). This type of perception is clearly common for acute, non-life-threatening illnesses (Lau & Hartman, 1983; Linz, Penrod, Siverhus, & Leventhal, Note 1) as well as for a chronic life-threatening disease such as cancer (Herzlich, 1973). People also attribute disease to more vague, external factors such as the "urban atmosphere" (Herzlich, 1973) and to externally induced stress (Prohaska, Leventhal, Leventhal, & Keller, in press). Stress may have many sources, such as work, economic need, family problems (with spouse or children), all of which demand different resources for coping (Pearlin & Schooler, 1978). Illness may also be attributed to internal factors or to one's own behavior, for instance, to poor health habits such as smoking, improper diet, inadequate sleep; to violation of rules of conduct; to excessive drive and ambition (Friedman & Rosenman, 1974, pp. 56–57); and to a somewhat more vague set of internal factors such as genetics and "aging" (Prohaska, Keller, Leventhal, & Leventhal, Note 3).

Differences in causal attribution may imply differences in the possibility for control of specific diseases (Prohaska, Keller, Leventhal, & Leventhal, Note 3; Lau & Hartman, 1983) and differences in blame for imposing the costs and stresses of illnesses on the family unit at an inappropriate age or time in the family's life course, as, for example, in the case of alcoholism (Jackson, 1956).

Consequences and time line are most frequently mentioned in the literature on illness and families. The more severe the illness the greater its impact on the individual and the family's economic resources, social life, choice of residential location, and on the ability of the family to maintain activities important for family solidarity and self-esteem (Klein, Dean, & Bogdonoff, 1967).

Coping with Illness. Coping involves planning and acting. This means collecting information; differentiating and prioritizing goals (Hamburg, 1974; Lazarus & Launier, 1978; Leventhal, 1970; Safer, Tharps, Jackson, & Leventhal, 1979); defining responses, that is, setting expectations to evaluate response effectiveness (Becker & Maiman, 1975; Mischel, 1973; Rotter, 1954); searching for models and expert assistance on how to execute specific responses (Bandura, 1977; Coelho, Solomon, Wolff, Steinberg, & Hamburg, 1969); taking initial steps; inhibiting premature responses; and sustaining the energy and strength needed to carry out the extended plan. Coping can be directed at goals set by any number of objective problems (for example, treatment, illness, economic needs), and by subjective emotion (Averill, 1973; Leventhal, 1970; Lazarus & Launier, 1978).

Appraisal. The appraisal of an action, even one as simple as taking two aspirins to relieve a headache, is more complex than meets the eye. The aspirin taker will, explicitly or implicitly, set criteria to define the success in the removal of the headache, judge the time for the therapy to work, develop hypotheses as to the meaning of success and failure, and detect "other" outcomes (e.g., gastric distress) that may influence taking aspirin in the future.

In addition, appraisals of illness are complex because they rely on expert social communication. A patient in chemotherapy for cancer must rely heavily on the oncologist for appraisal of the impact of the chemotherapy on the cancer, and the implications of the medical information may be ambiguous with respect to the patient's criteria for success, for example, although information of a drop in white cell count implies a serious problem, it may not have clear implications for the ultimate effectiveness of the treatment—the key concern of the patient and his or her family. But even if the physician's information is clearly understood, it may be inconsistent with changes in symptoms (tiredness, bone pain, changes in palpable tumors, etc.). For instance, about half our lymphoma patients with palpable tumors (Nerenz, Leventhal, & Love, 1982) found they could no longer feel their tumors after the first two or three treatment cycles. Rather than being joyful that their tumors had disappeared in a four week cure, these patients were highly distressed because treatment was to continue for another six to eight months even though they "felt" cured.

The individual's perception and appraisal of disease is also influenced by exposure to illness in friends and family; patients who have seen a mother die of breast cancer have a less optimistic view of treatment and a more malevolent view of the disease (Ringler, 1981). Indeed, every component of the illness control system, from the representation of the disease through the development and execution of coping to appraisal, is heavily influenced by interaction with the family and by its impact on the family unit.

Emotional Response.   Emotional responses will occur at many points over time and at many points in the sequence of representing, coping, and evaluating the illness and treatment. Symptoms such as blood in the urine or stools may be terrifying. The diagnosis of cancer may precipitate a catastrophic reaction (Meyerowitz, 1980). Coping with the seemingly endless and arduous battle against progression of a disease perceived as incurable (Aitken-Swan, 1959; Patterson & Aitken-Swan, 1954) may generate a constant state of fatigue and tiredness that gradually shifts into a state of despondency and depression (Peck, 1972). The manifestations of fear and disgust when a spouse views the scar of breast surgery may evoke self-depreciation, feelings of worthlessness and withdrawal from social contact (Bard & Sutherland, 1955; Friedenbergs et al., 1982; Meyerowitz, 1980). And each of these emotional responses has its impact and cost for the family as a unit.

Family System

Structure.   The two basic divisions to family structure are the generational divisions, consisting of the current nuclear family (the husband–

wife pair and one or more children), the prior nuclear family (parents and siblings) plus the extended family (grandparents, uncles and aunts, and cousins), and the biological-legal division (blood relatives and relatives by marriage). Although the popular press frequently claims that the traditional nuclear and extended family have undergone a radical transformation, the available empirical evidence spanning a 150-year period suggests that both are thriving with surprisingly little change in organization and behavior (Caplow et al., 1982).

Structural factors set the context for the family's response to illness in an adult member, but they are merely the beginning of the description of the family system. Concepts such as frequency of contact and role expectations within and across generations are essential as are the changes in these expectations over the life course of the family and the culture. For instance, although it is likely that there is still as frequent contact between parents and children today as 100 years ago, expectations regarding financial obligations are not the same. Although children now finish schooling at a later age than in the nineteenth century and are more fully dependent on parents during that time, they also move more quickly into the work force, thus freeing parents from the obligation for support (Caplow et al., 1982, p. 292). Not surprisingly, children are no longer expected to assist in the support of parents—or at least not while the parents are functional. What adult children do when their parents are aged, ill, and no longer functionally independent is less clearly prescribed—hence the availability of popular books on the topic (e.g., Silverstone & Hyman, 1982).

Roles, that is, status and behavioral expectations, are relatively well-defined and agreed upon in a well-organized family. Moreover, individual goals and ambitions are subordinated to or serve shared goals, and we can expect such a unit to be cohesive and effective in solving problems and reducing tensions that emerge from stressful life events and crises (Lewis, Beavers, Gossett, & Phillips, 1976; Rabkin, 1976). A poorly structured family, where individual behaviors are uncoordinated, will cope less well with crises requiring group action. Hence economic and illness threats will have a more severe and longer lasting impact on these families and their members (Hansen & Hill, 1964). But even a well-organized family will be affected by novel life stressors. The first experience of chronic illness in an adult may pose unanticipated demands and require coping responses that are not part of existent role expectations or skills. The ambiguities inherent in such novelty may bring to the forefront questions about the legitimacy of obligations and the legitimacy of requests for assistance and mutual action that are not typically considered in everyday family interactions. These questions are likely conditioned by the history of the family, whether the marriage is a first or second one, whether the children are the offspring of one or both of the marital partners, whether the husband or wife was accepted by the older generation at the time of the marriage, and so forth. Today's very high rate of marriage, the high expectations brought to marriage (Caplow et al., 1982), and the high rate of divorce make answers to these questions of great importance. If the main breadwinner feels no obligation to the spouse's parents or if a child is hostile toward a spouse in a second marriage, life-threatening disease in parents will have quite a different impact on the individuals within the family than might be the case under more "typical" conditions.

Expectations determining role behaviors during illness are also historically conditioned. These factors may be family specific, which is a likely occurrence in families with a high level of consciousness of family tradition, or they may be specific to particular religious or ethnic groups or defined by national or regional and local labels.

Family Functions.   Three broad classes of family functions likely to be influenced in different ways by illness in an adult family member are (1). the biological, (2). the psychological, and (3). the socioeconomic. Reproduction takes primary place in most sociological accounts of biological functions (Caplow et al., 1982). Equally important biological functions include the nurturing or physical care of family members; the feeding, cleaning, and tending to the growing infant; and the important tasks of tending to injury and illness in family members. The latter instance involves defining and preventing and curing health threats and deciding when expert help is needed.

The psychological functions of the family include the development and maintenance of the self-image or self-esteem—what I am and what I can do and what I am worth—for both children and adults. Emotional communication and training—expressing and sharing fear, anger, excitement, interest, and joy, thereby defining the conditions under which emotional expression is permitted, and providing models and instruction on how to control emotional expression—are clearly important family functions.

The family's social functions include establishing group solidarity and defining group boundaries and norms for in-group and out-group relationships (Boss, in press). The family is also a unit in relation to both informal and formal social institutions: it is a wage-earning, product-consuming, help-giving, tax-paying (i.e., legally defined and legally responsible) unit in our socioeconomic system.

Each of these functions defines an area for family assessment, that is, an estimate of how well the family is fulfilling biological, psychological, and social functions. Many subsidiary functions exist within each of these areas and some appear in all three. Communication, for example, is a critical component of successful interpersonal (systems) operation for child rearing, the maintenance of self-esteem, and participation in the religious life of the community. The type of information and success in communicating and developing a shared knowledge base will vary by problem. Assessment by direct observation is part of various family-therapy protocols, but little empirical evidence of this sort can be found in the area of the family and physical illness.

INTERACTION OF ILLNESS AND FAMILY SYSTEMS

The nature and severity of the impact of illness in adult members will vary as a function of (a) the biological type of illness (cancer, cardiovascular disease) and its natural history; (b) the stage of the illness in which the systems are observed, for example, prediagnostic, diagnostic and treatment, rehabilitation and control, recurrence; (c) the structure of the family; (d) the identity of the sick person (mother, father, grandparent); (e) the point in the individual's life span at which the illness occurs; and (f) the point in the life course of the family and culture at which the illness occurs. Given the several systems involved and the large number of factors operating in each system and that the stage of illness defines the problems for coping (Kaplan, Smith, Grobstein, & Fischman, 1977), we can limit our discussion by focusing on systems interactions at each stage.

The Impact of Chronic Illness in the Prediagnostic Phase

What are the effects of a chronic illness in an adult on families in the prediagnostic phase and how might they be studied? Although we know of no studies that have investigated this question directly, there are a number of investigations of factors such as delay in seeking care for cancer or cardiovascular disease that suggest that the anticipation or suspicion of disease threats may affect family structure and function (Hackett & Cassem, 1969; Matthews et al., 1983; Safer, Tharps, Jackson, & Leventhal, 1979). Clues from these and other studies suggest the possibility of major impact on family functions ranging from the biopsychological (e.g., diet, decisions to have children) to the social psychological (commitments to economic goals). These effects are a consequence of (a) the way the family represents and tries to cope with disease as an "objective" fact and (b) the way the illness threat alters the emotional reactions that may be part of the impact of the disease (threat) in the prediagnostic phase.

Representing and Coping with Disease Threat.   Retrospective reports can be used to address this issue, but they must be used cautiously as they are very likely influenced by reactions in the subsequent phase, the diagnosis itself. For example, it is sometimes reported that cancer patients wonder why they have become victims of so dread a disease (Bard & Sutherland, 1955) and blame themselves for falling ill. This way of representing cancer causation requires the individual to rewrite history by scanning his or her life situation to identify acts that the person believes merit punishment and then to identify the cancer as the punishment. Retrospective reports may also exaggerate emotional reactions to the news of disease onset. Espenshade (1984), for example, interviewed over 400 diabetics and found that ratings of emotional distress were more intense when diabetics reported their reactions to a previous diagnosis of retinal damage, whereas their reports of their current levels of distress actually matched those of a group of diabetics just diagnosed with retinal pathology. Although observations such as the above are interesting and important in respect to the way patient and family may perceive the illness and their own and one another's emotional reactions and role in the cause of the disease prior to diagnosis, they may not be relevant to the representation of illness and to mutual self-perceptions during the prediagnostic phase itself. To see how families deal with prospective threat, we must eventually obtain records of their thoughts and actions during the preillness time period.

The literature on delay in seeking care does provide clues that may be less subject to bias. For example, in their interviews of 100 randomly selected coronary patients, Hackett and Cassem (1969) found median delays of two hours for patients who acted on their own or consulted with friends as compared to a 12-hour delay for patients who consulted with family members. Given that anxiety about disease, for example, fear of cancer and the belief that it is incurable may increase delay (Goldsen, Gerhardt, & Handy, 1957; King & Leach, 1951), it seems reasonable to suggest that discussion with family members may encourage a defensive generalization of feelings of invulnerability and a failure to identify accurately warning signs in the prospective patient. This may be stimulated by a sense of personal threat, an increased awareness of the fragility of the family, or efforts to sustain and defend the belief that the family can maintain itself and achieve cherished goals or by a history of direct, fear-arousing encounters with cancer in the family (Cobb, Clarke, McGuire, & Howe, 1954). Family processes of this sort can be especially dangerous when the pathophysiology of disease involves slow and barely visible signs and symptoms that encourage "denial" or "normalization" of physical changes (Goldsen et al., 1957; Mechanic, 1972), whereas successful control of disease requires swift and dramatic intervention at the earliest possible stages. Studies of these processes could do much to enhance our understanding of the important role of interpersonal factors in processes such as denial that are typically conceptualized in an intrapsychic framework (Boss, in press; Janis, 1982).

Difficulty in defining illness in a spouse due to vague and fluctuating symptoms has been described for mental illness (Yarrow, Schwartz, Murphy, & Deasy, 1955) and alcoholism (Jackson, 1956). Jackson found that subtle changes, such as denial and withdrawal by wives and families, occurred in response to the asocial behavior of the husband prior to his being clearly labeled as alcoholic. Once diagnosis was clear and accepted, the wives began to reorganize the roles of each spouse, taking over themselves many of the roles of the husband and even refusing to allow their husbands' resumption of normal role functions after treatment and apparent "cure."

In a report of interviews by social workers with 1268 disability applicants, the great majority of whom suffered from cardiovascular disease

(33.7%), stroke (13.5%), and musculoskeletal disease (22.5%), Zahn (1973) found less disruption of family bonds when there was high clarity of the disabled person's status, for example, when the person was clearly not fit to work and the disability was more severe. It is likely, however, that role changes will be slight in the prediagnostic phase of most chronic illnesses unless the "well" member of the pair is motivated and feels competent to press for change in the face of ambiguous evidence and unless the disease consequences for chronicity and disability are clear. There may well be a sex bias in this case, with the well partner being more assertive if male than if female.

Comparing the behavior of families with members at risk for cancer with that of families where such risk is low or absent could help us to differentiate sources of response to perceived threat. The first step, of course, would be to determine whether differences in actual risk are related to perceived risk, that is, to examine whether individual representations of disease threats match the epidemiological data! Mismatches could reflect beliefs about the cause of the disease and preventive coping strategies. For example, a family might (accurately) perceive mother at risk because grandmother and sister had cancer and adopt a high-fiber, high-vitamin A diet in the belief it will protect the mother against disease. Or the family might push for low-stress vocations and less income to minimize disease threats to the father, whose own father and brothers died of coronary disease. Threat may be misjudged, however, due to defensiveness, ignorance, or inappropriate cognitive constructions. An example of the latter appeared in Espenshade's study (1984) where the adult members in a nuclear family did not perceive their diabetes as genetic because diabetes in their parent had followed rather than preceded the onset of their own. Had parental onset been earlier, it might have influenced the preventive health actions (diet, exercise) of the younger generation both for themselves and their children.

Failure to take preventive action due to mismatches between the psychological representation of a disease threat and its pathophysiology can, of course, result in failures to prevent or delay the onset or to control the spread of a chronic illness. Dent and Goulston (1982a) developed a simple ten-item test of knowledge about cancer and found that correct answers were given by less than 40% of 500 randomly selected respondents to six of the ten questions. The survey included 12 Likert-type attitude items and between one third and one half of the respondents agreed or were uncertain in response to three questions asking if cancer was preventable. A slightly higher percentage of respondents believed the disease cannot be controlled once it is contracted (Dent & Goulston, 1982b). Actions based on such erroneous beliefs could have important consequences for the family. Taking preventive action on the other hand can also have unintended consequences depending on how the behavior is understood. For instance, a father may communicate a sense of imminent doom or terror to his spouse and children by a too energetic pursuit of preventive measures; or a mother may lull her family into a false sense of security and into failure to monitor for disease changes by setting up an apparently invulnerable fortress of preventive actions through diet combined with reassurances of its effectiveness in eliminating disease. When coping overshoots the reasonable goals, it may enhance feelings of vulnerability and distress as in the first example above, or lead to surprise and a sense of victimization when feelings of invulnerability prove inaccurate. The consequences in either of the cases could be recriminations, outbursts of anger, feelings of mistrust, and breakdown in family solidarity at a later time.

Differences in the way family members represent the cause or consequences and the coping tactics needed for dealing with disease threats can influence family behavior on several levels and may even affect family structure. Parents may decide not to have children if they believe they are genetically susceptible to disease (Ben-Sira, 1977), and this causal interpretation may have different implications for each partner in a marriage. For example, the "carrier" may perceive the genetic factor to be a consequence of chance or the fault of his or her parents, whereas the observing spouse may see the genetic factor as a defect or fault in the carrier. Studies of attributions using actors and observers suggest that attributions in actual family units can be enhanced by role expectations (Leventhal, 1965) and lead to anger with the spouse and to divorce. Anger, anxiety, and depression have been recorded in both husband and wife following abortion because of a genetic disease (Blumberg & Golbus, 1975), although the anxiety and depression (but not the anger) can be reduced by therapeutic counseling (Antley & Hartlage, 1976). Willingness to consider other options such as adoption would obviously affect the outcome and these would have to be assessed. The growth of many new tests for susceptibility to diseases such as cancer opens a host of questions as to how individuals will respond to probabilistic information (Slovic, 1978) and how this response will be shaped by the individual's role in and interaction within the family. Studies of genetic counseling may provide clues to needs and to research problems in this area (Haan, 1979).

Emotional Reactions and the Family.   The actual or perceived threat of disease can also influence a variety of emotional processes. The experience of emotion and strategies for coping with emotions can affect relationships of family members to one another as well as the relationship of the family to its social context. An interesting and virtually unexplored issue is the effect of early, as yet undiagnosed, disease processes on the ill person's behavior and the impact of these behaviors on the family. For example, there may be hormonal changes associated with early stages of certain types of cancer or vascular changes associated with early stages of coronary disease that could lead initially to subtle, but increasingly frequent and salient, changes in emotional reactions such as feelings of fatigue, loss of hope, and passivity. These affective changes in the undiagnosed but ill spouse could make him or her feel unvalued or useless. This could influence the socialization of emotional responses in the children as well.

Barbara Anderson (1984) has reported data relevant to the above hypotheses in a study of 120 women, 40 of whom were eventually diagnosed with gynecological cancers (cervical, ovarian, endometrial, and vulvular). Anderson found substantial declines in sexual desire, which was distressing to these patients, in the time period before cancer was diagnosed and before they sought or received medical care. Evidence for such early change in sexual behavior did not appear in her study of two matched control groups—one that had benign gynecological disorders and the other that was healthy.

Emotional effects need not, however, be subtle, that is, feelings or emotional appraisals about illness may be expressed quite openly. For example, parents hypervigilant to a disease threat may openly express and communicate an intensified fear of the disease to children. Affective communications of this sort may be the basis for lifelong feelings of vulnerability to diseases such as cancer and may affect the child's ways of coping with such health threats or, depending upon other factors (e.g., the parents' survival without disease), may lead to the child's rejection of the parental model and a false sense of security. The available data suggest complex relationships between the health–illness behavior of parents and children. For example, Campbell (1975) found that mothers and their children agreed on the symptoms they would label as illness. The agreement held, however, only for group averages, that is, there was a normative view of the signs of illness, but there was no agreement when mother–child pairs were the basis for the analysis. Mechanic (1964) also found no relationship between illness behavior (perceived poor health, symptom complaints, adoption of sick role) of mothers and that of their children, although mothers dealt similarly with both themselves and their children. When Mechanic (1979a,b) studied these children 16 years later, their illness behavior as young adults was only slightly related to their own behavior 16 years earlier or to that of their mothers 16 years earlier. We cannot tell if this relationship is direct, if the mother's illness behavior influenced the child's, or indirectly, if other socializing experiences or similarities of constitutional makeup affected other factors (e.g., autonomic reactivity, attention to self) that direct illness behavior.

As we suggested before, families living with the anxiety of a disease threat may adopt specific strategies for minimizing this anxiety that encourage the problems of unwarranted delay in seeking care, which can lead to early fatality in an adult member and to disrupting the functional competence of the nuclear family in such a way as to limit their ability to survive as a productive unit. A family may also attempt to cope with fear by turning inward and trying to maximize the intensity of life experiences within the nuclear unit by segregating themselves from responsibilities to the extended family and community.

In summary, the mere possibility of disease may generate a threat that leads to a variety of changes in family behavior in the psychobiological domain (e.g., change in diet, change in job to reduce stress) and in the psychosocial domain (e.g., turning inward to reduce contact with others, not having children). These alterations may affect on individuals' sense of self, their feelings of esteem and beliefs about achievement of life goals within the family unit, thus placing strains on one another or on interpersonal cohesion. Finally, we suggested that the early stages of undetected illness may generate changes in moods and other emotional responses. The above changes could lead to enhancing family solidarity, which is an outcome that seems more likely if communication is open and there is congruence between the perception of the "objective" nature of the threat, the emotional response to it, and the role of each family member in minimizing danger. The enhanced congruity could firm the boundaries between the family and the outer world and, depending upon other factors, this could increase the family's ability to survive and fulfill its functions in relation to its social context or could increase its sense of alienation from this context. On the other hand, the result could be a reduction in family solidarity if the potential threat is differentially perceived, if some members feel alienated from the family's "defensive" life style, and if changes in mood alienate family members from the preclinically "ill" person.

Illness Impact During Diagnostic and Treatment Phase

Diagnosis and treatment are times of crisis (Moos & Tsu, 1977). A diagnosis of cancer is often described as a shock (Currier, 1966; Giacquinta, 1977), a numbing blow on the head (Parkes, 1972), as a state of siege (Kaplan, 1976), and the response to it as phobic (Lewis & Bloom, 1978–1979). The intensity of threat will vary as a function of the family's representation of the disease, especially its perceptions of the consequences, duration, and likelihood of successful coping (cure or control) of the disease. These attributes will vary by diagnosis. Diagnoses of diseases such as breast or colon-rectal cancer elicit far more threat than do diagnoses of diabetes, hypertension, arthritis, and so on. Each family member is likely to understand or represent an illness in different ways, and the degree of variation is likely to be greater within a relatively young nuclear family than in an older one. The members of the older unit are likely to share a greater number of experiences of chronic illness that occurred in their parents' generation as well as among their peers. But there is still little question that each member may have a somewhat different view of the dangers and feel more or less hopeless about the outcome.

Crisis conditions appear, however, to enhance group solidarity (Fritz & Mathewson, 1957; Kaplan, Smith, Grobstein, & Tischman, 1977). The focus of the family is on the consequence or implications of the disease threat, for example, does the cancer or heart attack mean an imminent or a slow death, a painful existence, and so on (Kaplan, 1976)? Many of these consequences are only remote possibilities of the individual and family time line until a positive diagnosis thrusts them abruptly forward in time and space (Cassileth & Hamilton, 1979). With death looming, all efforts are focused on its avoidance: The goal is the preservation of life.

In addition, both patient and family face numerous difficult decisions. For cancer care, treatments are in store, and choices must be made between radiation or surgery; chemotherapy may be strongly recommended both for metastatic conditions and as an adjuvant treatment to "ensure" the outcome of presumably successful surgery. Each choice requires the mastery of new information, the updating of the representation of the illness and treatment, and the preparation of coping and appraisal strategies. The difficulty of decision making will be compounded by shifts in attention of different family members from immediate to remote threats and back again, which lead to differences in the way the disease and its implications for the family are represented by different members. At times, the immediate threat of treatment can eclipse the more remote threats of illness as both patient and family attempt to perceive and understand the treatment alternatives and their consequences. Thus if surgery is to be performed, patient and family will have questions about the patient's survival, postsurgical status (mutilated, functional, etc.), the time it will take to return to normal, and how to distinguish the consequences of surgery from those of illness (e.g., will there be pain, what type and can we tell it apart from the pain of cancer or myocardial infarct) (Cassileth & Hamilton, 1979).

Each of the above questions raises issues for coping and appraisal. Each participant in the drama will represent the problem from one's own perspective and develop coping resources relevant to that perception. But as stated earlier, as long as the crisis is focused and well defined and as long as the medical staff facilitates this clarity with adequate communication, the representations formed by patient and family should show substantial overlap, thus facilitating the development of coping plans and actions that integrate individual roles into a relatively effective and harmonious whole (Kaplan et al., 1977). The ease of forming representations and coping plans will likely vary across generations. Young children and even young parents will be unfamiliar with the details of hospitals and medical procedures, with the treatment, and with potential changes for the patient. The level of anxiety and threat will be intensified by this uncertainty. The "out of time" nature of disease early in life may create added frustration, anger, and conflict with the medical staff. Despite these problems, the most likely outcomes are "heroic" actions, that is, strenuous efforts to learn about the threat and to acquire coping skills and favorable appraisals of oneself and other members of the group while the family supports the ill adult and holds itself together. Emotional communication is likely to be supportive as is assistance in coping with the immediate demands of the medical care system by attempts to minimize the varied costs of treatment, such as pain, and to maximize its benefits with hopes for cure or containment of the disease (Currier, 1966; Giacquinta, 1977).

Crisis conditions, however, are relatively short lived. As the drama of illness fades, as the threat of death recedes from days to weeks, months, or years, uncertainty about the permanence of cure develops and there is a major alteration in the family's position. There is a need to return to normal roles and routines, for Dad or Mom to return to work, to pick up the tasks of disciplinarian, housekeeper, and source of nurturance. Whatever the specifics, as the crisis ebbs and the family attempts to return to more or less normal functioning, there is a growing awareness of the need to define and cope with the impact of the illness on longer-term functioning. Will the disease wreck the family's financial dreams? Will it require selling the home? Does it mean giving up vacations, new cars, going away to school? Does it mean a permanent change in roles? Will Dad have to do all the heavy housework? Will Mother become the principal source of family support? As the family moves from crisis to normalcy, we believe that is the time when there is the greatest probability of the development of discord.

Rehabilitation and Resolution: Recovery, Disability, and Death

When treatment ends or becomes a predictable routine, the task is to "recover" or "rehabilitate," to regain one's strength, and to move toward normal social and emotional functioning. When treatment has a clear beginning and ending, social psychological problems are likely to be minimized. For example, when surgery is the only treatment, the family appears to return to normal social functioning within three to four months (Morris, Greer, & White, 1977; Palmore, Cleveland, Nowlin, Ramm, & Siegler, 1979). In an interview study of 36 couples (15 female patients and 21 male patients), Leiber, Plumb, Gertstenzang, and Holland (1976) report feelings of closeness and solidarity are often enhanced during the latter stages of cancer treatment although more for the female than for the male. Morris, Greer, and White (1977), however, report a decline in work adjustment. Their study is of interest as they managed to follow 110 of 168 patients for two years, slightly more than one half of whom were "controls" whose breast biopsies proved benign. We have virtually no data telling us how to predict which families will adjust successfully, and we know virtually nothing about how successful adjustment takes place. Indeed, successful adjustment may depend greatly upon the context, for example, upon the adequacy and extent of the family's social support and treatment network rather than upon "fixed" properties of the patient or the family (Wishnie, Hackett, & Cassem, 1971). Clear communication from medical practitioners about the disease course, relevant suggestions for coping ... eatment and illness from both practitioners and support networks, ... e availability of adequate health insurance may be good predictors of outcomes and factors susceptible to practical improvement. Janis has argued that situational factors are powerful determinants of posttreatment outcomes for the individual (Janis, 1958; Janis & Leventhal, 1965), and there is no reason to believe this will not be true for the family.

The return to "normal" functioning can lead to increased role conflict. This is particularly likely if family members are unaware of the major readjustments that occurred during the crisis period of diagnosis and treatment. Wives may have taken on the major role of organizing and maintaining the family finances. An older male child may have taken over a wide range of father's home tasks. If the wife is the patient, husband and children are likely to have moved into the role of housekeeper, with shopping, cooking, and cleaning apportioned out among them. Patterns of emotional sharing so critical for the sense of belonging and interpersonal value and self-esteem may have undergone important changes, with the father sharing thoughts and feelings with children in domains typically handled by the mother. The "patient" may be excluded from sharing in order to lessen the burdens of the "trivial" concerns of everyday life, concerns that the family perceives as causing stress, interfering with recovery, and perhaps bringing on recurrence because stress is often perceived as an important cause of disease, particularly in cardiovascular illness (Prohaska, Leventhal, Leventhal, & Keller, in press; Wishnie, Hackett, & Cassem, 1971). However, exclusion from this emotional give and take can reduce the patients' sense of participation and social value, damaging their self-esteem, increasing their feelings of distress, and leading to efforts to reassert their significance.

Return to normal role function is complicated by long recovery and rehabilitation periods. Treatment for cancer may lack a clear ending, which may promote uncertainty about the individual's status as ill or well. If the disease has spread and surgical treatment is incomplete, the patient will enter into a longer period of chemotherapy, a repetitive treatment in which daily life is disrupted about once every four weeks for injecting chemotherapy agents, followed by two weeks of oral medication and then by a two-week period that is medication free. Whether continued treatment such as chemotherapy increases or decreases the problems of a long recovery is unknown. The problem for the patient and the family unit is to adjust to the ambiguity of the "well–sick" role. The patient is returning to "wellness," where expectations are clear that he or she will perform everyday tasks, and yet is still living with the threat of cancer. Role ambiguity could be intense in the case of metastatic disease, for the patient is indeed sick, even though he or she may be able to handle a wide range of normal tasks for a considerable period of time. However, metastatic patients are generally very satisfied with the level of social support they receive from their families (Ringler, 1981). Zahn's (1973) analysis of social workers' interviews with 1268 disability applicants shows that family stress is low when the individuals have clearly recognized disabilities although more severe disabilities are related both to improved relationships and to greater distress in the family.

Continued treatment is recommended for many chronic illnesses that are otherwise seen as "cured." Extended chemotherapy is now recommended following successful breast cancer surgery with few signs of spread to lymph nodes, for it is known to enhance life expectancy (Bonadonna & Valagussa, 1981). Most patients see the treatment as preventive (Ringler, 1981), but we know little as to how it is seen by the family or how year-long treatment might affect return to normal family functioning. Lengthy rehabilitation following cardiovascular diseases such as stroke and myocardial infarct may provide a greater number of overt signs of the return of individual competence and facilitate role changes, but even here one half or more of the former patients report problems in resuming daily activities and family controversy over appropriate interpretations of medical regimens (Wishnie et al., 1971).

But even when cancer is not metastatic, or when recovery from stroke seems complete, the patient and family must live with the threat of recurrence. The family's willingness to revert to prior role organization and its need to maintain specific role changes—such as a wife's unwillingness to stop work; a spouse's unwilligness to resume close, dependent contact; or a child's desire to maintain emotional communication with the well adult—may depend upon perception and interpretation of the possibility of recurrence and loss of life. If chronic illness stimulates family members to think about and plan for the loss of the ill person, those who are well will need to develop clear representations and coping skills for dealing with tasks currently within the domain of the patient. They have to be able to do things alone. This independence may be perceived as rejection by the patient and by other family members who equate being independent or being ready for independence with being discarded and unneeded. These processes are probably similar to those experienced by parents of a growing child. Separation, however, in this latter instance comes at the expected time when the child's peers and their families are making similar transitions, undergoing the "empty nest" syndrome and establishing a set of norms appropriate for parental behavior.

Preparation for loss can be extremely complex when the chronically ill adult has been at the height of his or her physical and economic powers and there is discrepancy between the time of appearance of the crisis and the timing of this intrusion into the family's life span. Case reports suggest that the preparatory responses of an individual readying oneself for loss can be seen as a threat by others unable or unwilling to tolerate or think of loss (Fellner, 1973; Parkes, 1972). Just as preparing for loss may stimulate problems so too may family members accustomed to dependency on the sick person feel terror at the thought of abandonment by a strong, protective adult (Currier, 1966). Feelings of this sort may produce diffuse anger and hostility toward those who do not share the sense of terror at the likelihood of the patient's death. Accusations of callousness and not caring seem a likely outcome.

Many people appear to think in all-or-none terms—that is, the individual *is* sick or *is* well—rather than in graded terms, that is, the individual has *no* detectable disease but may still have a nondetectable disease that could progress to recurrence and *is* therefore at high risk. Such categorical thought could encourage extreme adaptations such as refusal to return to prior roles, or complete return and failure to prepare for recurrence, or conflict such as that elaborated above.

The strain placed on the family and its members because of ambiguities in fulfilling role tasks and changes in role enactments of other family members may greatly reduce the ability of both family and individuals to fulfill their functions for one another and for their context. The sick person carries the burden of disease, and debilitating treatments greatly reduce one's energy to undertake and sustain daily functions (Haylock & Hart, 1979). Other family members also feel the strain of worry and of enacting multiple roles, and they too report an increasingly large number of illness symptoms (Currier, 1966; Klein, Dean, & Bogdonoff, 1967). These feelings of tiredness and fatigue may substantially diminish the individual's sense of competence. New and even minor crises, either with the illness or in the socioeconomic sphere of family activity, could now appear as major and insurmountable as individuals wonder, "I'm exhausted! How can I handle this?" The feeling of threat and loss of esteem associated with these crises may provoke anger by well members of the unit toward one another or toward the patient. The probability of such dynamics may be increased if family members have expected that the "healthy" members of the unit should be able to bear any and all burdens. Inner feelings may have a profound effect on esteem, particularly in the absence of external justification (you're well, so stop acting put upon) and could stimulate considerable anger on the part of those members of the family prone to adopt and defend an heroic self-image.

Fatigue and mutual recrimination can disrupt emotional communication within the family, and failure in emotional sharing and mood maintenance could have an additional severe impact on people's sense of well-being and their self-esteem. Visual and physical contact, such as seeing one another's smiling faces, holding hands, touching, and sharing feelings during sexual acts, may be disrupted by the malaise and fatigue created by illness and the stresses and strains of new adaptations. When patient and family cease to provide the smiling faces and touches for mood maintenance, the family has ceased to create the emotional states that provide a context for being together and for being of value to one another.

It is clear from the above that role readjustments in the family may require a substantial degree of flexibility, for the patient is likely to demand both independence and support so that he or she will need help intermittently in the struggle to return to or preserve a "well self." Spouse and children may resist relinquishing newly acquired roles and the accompanying status, thus enhancing the patient's sense of worthlessness. If the patient expresses resentment or anger at the preemption of one's duties, there is abundant opportunity for feelings of injury on the part of the hardworking, self-sacrificing well members of the family.

Difficulties in adjustments internal to the family can be intensified by the need for readjustment in relationships to the outer world (Cassileth & Hamilton, 1979). Family members not only see one another as well or ill, as helpful and responsible, or as unhelpful and irresponsible, they also see themselves as viewed from the outside, as giving aid to the ill member and preserving the family or as failing to live up to the social expectations for a normal family member. A husband's need to usurp his wife's newly gained role as breadwinner can be intensified by the belief that he is perceived as inadequate by the community. Indeed, a case has been described to us where a husband maintained the sick role to justify himself in other people's eyes because his wife became the more aggressive and successful wage earner during his illness.

Chronic illness can also lead to rejection of the patient and family by colleagues and friends. Despite biomedical evidence to the contrary, many people appear to think and act as though cancer and other chronic illnesses were contagious (Currier, 1966). People may reject a "cancer patient" and family because contact stimulates anxiety about their own vulnerability, or they may avoid the family because they feel awkward and do not know how to respond, which is a phenomenon seen in interactions between the well and the physically disabled (Kleck, Ono, & Hastorf, 1966). Rejections of this sort may lower the esteem of all family members and engender especially strong feelings about the injustice of life among the well members of the family. The well members who feel victimized may even turn in anger on the patient, especially if they fail to communicate their feelings to one another and have no way of coping with the victimizing environment. Data are needed to appraise the frequency of such outcomes and to describe their determinants.

Despite the threat of severe chronic illness and the feeling it generates of a world collapsing, there is a reasonable amount of data suggesting that things return to normal and families adjust. Thus male myocardial infarction patients report little change from pre- to postillness (Croog & Richards, 1977); colostomy patients also report little change in families (Burnam, Eardley, Davids, & Schofield, 1976; Dyk & Sutherland, 1956); and there is a gradual acceptance of change by families of cancer patients (Parkes, 1972) as well as increased closeness of relationship reported by individuals with severe rather than mild disability (Zahn, 1973). Family integration and adaptation appear the rule rather than the exception. Indeed, in longitudinal study of reactions to one's own or a spouse's retirement, the children leaving the home, widowhood, and illness, Palmore, Cleveland, Nowlin, Ramm, and Siegler (1979) reported more substantial declines in life satisfaction and self-esteem and increases in psychosomatic symptoms with retirement than in response to major medical events. Although we must be cautious in accepting these findings, for there was a 52% refusal rate and only 375 of the 502 persons in the study continued to the end, the data certainly do contradict the commonly accepted idea that an on-time event (retirement) is more easily adjusted to than an unexpected event (major medical). Data clearly suggest, however, differences in the perception of the seriousness of the consequences of illness by the patient and other family members, for example, from data obtained on home visits with 570 homebound cancer patients, Wellisch, Landsverk, Guidera, Pasnau, & Fawzy (1983) found that patients were more likely to see their illnesses as creating difficulties with emotional relationships and economics—and these differences can be sources of role conflict unless the family negotiates a common perspective on its problems. Favorable outcomes in response to illness therefore suggest considerable psychological and physical work, dependent on the definition or interpretation of a chronic disease, the disability induced by treatment, and the ways of coping with that disease or disability, and thus the quality of adjustment. For example, ileostomy (resection of all of the colon) for ulcerative colitis requires a prosthesis and skills in self-management that are similar but not identical to those following colostomies (removal of a portion of the colon because of disease); yet the postoperative adjustment in the former case is typically positive, whereas in the latter it is often beset with problems in self-training for the management of the colostomy, the fear of odors, reduced sexual behavior, and withdrawal from social contacts (Druss, O'Connor, & Stern, 1969; Orback & Tallent, 1965; Sutherland, Orbach, Dyk, & Bard, 1952).

Although the differences in the surgery may be partially responsible for the differences in adjustment—removal of lymph nodes and the greater denervation that affect sexual performance in the cancer patient—a substantial portion of the difference appears to be due to the contrast between the preoperative and postoperative status and the psychological implications of these differences. The ileostomy patient has been suffering for years with a debilitating condition and has adjusted social behaviors to this condition. The colostomy patient moves from a state of wellness to one of illness, indeed one where there is a continuing threat to life. One cannot help but assume that these differences affect feelings about the ostomy and its implications for interpersonal relationships for both the patient and the family.

Impact of Chronic Illness on the Family Over the Life Course

From the biomedical perspective, the term *disease* has come to stand for the pathophysiology generated by a foreign agent or a failure in one of the body's physiological mechanisms that threatens normal functioning and life. The incompleteness of this perspective is clear from our discussion of the impact of chronic illness on the family. A bio-psycho-social definition of disease examines the full impact of the pathophysiology on individuals and their social setting (Engel, 1977; Fabrega, 1977). We have dealt with this broader range of phenomena from two perspectives: (1) that of inter-related and interacting biological, psychologicial, and social systems (i.e., multiple systems levels); and (2) that of the temporal unfolding of the systems interaction over phases (i.e., from the prediagnostic stage to the diagnosis and treatment, and through the rehabilitation to the resolution— recovery or demise—from the illness). One might summarize our analysis in the form of a matrix with systems (biological, psychological, social) as the columns and phases of illness the rows. Our discussion, however, did not follow such a neat pattern as it is impossible to remain within the cells of such a matrix if one is discussing systems interactions.

The goal of this section is to make salient yet another (set of) time dimension(s) that were introduced at various points in our prior discussions: These are dimensions defined by a life-course perspective on the family, the individual, and the illness. The individual and the nuclear family have a time-limited history and each changes in structure and function over time. Moreover, there is change in the social context in which the individual and family reside. These temporal dimensions are associated with processes that alter the impact of illness on the person and the family, and they influence (a) the representation and perception of disease and how it is coped with; (b) the type and intensity of emotional reactions to the perception of disease in an adult member; and (c) the type of communication patterns generated in response to the illness.

Life-Course Factors and the Representation of Illness.   As we have already indicated, the construction of the disease involves individual and group processes: It is the representation of the problem, the coping strategies employed to deal with it, the appraisals of coping outcomes, and the current and expected consequences of the illness for the individual and family. This social construction is influenced by the past history and current interactions of the sick person with the family and of both with the health care system and other social organizations with which they interact. These interactions are affected by the nature of the disease, the location of the family in the socioeconomic hierarchy, and the values of the social context.

Although there are undoubtedly many similarities in the types of response by individuals and families regardless of the time in the life course at which illness strikes, the processes affecting these responses will change over the history of each system. Cancer in an 80-year-old woman has a quite different meaning than the same disease in a 30-year-old woman with two young children. In the former instance, the illness is likely to be seen as striking at an appropriate or expected time in life, after the individual has lived many years, worked, raised children, enjoyed grandchildren, and perhaps lost parents, sibling(s), and husband. This is not to deny that the illness may have an impact on the economic, emotional, and social lives of her children or cause them emotional distress and grief. The quality of this impact, however, is likely to be vastly different for 50- to 60-year-old children who are economically independent and have formed attachments to their own children and grandchildren than for the three- to seven-year-old emotionally and economically dependent children of the younger mother. Cancer in the young mother is asynchronous with her roles and functions: It is a threat to the family unit.

Life-Course Effects on Emotional Reactions.   Chronic illness that is out of step with family and individual life-course processes is likely to generate powerful frustration and intense distress and anger. Emotional distress and anger appear more common among younger chronically ill patients than among older patients (Nerenz, Love, Leventhal, & Easterling, Note 2). These reactions may complicate the patient's and family's reaction to the health care system and to other social institutions; because it is out of step or temporally inappropriate, the illness is likely to be seen as unjust and victimizing. When others fail to share this anger and sense of injustice, or when they shy away from confrontation with the sick person and his or her family, they add to the feelings of injustice and the intensity of the sense of victimization and anger.

By contrast the emotional reactions of the older person are likely to be muted: Older persons strive to regulate or maintain their feelings within a relatively narrow range of intensity, thus adding strong feelings to the disease-produced distress (E. Leventhal, 1984; Prohaska, Leventhal, Leventhal, & Keller, in press). This does not mean that intense emotional reactions will not be seen in families where illness strikes an adult at an appropriate age. Rather it means that the emotional reactions will center about different issues. For example, chronic illness and death in an elderly grandparent or parent may be an occasion for bitter recrimination among adult children respecting the disposition of the deceased's estate. The less favored "child" who may have contributed most to the daily care of the ill and waning parent may receive relatively less than the "dashing, irresponsible" favored child. The resulting bitterness and anger are understandable even when the miniscule size of the estate suggests the response is unreasonable or inappropriate (Silverstone & Hyman, 1982).

Our observations of the representation of illness by ill people suggest that changes in the time perspective of an illness are a critical and an interesting factor for investigation. Regardless of the type of illness—for example, hypertension or cancer (Meyer, 1981; Nerenz, 1979; Ringler, 1981)—patients seem to fluctuate between construing the threat as an acute problem (one whose symptoms can be treated and for which there is a cure) and viewing it as a chronic (stable or worsening) condition. Substantial differences in emotional response appear to be contingent upon these differences in temporal perspective; the belief a disease is chronic is accompanied by a sense of despair and a failure to rehabilitate, and it is likely that both the time line and the affective changes are experienced by family members. We strongly suspect that time perspectives on an illness are affected by the point in the life course at which it strikes. Tracing variations in temporal perspective at different points in the life course and their impact on the psychological future and feelings of hope would likely yield important information about perceived stresses and changes in a family's coping patterns.

Life Course and Communication. Wortman and Dunkel-Schetter (1979) concluded in their survey of the literature that feelings of isolation and problems in communication were the main concerns of the cancer patient. Their conclusion is consistent with the finding by Meyerowitz, Heinrich, and Schag (1983) that 72% of 57 patients reported problems in communication with physicians and nurses and 86% reported problems in communication with family and friends. Whether communication is the most important problem or merely one of many, it is critical (very likely a part of the others). The intensity of such fears as mutilation from treatment, of death from disease, and of rejection due to physical impairment can be reduced or intensified by communication or by a lack of the same between patient and staff and patient and family. Communication problems may be equally as complex among the well members of the family as between patient and family (Krant & Johnston, 1978).

Communication problems therefore divide into a variety of more specific problems ranging from telling the doctor that one wants a second opinion, to the difficulty of getting and understanding information from the staff or of telling friends or relatives to leave when one is not feeling well, to concerns about the withholding of information and distress about excessive concentration on the disease (see Meyerowitz, Heinrich, & Schag, 1983; Krant & Johnston, 1978). Two interrelated problems seem of special importance: (a) double messages, or saying one thing and implying or nonverbally expressing another and (b) leaving things unsaid. Individuals' nonverbal expressions, their looks of gloom, anger, or despair often appear to contradict their words. Contradictions are most likely to arise when, for example, the family does not know what to say about cancer to the patient or to family friends, and when families are under stress, such as when the threats of death and family dissolution stimulate emotional reactions and expressions that may be at variance with their verbalized thoughts. Leaving things unsaid appears to be a common problem in dealing with illness in close relationships. A caretaker may resent the intrusions and criticisms of a sibling who implies that he or she is not doing enough for a dying parent, but the resentment may go unexpressed. A wife may avoid looking at the stoma of her husband to keep him from feeling upset about it and her avoidance may stimulate feelings of rejection and loss of worth, with neither party communicating about their actions. Silence can initiate a train of events that is difficult to reverse and that ultimately leads to the dissolution of the family. Data that trace communication problems over the course of an illness history could illuminate how the family copes with the disease and with its environment.

Ease of communication is clearly dependent upon life-course factors. Adult children may prove less communicative with an ill parent than with one another. A parent may have far greater difficulty in disclosing problems and asking for help with their own or their partner's illness if they need assistance from an adult child. The ability to ask may require acceptance of a role transition and require feeling emotional security, a sense of control, and esteem. On the other hand, communication may be easier in an elderly than in a younger couple, because years of practice enhance ease of emotional understanding. Such ease, however, may only be visible in well-adjusted marriages (Noller, 1980). Sensible advice and research ideas respecting communication problems across the generations can be found in Silverstone and Hyman (1982).

Communication is an area where data are available to document change both between and within cultures. Such information as a diagnosis of cancer is less likely to be communicated to patients and families in many traditional European and Middle Eastern settings than in the contemporary Western culture of the United States (Ley, 1977; Ray, 1980). But here too the change to more paternalistic frankness is relatively recent, having occurred over the past 30 to 50 years.

SUGGESTIONS FOR RESEARCH DESIGN

Many of the points we have made in the previous sections are speculative. This was unavoidable given the paucity of data. But where data are available, it is difficult to evaluate and use them. Indeed, we suspect that the gathering of data would be of less help than one might wish were the accumulation to continue in the form adopted in past studies that suffer from problems in design and measurement. We think it useful, therefore, to conclude with a few observations on research design.

Design Problems

Difficulties arise in using and interpreting existent data because of the absence of control groups, the lack of follow-up on cases over time, and the failure to cast investigations in a coherent theoretical framework. The first of these three problems is simple enough: It is difficult to interpret figures on family discord or percentages of patients and spouses reporting satisfactory sexual relationships without comparing these figures to those for well families and for families with other types of chronic (or acute) medical conditions. Comparisons with untreated controls are at the least essential. Comparisons with other illness conditions, such as that made between ileostomy and colostomy, begin to address the relative contribution of physical change and psychological interpretation to changes in the sexual and emotional relationships of spouses.

Although they are often difficult to conduct, we believe longitudinal investigations offer the possibility of greater insight into the impact of chronic illness on families. Ideally, one ought to assess critical variables at all three levels of process: (a) biological, (b) psychological (e.g., causal attributions and effects regarding illnesses), and (c) the social or family conditions prior to the onset of illness rather than relying on postdiagnostic reconstructions for base line assessments. This may prove possible in Health Maintenance Organizations and other such organizations that provide primary as well as secondary and tertiary care to a fixed panel of clients. It is extremely important to note, however, that any advantage of longitudinal data may be lost if researchers take measures at too few points in time or if they lack a theory to guide the temporal spacing of measures.

The relatively atheoretical nature of the existent literature is both problematic and understandable. Theory demands focusing attention, measuring some factors and ignoring others, in order to test the relationships important to theory. In the early stages of exploring a problem area, it may be unclear whether one or another theory is indeed applicable. A reading of recent "theory driven" papers by Taylor (1983) and Wortman and Dunkel-Schetter (1979) suggests that much contemporary social–psychological theory is either inapplicable to individual and social behavior during illness or that investigators have to learn how to test their concepts or to define other situationally specific propositions that modify their theoretically driven questions (Cacioppo, Petty, & Andersen, Note 4; Hempel, 1966). We believe the systems framework outlined here provides a reasonable alternative to both atheoretical descriptive approaches and to theoretical approaches developed for laboratory settings. The latter tend to ignore the subject's preexistent cognitive schemata—that is, the models of illness and models of parental role behaviors—brought to the setting and instead tend to study behavior over very brief time periods. The first factor leads these theories to place primary emphasis on variables such as cognitive biases (Nisbett & Ross, 1980; Kahneman & Tversky, 1973) and attributional rules (Abramson, Seligman, & Teasdale, 1978) and fails to tell us what produces the biases and what determines when they will be used. Studying behavior over very short periods of time creates the illusion of simple recursive (antecedent consequent) relationships and overlooks the nonrecursiveness (feedback from dependent to independent variable) of the behavioral system.

The systems approach has two distinct advantages. First, it requires the investigator to elaborate all variables of potential relevance to system function. This "exhaustive" aspect of the approach is consistent with the need for good descriptive data that is so much a part of the requirement in the early stages of investigating a phenomena. Second, the approach as defined here and elsewhere (Lazarus & Launier, 1978; Lazarus & Folkman, 1984; Leventhal, 1970; Leventhal, Meyer, & Nerenz, 1980; Leventhal & Nerenz, 1982; Leventhal, Nerenz, & Leventhal, 1982; Nerenz & Leventhal, 1983), requires that the investigator examine the situation from the perspective of the patient and the family. Variables need to be identified from the participant's perspective and not simply from that of an external observer. This does not mean that measurement is entirely subjective, although it rightly emphasizes the need to assess how the individual perceives the cause, duration, and consequences of an illness for oneself and for the family. Once variables are defined from the perspective of the patient it is appropriate to search for, identify, and assess those situational factors (e.g., spouse and practitioner communications in the verbal and nonverbal domain) that initiate and sustain specific patient and family definitions of problem situations. In short, focus on the subject's perspective provides a route for the operational statement of both subjective and objective environmental factors affecting the patient–family system. This approach has much in common with that of investigators of coping who work in a "problem-centered" (D'Zurilla & Goldfried, 1971) or transactional framework (Lazarus & Launier, 1978; Lazarus & Folkman, 1984). Meyerowitz and her colleagues (Meyerowitz, 1980; Meyerowitz, Heinrich, & Schag, 1983) as well as Turk and his colleagues (Turk, 1979; Turk, Sobel, Follick, & Youkilis, 1980) have also clearly recognized the value of the approach in the study of adaptation to health threats.

Assessment of General Properties and Situationally Specific Factors.   The need for generalized assessment of family and individual adaptation on the one hand and the specification of the way patient and family represent, cope, and appraise outcomes on the other hand generate two seemingly contrasting demands for the investigator. The first more generalized need creates pressure for the assessment of family cohesion, boundary setting, interfamily communication, and so forth, with respect to a wide range of problems over a relatively long period of time. The second need is to specify coping and appraisal with respect to particular problems and requires intensive focusing on specific situations, for example, diagnosis, surgery, and on defining the attributes of the problems and their interpretation and coping within the family system. Few investigators can satisfy both demands in a single study. One possible way to do so is to adopt a "double longitudinal design" in which generalized assessments are made at defined intervals (yearly, at study intake, and at six months and one and one half years after surgery) and specific assessments made when particular problems arise in the cohort (e.g., at point of diagnosis, immediately postsurgery, and one or two months later). This type of design would trace the pattern of change in both the general measures of adaptation and in the response to specific problems. It could also allow us to identify variables that affect how the feedback from specific episodes influence the more general measures.

CONCLUSION

Two decades ago social researchers were groping toward a better understanding of the complex interrelationships among individuals, family, health, and society (Hanson & Hill, 1964). Systematic attention to the impact of individual illness on the total family is still recent in its origin (Litman, 1974), and investigators are taking their first major steps toward this goal. Few studies have focused on complex interrelated variables, such as analysis of patient and family variables in conjunction with one another. More specifically, research on family coping with chronic illness in an adult member has been guided by a metatheoretical perspective that ignores the cybernetic aspects of family interactions and the social context of these interactions (Burr, Hill, Nye, & Reiss, 1977).

In this chapter we have suggested that systems theory offers a possible framework to the study of family response to chronic illness in an adult member if its variables are operationalized in a longitudinal design, preferably with built-in sequential strategies (Nesselroad & Baltes, 1979). The systems model is interactional, focusing on family dyads and triads (Parke, Power, & Gottman, 1979; Lewis & Feiring, 1982) rather than on the individual patient. Family response to crises is dynamic and interactive and should be assessed in all members if we are to understand the unit and its individual members. In fact, chronic illness behavior in an adult member and family response are aspects of a coping dialogue of people actively striving to control their environment, to meet their responsibilities, and to make their everyday circumstances more tolerable and less uncertain.

Finally, the life-course approach proposed in this chapter suggests not only that we examine the synchronization of the behavior of the chronically ill person with that of the behavior of the family but also that we consider the family unit in its historical context and in the context of the history of its culture. Many of the processes and phenomena we see in chronic illness may be a product of factors related to the time in the life of the ill person, the family, and the culture, that is, they may be "facts" of social history. The only way we can tell if the phenomena generalize over time or are historical facts is to examine the interaction between "individual time," "family time," and "historical time."

The systems framework and the life-course perspective in the study of family response to chronic illness in an adult member constitute an uncharted frontier, but they may bring rich rewards including the development of a systems theory able to account for the social nature of individual cognition and action, and the social–cultural factors regulating primary, face-to-face groups. Rewards may also appear in the development of new techniques for intervention where various forms of interpersonal power—such as, expert and referrent (Janis, 1983)—are used to enhance role clarity, family cohesion, and individual competence in coping with chronic illness.

NOTES

1. Linz, D., Penrod, S., Siverhus, S., & Leventhal, H. *The cognitive organization of disease and illnesses among lay persons*. Manuscript in preparation.
2. Nerenz, D. R., Love, R. R., Leventhal, H., & Easterling, D. V. *Psychosocial consequences of chemotherapy for elderly patients*. Manuscript in preparation.
3. Prohaska, T. R., Keller, M., Leventhal, E., & Leventhal, H. *Health behaviors and beliefs across the adult life span*. Manuscript in preparation.
4. Cacioppo, J. T., Petty, R. E., & Andersen, B. L. *A theory of psychophysiological comparison processes*. Unpublished manuscript.

REFERENCES

Abramson, L. Y., Seligman, M. E. P., & Teasdale, J. D. (1978). Learned helplessness in humans: Critique and reformulation. *Journal of Abnormal Psychology, 87*, 49–74.

Aitken-Swan, J. (1959). Nursing the late cancer patient at home. *Practitioner, 183*, 64–69.

Anderson, B. (1984). *Longitudinal study of psychological responses to cancer*. Invited paper at the fifty-sixth annual meeting of the Midwestern Psychological Association, Chicago.

Antley, R. M., & Hartlage, L. C. (1976). Psychological response to genetic counseling for Down's syndrome. *Clinical Genetics, 9*, 257–265.

Arbib, M. A. (1972). *The metaphorical brain*. New York: Wiley.

Aschoff, J. (1965). Circadian rhythms in man. *Science, 148*, 1427–1432.

Averill, J. R. (1973). The disposition of psychological dispositions. *Journal of Experimental Research in Personality, 6*, 275–282.

Baltes, P. B., & Nesselroade, J. R. (1973). The developmental analysis of individual differences on multiple measures. In J. R. Nesselroade & H. W. Reese (Eds.), *Life-span developmental psychology: Methodological issues*. New York: Academic Press.

Bandura, A. (1977). Self-efficacy: Toward a unifying theory of behavioral change. *Psychological Review, 84*, 191–215.

Bard, M., & Sutherland, A. M. (1955). Psychological impact of cancer and its treatment: IV. Adaptation to radical mastectomy. *Cancer, 8*, 656–672.

Becker, M. H., & Maiman, L. A. (1975). Sociobehavioral determinants of compliance with health and medical care recommendations. *Medical Care, 13*, 10–24.

Ben-Sira, Z. (1977). Involvement with a disease and health-promoting behavior. *Social Science and Medicine, 11*, 167–173.

Blumberg, B. D., & Golbus, M. S. (1975). Psychological sequelae of elective abortion. *Western Journal of Medicine, 3*, 158–193.

Bonadonna, G., & Valagussa, P. (1981). Dose-response effect of adjuvant chemotherapy in breast cancer. *New England Journal of Medicine, 304*, 10–46.

Boss, P. (in press). Family stress: Perception and context. In M. B. Sussman & S. Steinmetz (Eds.), *Handbook on marriage and the family*. New York: Plenum Press.

Brown, F. A. (1972). The clocks timing biological rhythms. *American Scientist, 60,* 756–766.

Buckley, W. (1967). *Sociology and modern systems theory.* Englewood Cliffs, NJ: Prentice-Hall.

Burnam, W. R., Eardley, A., Davids, F. N., & Schofield, P. F. (1976). Problems of a permanent colostomy. *Gut, 12,* 391–392.

Burr, W. R., Hill, R., Nye, F. I., Reiss, I. L. (Eds.), (1977). *Contemporary theories about the family* (Vol. 2). New York: Free Press.

Calne, D. B., & Langston, J. W. (1983). Aetiology of Parkinson's disease. *Lancet, 8365,* 1457–1459.

Campbell, J. D. (1975). Attribution of illness: Another double standard. *Journal of Health and Social Behavior, 16,* 114–126.

Caplow, T., Bahr, H. M., Chadwick, B. A., Hill, R., & Williamson, M. H. (1982). *Middleton families.* Minneapolis: University of Minnesota Press.

Carver, C. S., & Scheier, M. F. (1982). Control theory: A useful conceptual framework for personality-social, clinical, and health psychology. *Psychological Bulletin, 92,* 111–135.

Cassileth, B. R., & Hamilton, J. N. (1979). The family with cancer. In B. R. Cassileth (Ed.), *The cancer patient.* Philadelphia: Lea & Febinger.

Cobb, B., Clark, R. L., McGuire, C., & Howe, C. D. (1954). Patient-responsible delay in cancer: A social psychological study. *Cancer, 7,* 920–926.

Coelho, G. V., Solomon, F., Wolff, C., Steinberg, A., & Hamburg, D. A. (1969). Predicting coping behavior in college. *Journal of Nervous and Mental Disease, 149,* 386–397.

Croog, S. H., & Richards, N. P. (1977). Health beliefs and smoking patterns in patients and their wives: A longitudinal study. *American Journal of Public Health, 67,* 921–930.

Currier, L. M. (1966). The psychological impact of cancer on the cancer patient and his family. *Rocky Mountain Medical Journal, 63,* 43–68.

Dent, O., & Goulston, K. (1982a). A short scale of cancer knowledge and some socio-demographic correlates. *Social Science and Medicine, 16,* 235–40.

Dent, O., & Goulston, K. (1982b). Community attitudes to cancer. *Journal of Biosocial Science, 14,* 359–372.

Deutsch, K. W. (1948–1949). Some notes on research on the role of models in the natural and social sciences. *Synthese, 7,* 506–533.

Druss, R. G., O'Connor, J. R., & Stern, L. (1969). Psychologic response to colectomy: II. Adjustment to a permanent colostomy, *Archives of General Psychiatry, 20,* 419–427.

Dyk, R. B., & Sutherland, R. M. (1956). Adaptation of the spouse and other family members to the colostomy patient. *Cancer, 9,* 123–138.

D'Zurilla, T., & Goldfried, M. (1971). Problem-solving and behavior modification. *Journal of Abnormal Psychology, 78,* 107–126.

Engel, G. L. (1977). The need for a new medical model: A challenge for biomedicine. *Science, 196,* 129–136.

Espenshade, J. (1984). *Diabetics' perceptions of their illness and responses to evaluation for retinopathy.* Unpublished master's thesis, University of Wisconsin, Madison.

Fabrega, H., Jr. (1973). Toward a model of illness behavior. *Medical Care, 9,* 470–484.

Fabrega, H., Jr. (1975). The need for an ethnomedical science. *Science, 189,* 969–975.

Featherman, D. L. (1984). Individual development and aging as a population process. In J. Nesselroade & A. V. Eye (Eds.), *Individual development and social change: Explanatory analysis.* New York: Academic Press.

Fellner, C. H. (1973). Family disruption after cancer care. *American Family Physician, 8,* 169–172.

Frei, E. (1978). Cancer. In H. Wechsler, J. Gurin, & G. F. Cahill (Eds.), *The horizons of health.* Cambridge, MA: Harvard University Press.

Friedenbergs, I., Gordon, W., Hibbard, M., Levine, L., Wolff, C., & Diller, L. (1982). Psychosocial aspects of living with cancer: A review of the literature. *International Journal of Psychiatry in Medicine, 11*, 303–329.

Friedman, M., & Rosenman, R. H. (1974). *Type A behavior and your heart.* New York: Knopf.

Fritz, C. E., & Mathewson, J. H. (1957). *Convergence behavior in disasters: A problem in social control* (Disaster study No. 9). Washington, D.C.: National Academy of Sciences—National Research Council.

Giacquinta, B. (1977). Helping families face the crisis of cancer. *American Journal of Nursing, 77*, 1585–1588.

Goldsen, R. K., Gerhardt, P. R., & Handy, V. H. (1957). Some factors related to patient delay in seeking diagnosis for cancer symptoms. *Cancer, 10*, 1–7.

Haan, N. G. (1979). Psychosocial meanings of unfavorable medical forecasts. In G. C. Stone, F. Cohen, & N. E. Adler (Eds.), *Health psychology—A handbook.* San Francisco: Jossey-Bass.

Hackett, T. P., & Cassem, N. H. (1969). Factors contributing to delay in responding to the signs and symptoms of acute myocardial infarction. *The American Journal of Cardiology, 24*, 651–658.

Hamburg, D. A. (1974). Coping behavior in life-threatening circumstances. *Psychotherapy and Psychosomatics, 23*, 13–25.

Hansen, D. A., & Hill, R. (1964). Families under stress. In H. T. Christensen (Ed.), *Handbook of marriage and the family.* Chicago: Rand-McNally.

Hayes-Bautista, D. E. (1976). Modifying the treatment: Patient compliance, patient control and medical care. *Social Science and Medicine, 10*, 233–238.

Haylock, P. J., & Hart, L. K. (1979). Fatigue in patients receiving localized radiation. *Cancer Nursing, 2*, 461–467.

Hempel, C. G. (1966). *The philosophy of natural science.* Englewood Cliffs, NJ: Prentice-Hall.

Herzlich, C. (1973). *Health and illness: A social psychological analysis.* New York: Academic Press.

Jackson, J. K. (1956). The adjustment of the family to alcoholism. *Marriage and Family Living, 18*, 361–369.

Janis, I. L. (1958). *Psychological stress.* New York: Wiley.

Janis, I. L. (1962). Psychological effects of warnings. In G. W. Baker & D. W. Chapman (Eds.), *Man and society in disaster.* New York: Basic Books.

Janis, I. L. (1982). *Stress, attitudes, and decisions: Selected papers.* New York: Praeger.

Janis, I. L., & Leventhal, H. (1965). Psychological aspects of physical fitness and hospital care. In B. B. Wolman (Ed.), *Handbook of clinical psychology.* New York: McGraw-Hill.

Janis, I. L., & Leventhal, H. (1968). Human reactions to stress. In E. F. Borgatta and W. W. Lambert (Eds.), *Handbook of personality theory and research.* Chicago: Rand-McNally.

Kahneman, D., & Tversky, A. (1973). On the psychology of prediction. *Psychological Review, 80*, 237–251.

Kaplan, D. M. (1976). Family reaction matters a lot in cancer therapy. *Journal of the American Medical Association, 235*, 2067–2072.

Kaplan, D. M., Smith, A., Grobstein, R., & Fischman, S. E. (1977). Family mediation of stress. In R. H. Moos (Ed.), *Coping with physical illness.* New York: Plenum Press.

King, R. A., & Leach, J. E. (1951). Habits of medical care. *Cancer, 4*, 221–225.

Kleck, R., Ono, H., & Hastorf, A. H. (1966). The effects of physical deviance upon face-to-face interaction. *Human Relations, 19*, 425–436.

Klein, R. F., Dean, A., & Bogdonoff, M. D. (1967). The impact of illness upon the spouse. *Journal of Chronic Disease, 20*, 241–248.

Kleinman, A. (1980). Healers and patients in the context of culture: The interface of anthropology, medicine and psychiatry. Berkeley: University of California Press.

Krant, M. J., & Johnston, J. (1978). Family member's perceptions of communications in late stage cancer. *International Journal of Psychiatry in Medicine, 8,* 203–216.

Lau, R. R., & Hartman, K. A. (1983). Common sense representations of common illnesses. *Health Psychology, 2,* 167–185.

Lazarus, R. (1966). *Psychological stress and the coping process.* New York: McGraw-Hill.

Lazarus, R. S., & Folkman, S. (1984). *Stress, appraisal, and coping.* New York: Springer.

Lazarus, R. S., & Launier, R. (1978). Stress-related transactions between person and environment. In L. A. Pervin & M. Lewis (Eds.), *Perspectives in interactional psychology.* New York: Plenum Press.

Leiber, L., Plumb, M. M., Gerstenzang, M. C., & Holland, J. (1976). The communication of attention between cancer patients and their spouses. *Psychosomatic Medicine, 38,* 379–389.

Leventhal, E. (1984). Aging and the perception of illness. *Research on Aging, 6,* 119–135.

Leventhal, H. (1965). Fear communications in the acceptance of preventive health practices. *Bulletin of the New York Academy of Medicine, 2,* 20–29.

Leventhal, H. (1970). Findings and theory in the study of fear communications. In L. Berkowitz (Ed.), *Advances in experimental social psychology.* New York: Academic Press.

Leventhal, H. (1983). Behavioral medicine: Psychology in health care. In D. Mechanic, (Ed.), *Handbook of health, healthcare, and the health professions.* New York: Free Press.

Leventhal, H., Meyer, D., & Nerenz, D. (1980). The common sense representation of illness danger. In S. Rachman (Ed.), *Medical psychology* (Vol. II). New York: Pergamon Press.

Leventhal, H., & Nerenz, D. R. (1982). A model for stress research and some implications for the control of stress disorders. In D. Meichenbaum & M. Jaremko (Eds.), *Stress reduction and prevention.* New York: Plenum Press.

Leventhal, H., Nerenz, D. R., Leventhal, E. (1982). Feelings of threat and private views of illness: Factors in dehumanization in the medical care system. In J. Singer & S. Baum (Eds.), *Environment and health: Advances in environmental psychology* (Vol. 4). Hillsdale, NJ: Erlbaum.

Leventhal, H., Nerenz, D. R., & Steele, D. (1984). Disease representations and coping with health threats. In A. Baum and J. Singer (Eds.), *Handbook of psychology and health.* Hillsdale, NJ: Erlbaum.

Lewis, F. M., & Bloom, J. R. (1978–1979). Psychosocial adjustment to breast cancer: A review of selected literature. *International Journal of Psychiatry in Medicine, 9,* 1–17.

Lewis, J. M., Beavers, W. R., Gossett, J. T., & Phillips, V. A. (1976). *No single thread: Psychological health in family sysytems.* New York: Brunner/Mazel.

Lewis, M., & Feiring, C. (1982). Direct and indirect interactions in social relations. In L. Lipsitt (Ed.), *Advances in infancy research,* (Vol. 1). Norwood, NJ: Ablex.

Ley, P. (1977). Psychological studies of doctor-patient communication. In S. Rachman (Ed.), *Contributions to medical psychology,* (Vol. 1). Oxford, England: Pergamon Press.

Litman, T. J. (1974). The family as a basic unit in health and medical care: A social behavioral overview. *Social Science and Medicine, 8,* 495–519.

Matthews, K. A., Siegel, J. H., Kuller, L. H., Thompson, M., & Varat, M. (1983). Determinants of decision to seek medical treatment by patients with acute myocardial infarction symptoms. *Journal of Personality and Social Psychology, 44,* 1144–1156.

McCubbin, H. I., McCubbin, M. A., Patterson, J. A., Cauble, A. E., Wilson, L. R., & Warwick, W. (1983). CHIP—Coping Health Inventory for Parents: An assessment of parental coping patterns in the care of the chronically ill child. *Journal of Marriage and the Family, 45,* 359–370.

McCubbin, H. I., & Patterson, J. M. (1981). *Systematic assessment of family stress, resources and coping: Tools for research, education, and clinical intervention.* St. Paul, MN: Family Social Science.

Mechanic, D. (1964). The influence of mothers on their children's health attitudes and behaviors. *Pediatrics, 33,* 444–453.

Mechanic, D. (1972). Social psychological factors affecting the presentation of bodily complaints. *New England Journal of Medicine, 286,* 1132–1139.

Mechanic, D. (1979a). The stability of health and illness behavior: Results from a 16-year follow-up. *American Journal of Public Health, 69,* 1142–1145.

Mechanic, D. (1979b). Development of psychological distress among young adults. *Archives of General Psychiatry, 36,* 1233–1234.

Meyer, D. (1981). *The effects of patients' representation of high blood pressure on behavior in treatment.* Unpublished doctoral dissertation, University of Wisconsin, Madison.

Meyerowitz, B. E. (1980). Psychosocial correlates of breast cancer and its treatments. *Psychological Bulletin, 87,* 108–131.

Meyerowitz, B. E., Heinrich, R. L., & Schag, C. C. (1983). A competency-based approach to coping with cancer. In T. G. Burish, & L. A. Bradley (Eds.), *Coping with chronic disease.* New York: Academic Press.

Miller, G. A., Galanter, E., & Pribram, K. H. (1960). *Plans and the structure of behavior.* New York: Holt, Rinehart and Winston.

Mischel, W. (1973). Toward a cognitive, social learning reconceptualization of personality. *Psychological Review, 80,* 252–283.

Moos, R. H., & Tsu, W. D. (1977). The crisis of physical illness. In R. H. Moos (Ed.), *Coping with physical illness.* New York: Plenum Press.

Morris, T., Greer, H. S., & White, P. W. (1977). Psychological and social adjustment to mastectomy. *Cancer, 40,* 2381–2387.

Nerenz, D. R. (1979). *Control of emotional distress in cancer chemotherapy.* Unpublished doctoral dissertation, University of Wisconsin, Madison.

Nerenz, D. R., & Leventhal, H. (1983). Self-regulation theory in chronic illness. In T. Burish & L. Bradley (Eds.), *Coping with chronic disease: Research and applications.* New York: Academic Press.

Nerenz, D. R., Leventhal, H., & Love, R. R. (1982). Factors contributing to emotional distress during cancer chemotherapy. *Cancer, 50,* 1020–1027.

Nesselroade, J. R., & Baltes, P. B. (Eds.). (1979). *Longitudinal research in the study of behavior and development.* New York: Academic Press.

Nisbett, R. E., & Ross, L. (1980). Human inference: Strategies and shortcomings of social judgment. Englewood Cliffs, NJ: Prentice-Hall.

Noller, P. (1980). Misunderstanding in marital communication: A study of couples' nonverbal communication. *Journal of Personality and Social Psychology, 39,* 1135–1148.

Orback, C. E., & Tallent, N. (1965). Modification of perceived body and of body concepts. *Archives of General Psychiatry, 12,* 126–135.

Palmore, E., Cleveland, W. P., Nowlin, J. B., Ramm, B., & Siegler, I. C. (1979). Stress and adaptation in later life. *Journal of Gerontology, 34,* 841–851.

Parke, R. D., Power, T. G., & Gottman, J. (1979). Conceptualizing and quantifying influence patterns in the family triad. In M. E. Lamb, S. J. Soumi, & G. R. Stephenson (Eds.), *Social interaction analysis: Methodological issues.* Madison: University of Wisconsin Press.

Parkes, C. M. (1972). The emotional impact of cancer on patients and their families. *Journal of Laryngology and Otology, 89,* 1271–1279.

Patterson, R., & Aitken-Swan, J. (1954). Public opinion on cancer. *Lancet, 6843,* 857.

Pearlin, L. I., & Schooler, C. (1978). The structure of coping. *Journal of Health and Social Behavior, 19,* 2–21.

Peck, A. (1972). Emotional reaction to having cancer. *American Journal of Roentology, Radium Therapy, and Nuclear Medicine, 114,* 591–599.

Pengelley, E. G., & Asmundson, S. J. (1971). Annual biological clocks. *Scientific American, 224,* 72–79.

Pitot, H. C. (1981). *Fundamentals of oncology* (2nd ed). New York: Dekker.

Powers, W. T. (1973). *Behavior: The control of perception.* Chicago: Aldine.

Prohaska, T. R., Leventhal, E. A., Leventhal, H., & Keller, M. L. (In press). Health practices and illness cognition in young, middle-aged and elderly adults. *Journal of Gerontology.*

Rabkin, L. Y. (1976). The institution of the family is alive and well. *Psychology Today,* (February), 66–73.

Raskin, P. (Ed.). (1982). *Medical clinics of North America: Symposium on Diabetes Mellitus* (Vol. 6). Philadelphia: Saunders.

Ray, C. (1980). Psychological aspects of early breast cancer and its treatment. In S. Rachman (Ed.), *Contributions to medical psychology* (Vol. 2). New York: Pergamon Press.

Ringler, K. (1981). *The process of coping with cancer chemotherapy.* Unpublished doctoral dissertation, University of Wisconsin, Madison.

Rotter, J. B. (1954). *Social learning and clinical psychology.* Englewood Cliffs, NJ: Prentice-Hall.

Safer, M. A., Tharps, Q., Jackson, T., & Leventhal, H. (1979). Determinants of three stages of delay in seeking care at a medical clinic. *Medical Care, 17,* 11–29.

Schwartz, G. (1979). The brain as a health care system. In G. C. Stone, F. Cohen, & N. E. Adler (Eds.), *Health psychology.* San Francisco: Jossey-Bass.

Scott, R. E., Wille, J., Jr., & Wier, M. L. (1984). Mechanisms for the initiation and promotion of carcinogenesis: A review and a new concept. *Mayo Clinic Proceedings, 59,* 107–117.

Silverstone, B., & Hyman, H. K. (1982). *You and your aging parent.* Mount Vernon, NY: Consumers Union.

Slovic, P. (1978). The psychology of protective behavior. *Journal of Safety Research, 10,* 58–68.

Speer, D. C. (1970). Family systems: Morphostasis and morphogenesis, or "Is homeostasis enough?" *Family Process, 9,* 259–279.

Suchman, E. A. (1965). Stages of illness and medical care. *Journal of Health and Social Behavior, 6,* 114–128.

Sutherland, A. M., Orbach, C. E., Dyk, R. B., & Bard, M. (1952). The psychological impact of cancer and cancer surgery: I. Adaptation to the dry colostomy; preliminary report and summary of findings. *Cancer, 5,* 857–872.

Tanner, J. M. (1973). Growing up. *Scientific American, 229,* 35–43.

Taylor, J. A. (1983). A personality scale of manifest anxiety. *Journal of Abnormal and Social Psychology, 48,* 285–290.

Todaro, G. J. (1977) RNA tumor virus genes (virogenes) and the transforming genes (oncogenes): Genetic transmission, infectious spread and modes of expression. In H. Hiatt, J. D. Watson, & J. A. Winsten (Eds.), *Origins of human cancer. Book B: Mechanisms of carcinogenesis.* Cold Spring Harbor Conferences on Cell Proliferation. Cold Spring Harbor, NY: Cold Spring Harbor Laboratories.

Turk, D. C. (1979). Factors influencing the adaptive process with chronic illness: Implications for intervention. In I. G. Sarason & C. D. Spielberger (Eds.), *Stress and anxiety* (Vol. 6). Washington, D.C.: Hemisphere.

Turk, D. C., Sobel, H. J., Follick, M. J., & Youkilis, H. D. (1980). A sequential criterion analysis for assessing coping with chronic illness. *Journal of Human Stress, 6,* 35–40.

Wellisch, D., Landsverk, J., Guidera, K., Pasnau, R. O., & Fawzy, F. (1983). Evaluation of psychosocial problems of the homebound cancer patient: I. Methodology and problem frequency. *Psychosomatic Medicine, 45,* 11–21.

Wikler, L. (1981). Chronic stresses of families of mentally retarded children. *Family Relations, 30,* 281–288.

Wishnie, H., Hackett, T. P., & Cassem, N. H. (1971). Psychological hazards of convalescence following myocardial infarction. *Journal of the American Medical Association, 215,* 1292–1296.

Wortman, C. B., & Dunkel-Schetter, C. (1979). Interpersonal relationships and cancer: A theoretical analysis. *Journal of Social Issues, 35,* 120–155.

Yarrow, M. R., Schwartz, C. G., Murphy, H. S., & Deasy, L. L. (1955). The psychological meaning of mental illness in the family. *Journal of Social Issues, 11,* 12–24.

Zahn, M. A. (1973). Incapacity, impotence, and invisible impairment: Their effects upon interpersonal relations. *Journal of Health and Social Behavior, 14,* 115–123.

=6

A Biopsychosocial Approach to Illness and the Family: Neurological Diseases Across the Life Span

Robert D. Kerns

Alison D. Curley

Despite recent major medical advances in the diagnosis, prevention, treatment, and rehabilitation of neurological disorders, this widely varied group of disorders continues to have a devastating impact on our

Support for completion of this chapter was provided by a Veterans Administration Merit Review grant.

society. For example, advances in anticonvulsant therapy have resulted in dramatic improvements in seizure control, but epilepsy remains a highly stigmatized disorder that has major negative psychological and social concomitants for the more than one million Americans afflicted (Hauser & Kurland, 1975). The past 20 years have seen a dramatic increase in the survival rate from traumatic brain injury (TBI) that is related to the development of urban trauma centers and surgical advances (Thomsen, 1974; Trunkey, 1983); yet TBI remains a major cause of death and disability especially in the age group between one and 44 years (Timming et al., 1980; Trunkey, 1983).

Although the frequency of cerebrovascular accident (CVA), or stroke, is on the decline in the United States related to increased attention to the identification and treatment of primary risk factors such as hypertension, stroke still remains the third leading medical cause of death (Adams & Victor, 1981). Over one million Americans are thought to suffer from Alzheimer's disease, the most common form of senility in the United States (Katzman, 1976; National Institute on Aging Task Force, 1980). These are only four examples of the variety of central nervous system disorders that affect individuals across the life span.

It goes without saying that the overall cost of neurological disorders to society, in terms of lost productivity, health care costs, and the social burden of caring for many neurologically impaired individuals, is immense. These costs are greatly multiplied when the potential impact on the families of neurologically impaired individuals is considered. The impact on the family may be measured in terms of restricted social and vocational roles as they relate to increased time spent caring for the impaired family member, negative emotional reactions, financial burden, social stigma, the need to attend to a variety of important decisions (e.g., institutionalization of the family member), increased stress within the family system, and so forth. Furthermore, Blumenthal (1979), in describing a transactional model involving the Alzheimer's disease patient and his or her family, proposed that increased family dysfunction and associated distress may lead to further behavioral decompensation in the patient. The transactional model highlights the relevance of the social context of the neurologically impaired individual and the importance of considering this context in evaluating the full impact of the disease process.

The past decade has seen a rapidly expanding interest in multidimensional and integrative models of health and illness (Engel, 1977; Lipowski, 1977; Pomerleau, 1979; Schwartz & Weiss, 1977). One function of these developments has been a growing awareness of the relevance of the social context, in addition to biological and psychological dimensions, in determining or predicting a variety of health-related outcomes. Of central importance in considering the social influences on health and illness issues is the role of the family (Friedman & DiMatteo, 1979; Litman, 1974).

Given the complex nature of neurological diseases and their impact on psychological and interpersonal functioning, it is interesting, but perhaps not surprising, that little attention has been paid to the family of the neurologically impaired individual. Although the past ten years has seen a rapid growth of empirically derived information about neurological disease processes and their impact on cognitive, affective, and sensorimotor functioning, an understanding of the impact of neurological disease on social/familial functioning, or even more so on social/familial influences on the neuropsychological functioning of the impaired individual, has lagged far behind. Review of the literature reveals a wide range of anecdotal and clinical reports and an articulation of potentially important areas for investigation. However, the empirical literature is sparse, and with few exceptions, methodologically weak. Attention to family variables in the rehabilitation medicine literature and in the developing psychological literature addressing the application of behavioral strategies in cognitive remediation and other aspects of neurological disease provides optimism for future investigation (e.g., Diller, 1976; Horton, 1978; Mostofsky & Balaschak, 1977).

APPLICATION OF A BIOPSYCHOSOCIAL MODEL

In order to begin to integrate and summarize the literature on the neurologically impaired individual and the family, it is crucial to elaborate a model and context in which to work. The model we will apply is a biopsychosocial one espoused by Engel (1977, 1980). Although there are a variety of important aspects to the model that apply to the issue at hand, we will focus on the simplest model and perhaps the most intuitively obvious aspect of the model that articulates the complex interaction between biological (in this case primarily neurological), psychological, and social dimensions of the phenomenon of "neurological" disease. It is assumed that a variety of clinical and research issues are critically important to consider in reaching an understanding of each of these three dimensions separately and in interaction with one another. However, an exhaustive review of the relevant variables within any of these dimensions is clearly beyond the scope of this chapter. The following discussion is included merely to emphasize the complex nature of the problem and a few of the more salient subdimensions or factors that are important for consideration.

Biological/Neurological Dimension

Discussion of neurological disease as a single-disease category fails to address important differences related to biologically significant variables. Lishman (1978) has enumerated several variables that are important in understanding the psychological and social consequences of cerebral disorder. One important factor is the acute versus chronic nature of the cerebral dysfunction. Relatively slow, intermittent, and/or chronic progression of a neurological disease process, as may be the case in multiple sclerosis (MS) or senile dementia-Alzheimer's type (SDAT), may permit adaptive adjustment to cognitive and sensorimotor deficits and a "masking" of symptoms and signs from others' observations. On the other hand, dramatic changes in functioning associated with an acute or sudden brain lesion, for example, in the cases of CVA (stroke) or TBI, are likely to be obvious to others and an extreme threat to the adaptive and coping abilities of the individual.

A second factor to be considered is the focal versus diffuse nature of the neurological impairment. Neuropsychological investigation has provided a large body of information related to the functional localization and organization of the brain. Although great variability is the rule rather than the exception, it is clear that focal disruption of central nervous system (CNS) functioning may be predicted by relatively specific cognitive, sensorimotor, and affective changes. Thus localization of the disease process may have important implications for psychological and social concomitants.

Related to these first two factors is the evolving versus resolving nature of the neurological process. The stroke victim, for example, may suffer a dramatic and sudden decline in functioning associated with an acute ischemic events. However, among those stroke patients surviving the acute phase of recovery from the event, many individuals continue to experience recovery of functioning over the course of several months. This outlook is quite different from the individual with one of several dementing extrapyramidal disorders such as Huntington's chorea or Parkinson's disease. Individuals suffering from these disorders may expect continued deterioration of functioning associated with a progression of the disease.

A variety of other disease-specific variables are important to consider for obvious reasons. Age at onset of the neurological insult is particularly important. In most cases, the age of onset is directly associated with the type of problem. Stroke and SDAT, for example, are most often associated with late middle-aged and older individuals. Multiple sclerosis typically develops between the ages of ten and 50 years. Epilepsy is most common among children and adolescents, and if its onset is later in life it is most often indicative of tumor, stroke, toxicity, or some other insult to the CNS (Adams & Victor, 1981). In the case of TBI, age, as an index of level of CNS maturity, may have important implications for the long-term effects. Among children suffering TBI, the adaptive and flexible nature of the CNS may promote optimal recovery and minimal residual deficits. Among middle-aged individuals, the same injury may result in relatively devastating and permanent disabilities. Other disease-specific variables are associated with similarly important implications. These include the severity of cognitive, affective, and sensorimotor impairment, the availability of adequate diagnosis, the availability of medical and/or surgical intervention, genetic involvement and implications.

Psychological Dimension

In a manner analogous to the discussion of the biological or neurological dimension, it is important to define subcomponents or factors of the psychological dimension that are potentially relevant to a discussion of the family's role in neurological illness. In this context, three major factors appear important: (a) the psychological functioning of the individual premorbidly, (b) the nature and severity of deficits in psychological functioning associated with the neurological disease; and (c) the individual's residual abilities to evaluate, adapt, and cope with the psychological, neurological, and social changes and resulting deficits as a function of the illness. In the context of discussing these primary factors, it is important to recognize the variety of abilities or functional capacities that may be represented within the framework of the psychological or behavioral sphere. These functional capacities include basic cognitive/intellectual capacities such as encoding, memory, reasoning, judgment, affective functioning, and complex sensorimotor integrative abilities.

The premorbid psychological functioning of the individual appears to have been particularly neglected in considering the social impact of neurological illness. The individual's premorbid cognitive, affective, and behavioral functioning greatly influences the extent and meaning of perceived psychological and social losses as well as the individual's and the social environment's ability to cope with or adapt to these losses. Some examples illustrate this point.

The nondominant (right) hemisphere lesions in most adults may be expected to be associated with disruption of spatial abilities and left-sided sensorimotor functioning. Although one cannot minimize the catastrophic effect of these losses for many individuals, the impact on an artist, who might experience the loss of unusually keen perceptual abilities, or a plumber, who is unable to work without full use of both hands, might be relatively more significant than, for example, a right-handed writer, who could continue his or her work with a minimal experience of decline in functioning.

Related more specifically to the present discussion on the family, there is reason to believe that individuals who have achieved relatively higher levels of psychological functioning (e.g., bright, affectively stable, behaviorally skilled) may also be individuals who achieve relatively higher levels of social functioning as manifested by the acquisition of social supports (e.g., family, friends, and work colleagues). Thus premorbid psychological adaptation, to a certain extent, may predict premorbid social functioning and, subsequently, the availability of social resources following the onset of neurological illness.

The nature and severity of deficits in cognitive/intellectual, affective, and sensorimotor functioning also clearly have important implications for transactions with social/familial variables. Besides potential problems in self-care behaviors and activities of daily living as a function of these deficits, declines in a variety of social roles further compromise the individual's adaptive functioning and psychological well-being. To the extent that social influences on rehabilitation, medical management, and self-management of the disorder are disrupted (e.g., the environment loses its potential as a mediator of management strategies) problems secondary to the disorder and the disorder itself may be exacerbated. Conversely, the impact of specific psychological deficits on the social network and particularly the family may be expected to vary widely. For example, loss of communicative functioning following a dominant hemisphere stroke may leave a spouse feeling functionally alone. A similar-sized stroke in the non-dominant hemisphere may result in declines in spatial reasoning, but may only have marginal impact on marital communication.

Social Dimension

The preceding discussion has been presented to emphasize the widely varied factors related to the neurological disorder itself and the psychological functioning of the neurologically impaired individual that may interact in relatively idiosyncratic ways with family variables. The process of understanding the family of the neurologically impaired individual becomes even more complicated when one attempts to articulate (a) the social organization of the individual (e.g., family and social background, present social and family roles, future family and social aspiration); and (b) the bidirectional transaction between the individual and the social and family environment.

In the following section we will develop an historical perspective to investigation of the family of the neurologically impaired individual. From this perspective we will attempt to articulate relevant family factors, issues, and questions that can be more precisely addressed within the context of discussions of specific neurological disease categories. Thus after providing an historical overview, we will present a more thorough review of the current state of knowledge related to three specific disease categories. These categories, childhood epilepsy, traumatic brain injury (TBI), and senile dementia-Alzheimer's type (SDAT), have been selected in keeping with the life-span perspective taken by this volume, and because these disease categories represent some of the major neurological and psychological variables already outlined. Finally, major methodological issues and future directions for research will be described.

HISTORICAL PERSPECTIVE

A voluminous literature describing the psychological or neuropsychological sequelae of neurological disease has developed over the past century. A primary objective of this literature has been to articulate causal associations between the focus, extent, and specific type of structural CNS lesion and psychological or functional changes. This literature has led to a variety of hypotheses regarding the functional organization of the brain based primarily on analyses of functional deficits concomitant with discrete lesions. Within this context attention has been paid to personality change and attempts have been made to describe categories of personality disorder that may likely occur in conjunction with focal lesions (e.g., prevalence of psychosis in patients with epilepsy emanating from the left himisphere; see Sherwin, 1982). Nevertheless, it seems abundantly clear from a wide range of research that the relative importance of a physiogenic element is eclipsed by a variety of psychological and social determinants (Lishman, 1968). These factors include premorbid intellectual functioning (Dencher, 1958); premorbid personality (Kozol, 1945); the cognitive appraisal and emotional reaction to the injury itself (Denny-Brown, 1945; Guttman, 1946); the psychological response to intellectual and sensorimotor impairments (Goldstein, 1952); environmental difficulties (Adler, 1945); factors of compensation or litigation (Miller, 1961); and social class (Crandell & Dohrenwend, 1967).

More recently, increasing attention has been paid to the mediational role of social variables in understanding the relationship between psychological symptoms and, in particular, the affective distress of the individual and neurological disease variables. For example, although researchers continue to pursue an hypothesis suggesting a relationship between symptoms of depression and locus of the lesion among stroke patients (Gainotti, 1972; Robinson & Szetela, 1981), recent studies have demonstrated that severity of depression may be most highly predicted by loss of social roles and activities (Feibel & Springer, 1982; Gresham et al., 1979; Hyman, 1972; Labi, Phillips, & Gresham, 1980). Along a similar vein, Thomsen (1974) found that a group of TBI patients reported that among a wide range of physical and psychological problems they experienced, lack of social contact and resulting loneliness was the most troubling. It is also interesting to note that Blumental (1979) had suggested that identification and diagnosis of Alzheimer's disease are more related to a variety of social/environmental factors than to disease-specific factors.

Thus far specific attention to family-relevant factors has been limited. Evaluation of the transaction between the neurologically impaired individual and the family has typically been limited to evaluations of only one direction of the relationship (i.e., evaluation of the impact of the neurological impairment on the family *or* evaluation of the family's influence on the neurologically impaired individual) within the consideration of any one disease process. For example, the bulk of the research on childhood epilepsy has focused almost exclusively on parental influences on seizure control and the affective, intellectual, and behavioral maturity of the child. Conversely, a review of the literature on TBI reveals a developing understanding of the family's distress and variables that are associated with increased distress. Excluded from this literature is even a rudimentary awareness that the family may influence the course of recovery from TBI.

As will be seen when reviewing the growing literature on SDAT, increasing attention is being paid to issues other than a description of the affective distress of the family of neurologically impaired individuals. For example, within the SDAT literature studies have begun to investigate family factors that may be associated with identification and labeling of the disorder (Blumenthal, 1979; Brody, 1974; Brody, Poulshock, & Masciocchi, 1978); family decision making related to institutionalization (Sanford, 1975); and factors that may affect the perceived burden on the family (Wells, 1977; Zarit, Reever & Bach-Peterson, 1980). Attention to these and simularly important issues are, however, clearly lacking in other areas. For example, although attention has been paid to family influences on adherence to medical regimens for other childhood disorders (e.g., for childhood diabetes, see Baranowski & Nader, Chapter 3, and Johnson, Chapter 8, this volume), no research has evaluated parental influences on adherence to anticonvulsant medication schedules among children with epilepsy. As already noted, although rehabilitation specialists appear cognizant of the important role that some families play in the optimal rehabilitation of the impaired individual, little empirical work has been initiated to delineate this role or relevant family factors that may influence rehabilitation outcome. These shortcomings in the literature will be further emphasized in the next section.

One final development in the area has been the clinical, anecdotal, and occasional empirical description of intervention strategies applied to families of the neurologically impaired. The efficacy of support groups for the families of MS, stroke, and SDAT patients among others have now been described. Targets for these groups have been primarily the affective distress, lack of information, and declining social support of the families. Again, it will be incumbent upon future investigators to more adequately evaluate these intervention strategies.

CURRENT STATE OF KNOWLEDGE

Childhood Epilepsy

Epilepsy has long been a misunderstood and feared disorder, primarily because of the often frightening manifestation of seizure activity. It is a disorder of unknown etiology, but a major neurological disorder, second only in frequency to stroke (Adams & Victor, 1981). Conservative estimates suggest that more than one million Americans experience recurrent seizures (Hauser & Kurland, 1975), with approximately 80% of individuals experiencing their initial seizure before they reach the age of 20 (Ziegler, 1982). Prevalence estimates of epilepsy in childhood range from 3.5 per 1000 (McMullin, 1983) to 18 per 1000 (Rose, Penry, Markush, Radloff, & Putnam, 1973), or roughly one child in every three or four classrooms (National Epilepsy League, 1958).

Seizure activity may best be described as an intermittent, excessive discharge of electrical activity from cerebral neurons that results in a temporary disturbance in the integrity of the nervous system. Consciousness may or may not be lost, depending on the type of seizure experienced. The frequency with which seizures occur is unique to each individual, with some experiencing seizures daily, whereas others experience them monthly or yearly. Some seizures are preceded by an aura, or warning signal, to the individual that allows precautionary measures to be taken before the seizure occurs; others occur without warning. Also, some individuals may have their seizure activity eliminated entirely by anticonvulsant medication; yet the possibility of having a seizure is ever present. Thus the unpredictability of seizure onset makes epilepsy a particular problem for patients and their families.

Unlike many other neurological conditions, epilepsy is not a condition that is apparent through casual contact with an individual. In the vast majority of cases, there are no physical deformities or disabilities apparent, no language problems, no outward signs of anything amiss. Except in severe cases where the seizures cannot be adequately controlled by anticonvulsant medication (approximately 20% of cases) or where a deteriorative process is in progress (e.g., Lennox-Gastaut syndrome), the presence of the disorder will be known only to the individual, his or her family, and those in whom the patient has chosen to confide.

Compared with the medical attention directed toward understanding and treating this disorder, few psychological investigations have been conducted. A relatively new line of research is examining how seizure activity can be reduced through psychological intervention (Mostofsky & Balaschak, 1977). Another and older avenue of investigative pursuit has attempted to identify the variables responsible for the high prevalence of behavior disorders in children with seizures (e.g., Grunberg & Pond, 1957; Nuffield, 1961). Children with seizure disorders have been repeatedly shown to exhibit more behavior problems than other children. For example, in a systematic survey of all of the schoolchildren on the Isle of Wight, England, Rutter, Graham, and Yule (1970) demonstrated that four times as many children with seizures exhibited psychiatric disorder as compared to healthy controls. However, a behavior disorder unique to epilepsy (i.e., the "epileptic personality") has not been shown to exist (Stores, 1981). Recent systematic investigations into the relationship between seizure-related variables (e.g., seizure type, frequency of seizures, and others) and behavior disorders have not been able to demonstrate that these "biological" variables account for a significant proportion of the variance (e.g., Whitman, Hermann, Black, & Chhabria, 1982). Whitman and his colleagues, in particular, call for more research to be directed at understanding the psychological impact of parent, family, and peer reactions on the child who has seizures.

Only recently have researchers begun to investigate how the child influences family or parental functioning, or considered the possible reciprocal influence that each may have on the other. In the following sections we will review the available literature that addresses itself to the influence of the family on the epileptic child, the impact of the child on parental and family functioning, and interventions developed for the treatment of family disturbances in the presence of epilepsy.

Influence of the Family. Research examining the association between family functioning and behavior disorders in children with epilepsy began in the late 1940s, when Jensen (1947) and Bridge (1949) described groups of epileptic children and their families. They noted such factors as "broken homes," "family tension," "marital discord," and "family incompetence or irresponsibility" as commonplace in the children with the most disturbed behavior. Pond (1952), relying on his observations and clinical impressions, noted that "disturbances at home (and secondarily at school) were the most common reasons for recommending a child be sent to an epileptic colony, and not the actual seizures!" (p. 407).

Descriptive studies of psychological variables associated with childhood epilepsy, most often relying on the subjective impressions of a psychiatrist or the mother, appear throughout the literature. Unfortunately, few studies employed control groups for comparative purposes (e.g., Pond. 1952), or if they did, failed to operationalize their variables of interest (e.g., family tension). As a result, we are left with few studies from which we can draw conclusions. Three subtopics are worthy of elaboration, however: (a) how the family functions when a child has seizures; (b) the potential influence of family discord; and (c) the parent's role in medication compliance and its effectiveness.

Ziegler's Model of Family Functioning. Ziegler (1981) presents an interactive model of family functioning to explain how the family responds when a child has a seizure disorder. Central to his model is the patient's and his or her parents' disruption in feelings of control and competence and the primary causative role these feelings have in creating the unique, and often detrimental, style of family functioning seen in families of children with seizures. Although not explicitly presented by Ziegler as a biopsychosocial model, his model clearly contains all the necessary components.

In this model, the child's first seizure can change the nature of family functioning. Over time, the family's reaction to the seizure disorder "sets the stage" for whether or not the child interprets his or her seizure disorder as catastrophic or simply inconvenient, and these reactions in turn have major implications for the child's sense of self and self-esteem. Thus the child and family form a "reverberating circuit, within which fears of loss of control can be magnified or contained" (Ziegler, 1981, p. 339, citing Hoffman, 1971). As Ziegler (1982) notes in a later paper, the primary reaction of the child does not appear to be related to the diagnosis of epilepsy per se, particularly in younger children. Many of the reactions and concerns of the child are related to the "consequences of epilepsy which make one different" (p. 169).

Ziegler's model for family functioning, that is, that there is a "reverberating circuit" that determines how all family members, but especially the child with seizures function, receives some support from other investigators. Green and Hartlage (1971), for example, found that epileptic children and adolescents functioned below expectany levels on tests of academic and social skills. They suggested that the parents' overprotective attitudes and their acceptance of lower levels of performance seemed to be related to the children's underachievement, thus suggesting the presence of a downward spiral. Indeed, Ferrari, Matthews, and Barabas (1983) suggest that poor self-concept in a child with epilepsy is related to low parental expectations.

Family Discord.   To date, the relationship between marital discord, separation, or divorce among parents of epileptic children and the nature of their seizure disorder or behavioral abberation has not been examined in a systematic fashion. This area of empirical neglect is particularly interesting in light of the consistent, positive relationship that has been demonstrated between marital discord and behavior problems in other populations of children (see Emery, 1982, for a review). Similarly, no data are available on what percentage of victims of child abuse have epilepsy, although handicapped and physically ill children have consistently been overrepresented in surveys of populations of abused and neglected children (Friedrich & Boriskin, 1976; Lynch, 1975). The clinical literature that emphasizes the stress to the family that occurs when a child has seizures at least raises the suspicion that these children may be at risk for child abuse.

Family and the Therapeutic Regimen.   Whether or not the appropriate blood plasma levels of anticonvulsant medication are maintained in the patient's bloodstream for controlling or eliminating seizure activity is one of the major, if not *the* major, concern for medical professionals treating individuals with epilepsy. Although there are many drug interactions (e.g., between anticonvulsants and psychotrophic medications) that will depress the amount of circulating or free anticonvulsant medication that is available for seizure suppression, the major cause of low blood drug levels is from not taking the pills in the first place (Masland, 1982).

Parents have a crucial role in the life of a child when it comes to medication compliance (see Baranowski & Nader, Chapter 3, this volume). Because children who have seizures must rely on their parents for drug treatment of seizure control, medication compliance in childhood epilepsy is a family issue. At least one set of investigators (Wolf et al., 1977) have noted as an aside that *parental* noncompliance was responsible for at least 10% of the children they studied having either low or nonexistent circulating anticonvulsant medication blood levels. The reasons for noncompliance, however, have not been investigated by any researchers to date.

In an attempt to understand how parenting attitudes and seizure control may interract, Hauck (1972) surveyed parents of 160 children with seizures in the Epilepsy Clinic of the Children's Hospital of Heidelberg University for investigating "autocratic" (obedience, respect, and authority) and "repressive" (tendency to use physical punishment) components of authoritarianism. An autocracy scale was drawn up based on parent's answers to two questions concerning their view of the role of obedience, respect, and authority in education. They then compared children who were currently not having seizures with those who had seizures in the year preceding the survey despite three years of outpatient anticonvulsant medication treatment. Of the autocratic parents, 61% of their children on adequate medication still had seizures. Of the nonautocratic parents, 61% of the children were seizure free. The difference is statistically significant. When parents are divided according to whether their tendency to use punishment is weak or strong, the following similar pattern emerges: Of parents with a strong tendency to use physical punishment, 60% of the children continued to have seizures compared with 31% when the parents were reluctant to punish physically.

When the results from these two components are combined to yield a measure of the basic variable "authoritarianism," an even closer relation to successful control is found than with either component alone. When the parents are strongly authoritarian, 71% of their children continued to have seizures as compared with 36% when the parents were less markedly authoritarian. Thus an authoritarian parenting attitude may result in an inability to control seizure activity even when medication is adequate.

Impact on the Family.   Having a child with epilepsy in the family impacts not only on the child and his or her parents but on the entire immediate and extended family. Only recently has research emerged to support this contention. A few investigators have attempted to examine family functioning to determine whether or not children with epilepsy assume a different role in the family relative to their siblings and to what extent siblings are negatively affected. Overall family functioning has been the most systematically examined, whereas the impact of extended family members on the child and the nuclear family has received virtually no attention. The handful of studies available for review will be presented below.

As noted above, research on the impact of a seizure disorder on the child's sibling has been sparse. The only study to systematically report on siblings of epileptic children was that by Long and Moore (1979). Parents of 19 children (aged six to 16 years) who had seizures were evaluated to examine the psychological adjustment of the child with epilepsy relative to his or her sibling nearest in age as well as the intrafamilial parenting styles. Looking at their data for the sibling controls, Long and Moore (1979) report that healthy siblings are perceived by their parents to have fewer emotional problems, to be more predictable, and to be less "high strung" than their sibling who has epilepsy. In addition, they are expected to perform better in school, to play in more sports, to have better concentration, and to have a wider range of occupational choices than their sibling with seizures. All these findings are, of course, relative to the child with epilepsy, so there is no way of knowing how these healthy siblings compare with other healthy children their age. In addition, parents report placing fewer restrictions on the healthy sibling than on the child with seizures. In short, these findings suggest that children who have seizures and their healthy siblings are regarded differently by their parents and receive differential treatment from them.

Richardson and Friedman (1974) also report on siblings of adolescents with epilepsy. Although most of the families they evaluated reported more problems with the child who has seizures, three families out of 17 reported that the sibling had more problems than the epileptic child in areas of health, school, and family.

One cannot help but wonder whether there is increased pressure placed on the healthy sibling to "make up" for the deficits of their sibling with epilepsy. Binger (1973) reports that 64% of siblings of children with leukemia have emotional or behavioral disturbances. Berggreen (1971) reports such a finding in 25% of siblings of multihandicapped children. In contrast, Breslau, Weitzman, and Messenger (1981) report that few siblings of disabled children suffer from any behavioral or emotional difficulties.

Exactly how siblings of children with epilepsy fare psychologically and the extent to which they are negatively or positively impacted as a result of their brother's or sister's seizure disorder is as yet unknown. Their adjustment can, of course, influence the adjustment of the epileptic sibling. Clearly, more research is necessary before we can begin to appreciate the potentially adverse effect a seizure disorder can have on the adjustment of the child's sibling, and how this could in turn affect the epileptic child.

Only one study has reported on an examination of the extended families of children with epilepsy and their reactions to the disorder (Romeis, 1980). Although solely descriptive in nature, this study raises the interesting issue that the extended family environment is not always supportive and understanding. Seventy-eight percent of grandparents of 32 children with epilepsy were identified as "least helpful and a consistent source of stress and adjustment difficulty," whereas two thirds of teachers were rated as "most helpful" (pp. 39–40). Romeis viewed the negative attitudes held by grandparents to reflect the prejudice commonly held in the past toward individuals with epilepsy. As Reis (1977) points out, older age is the strongest predictor of intolerance and social distance for individuals with epilepsy. Thus even within the family, misinformation and prejudice may be working to undermine the self-esteem and confidence of an epileptic individual, and may adversely affect overall family functioning.

The notion that the family functions differently as a unit when a member of the family has epilepsy has only received attention from researchers since 1981 when Ritchie (1981) first systematically examined this issue. She videotaped structured family problem-solving sessions of 15 families with a child with epilepsy and 15 healthy control families. In all families there were four members—mother, father, and older and younger siblings. In every case the epileptic child was the oldest of the two siblings, was on monodrug (Dilantin or phenytoin) therapy to control seizures, and had been seizure free for at least six months. Videotapes of the family problem-solving sessions were rated by two undergraduates who simultaneously viewed the tapes, but who were separated by a wooden screen to reduce interrater influence. Raters categorized the verbal behavior of the family members and coded the frequency of occurrence. Interrater reliability coefficients for each of the interaction variables were computed, and varied between .84 and 1.00.

Ritchie found that communication styles in families with children who have seizures were significantly different from controls. In 12 out of 15 of the families who have children with seizures, the mother assumed a much more prominent position than control mothers, as determined by the number of times they spoke. They also made significantly more "speeches" than their husbands, who did not differ from control fathers. The epileptic child was not as involved in the decision-making process as the eldest child in the control families; younger siblings, however, in the two groups of families did not differ. Families with children who had seizures, on average, solved more problems than controls. They did this by "minimizing disagreements and interruptions between family members and by a greater tendency to change individual opinions in the direction of group consensus" (p. 70).

Although these families tended to be much better "problem-solving units" than control families, Ritchie questions the need for such efficiency. She notes that this kind of interactive style is similar to that found by O'Connor (1969) with regard to families with a mentally retarded child. O'Connor postulated that family members behaved in such a manner in order to "protect the family against the potentially disruptive effect of the child's handicap" (p. 70). As Ritchie points out, however, none of these children had had any seizures for at least six months, so the continued adherence to this kind of family problem-solving style could ultimately be detrimental to the child's social development. She additionally noted that this interactive style has also been found to differentiate nonepileptic children who behave abnormally from those without behavior problems (Hetherington, Stouwie, & Ridberg, 1971), and suggests this kind of interactive style, although adaptive for dealing with short-term crises, may create problems if maintained.

Finally, in a first attempt to evaluate whether epilepsy, and the family's reaction to it, is unique from other chronic disorders of childhood, Ferrari, Matthews, and Barabas (1983) evaluated parents of children who had seizures (n = 15), those who had juvenile diabetes (n = 15), and those without chronic illness (n = 15). The diabetes control group was included to control for the possibility that a "chronic physical problem requiring a daily regimen of medication (and thus serving as a constant reminder to the child and family of the child's illness) could account for the intrafamilial psychosocial difficulties" (p. 54). All parents were administered the Rochester Adaptive Behavior Inventory (RABI). The RABI is a two- to three-hour clinical interview instrument consisting of open and closed questions pertaining to the child's behavior and adjustment at home with family members and peers, and the overall functioning of the family. Interrater reliability was assessed on two occasions with a resultant agreement of scoring on 88% of items. They also administered the Piers-Harris Children's Self-Concept Scale (Piers & Harris, 1969) to all children.

Significant differences between children with seizures and the two control groups of children (as rated by their parents) were found on the following items: history of assaultive behavior toward parents; more likely to be a "follower" than a "leader"; to complain about self more often (e.g., "everybody picks on me"; "nobody loves me"); to laugh or smile at serious events such as death or illness or accidents; to be more likely to act babyish or immature; and more prone to periods of particular emotional upset (extracted from Table I, p. 55). Further, families with children who have seizures report themselves to be significantly less close than the controls, and the quality of communications is different. Children with epilepsy communicate with their parents about specific problems or potential problems (e.g., someone telling secrets about them) more frequently than the other two groups of children, who tend to discuss more general topics (e.g., what they have done during the day). Additionally, the children perceive themselves as more problematic to their families than do controls, endorsing such items as "I cause trouble to my family" and "My family is disappointed in me" much more frequently than controls. Mean total scores on the Piers-Harris study revealed children with epilepsy to have lower self-concepts than the children with diabetes who obtained lower scores than healthy children. The overall difference between groups on this measure was significant.

From these findings Ferrari et al. (1983) conclude that the presence of epilepsy in children "places the family at risk for problems involving family communication, cohesion, and integration," further noting that their hypothesis of "a distinct familiar adjustment pattern in seizure disorders as compared with the chronic illness of diabetes can clearly be supported from the data" (p. 57). Diabetic children and their families were not differentiated from healthy children and their families on the RABI. In addition, they suggest that the lack of cohesion, communication difficulties, and poor integration may be the "tip of the proverbial iceberg" of marital discord in families dealing with epilepsy, and call for an epidemiological study of marital discord in these families.

Although this study represents a significant step forward in its incorporation of appropriate control groups, its reliance on self-report measures that do not have established validity or reliability data compromise full support for the conclusions of the authors. Their findings do raise some interesting questions about differential family functioning vis-à-vis chronic childhood illness. However, further research will be necessary in order to validate and support their conclusions.

In sum, there are few broad assertions that can be derived from this body of literature. The most recent data (Ferrari et al., 1983; Ritchie, 1981) suggest that a significant proportion of families in which there is a child who has seizures might have a different style of interaction than those without such a child. This interactive style is marked by the presence of a "take-charge" attitude on the part of the mother relative to mothers of healthy children. Marital disharmony may be present to a significant degree, but this has yet to be empirically demonstrated. Also, reactions or adjustment to seizures may be quite different relative to other chronic disorders such as diabetes. Findings by Ferrari and his colleagues suggest that familial reactions to different chronic illnesses are not equal, and that seizures may pose unique problems because of the unpredictable and frightening manifestations of its symptoms. This conclusion, however, requires further validation.

Intervention.   Epileptic seizures, because of their dramatic presentation, tend to evoke concern and distress in those who witness them. For this very reason, seizure activity can become functional for the person with epilepsy and take on a manipulative quality or may even be feigned for attention-getting or avoidance purposes. In many cases, the epileptic seizure acitvity takes on secondary gain in the family setting.

Libo, Palmer, and Archibald (1971) report on a striking functional component of seizure activity for two children from different families with photosensitive seizures. The children could induce seizures by waving their hands, fingers outstretched in front of their faces in the sunlight, or by standing in front of a flickering television set. Their parents were terrified of the seizures, and the children had independently developed a manipulative pattern of interaction whereby each would induce a seizure whenever they anticipated not getting their way. Intervention was accomplished by involving the families of both children in group family therapy and delineating the rules under which the families and children were operating. Setting limits on the children's behavior, providing meaningful contact between parent and child, and teaching the parents effective parenting skills were crucial to their intervention. At the end of approximately one year of family intervention, one child had been seizure-free for four months and the other child's frequency of self-inducing seizures had diminished but not disappeared.

Unfortunately, the study described above did not incorporate treatment reversal into its design, nor were there any nontreatment controls, and multiple interventions were employed. Thus we are left to speculate about the exact mechanism for seizure reduction. Only four-month follow-up data are provided, leaving the duration of the effect unknown. Nevertheless, this study illuminates the degree to which a neurological disorder can take on secondary gain in the family and the degree to which seizure activity can be reduced by psychological intervention.

More research is needed to understand and treat the unique problems that arise in families when one member has seizures. This area of research holds great promise from a prevention viewpoint because the psychological aspects of having epilepsy appear to be closely intertwined with the neurological. The possibility exists that early family intervention when a child is diagnosed with a seizure disorder could ultimately result in less severe or better controlled seizure activity, fewer behavior problems in the child, and better family functioning.

Traumatic Brain Injury

Damage to the central nervous system as a function of head trauma can occur at any stage of life cycle and is a major cause of death and disability in the age range from one to 44 years (Trunkey, 1983). A variety of important variables related to the individual's biological, psychological, and social functioning at the time of traumatic brain injury (TBI) may be expected to influence interactions with relevant family variables. For example, within the biological/neurological domain, researchers have focused on such variables as the specific type of injury (e.g., closed head injury, hematoma, open skull fractures, or severe anoxia), the locus of the lesion (e.g., dominant hemisphere, nondominant hemisphere, brainstem, or diffuse), and severity as indexed by "posttraumatic amnesia" (PTA) duration. Psychological variables of relevance include cognitive/intellectual changes (e.g., presence or absence of language problems, memory problems, and deficits in reasoning and judgment), personality changes (e.g., irritability, dependency, and talkativeness), and other affective changes, as well as the premorbid psychological functioning of the individual. Finally, researchers have addressed the social context of the injured individual (e.g., marital status, employment status, and availability of social support).

The majority of the published reports in this area have clearly focused on the impact of TBI on the family. In particular, researchers have focused on describing the experience of affective distress, burden, and social changes of the family and the extent to which variables related to the individual, such as those just described, may influence the impact on the family. Furthermore, researchers have attempted to evaluate the degree to which disruption in the family following TBI is specific to some aspect of the TBI or to other nonspecific variables. Little research but considerable speculation has focused on evaulating family variables and how they may affect the adjustment and rehabilitation of the TBI patient. Finally, the few available descriptions of family-relevant interventions generally support their efficacy and emphasize the apparent need for further family involvement, but little has been done to articulate targets for intervention, optimal intervention strategies, the timing of family intervention, and other important variables.

Impact on the Family. A review of the literature clearly supports the notion that TBI to a family member will have both acute and potentially chronic influences on family members and the family system. The primary influences appear to be negative affective changes (McKinlay, Brooks, Bond, Martinage, & Marshall, 1981; Oddy, Humphrey, & Uttley, 1978a; Rosenbaum & Najenson, 1976), increased experience of subjective burden (Brooks & McKinlay, 1983; McKinlay et al., 1981), disruption of family relationships (Rosenbaum & Najenson, 1976), and shifting social roles within the family (Brooks, 1980; Najenson et al., 1974; Rosenbaum & Najenson, 1976). Variables related to the TBI patient's impairments have drawn the most attention as the primary sources for these negative influences on the family (Brooks & McKinlay, 1983; McKinlay et al., 1981; Oddy et al., 1978a,b; Rosenbaum & Najenson, 1976; Thomsen, 1974; Weddell, Oddy, & Jenkins, 1980). Variables related to family structure and family interaction are just beginning to be addressed in terms of their influence on family distress (Bicknell, 1982; Brooks & McKinlay, 1983).

As might be expected, clinicians and researchers alike have relied primarily on the report of family members when assessing the impact of TBI on functional capacities including social and vocational functioning, personality changes, and language, memory, reasoning and judgment, and other cognitive changes. In this context investigators have attempted to assess the differential impact on the family of a variety of changes related to TBI. A consistent finding is that the report of personality changes is the most common complaint among close relatives. Thomsen (1974) interviewed relatives of 50 TBI patients with varying levels of language dysfunction and reported that complaint of personality change (e.g., irritability, hot temper, spontaneity, restlessness, emotional liability, stubbornness) was mentioned by 42 relatives, second in frequency only to memory loss. Interestingly, no relatives complained of physical limitations nor associated burden with motor dysfunction, and only a few complained that communication was a problem.

Brooks, McKinlay, and their colleagues (Brooks & McKinlay, 1983; McKinlay et al., 1981) similarly interviewed relatives of 55 TBI patients at three, six, and 12 months after the injury. Over 50% of the sample noted significant emotional changes (e.g., irritability, anger with control problems, low mood, anxiety, impatience) and other subjective problems (e.g., slowness, tiredness, headaches) on a problem checklist. Finally, Weddell, Oddy and Jenkins (1980) also noted that personality change and, in particular, increased irritability were the most common complaints of a group of 44 relatives of TBI patients.

These authors, among others, have discussed the significance of these personality changes by noting the disruptive nature of these changes both within the family and in other social contexts. It is hypothesized that affective and behavioral changes associated with the TBI such as increased irritability, emotional lability, a pervasive lack of spontaneity, and restlessness are specifically disruptive of interpersonal communication and social role functioning. Such changes are thought to lead to increased social isolation of the TBI individual as family and friends withdraw from increasingly aversive or at least increasingly less positive interactions. Consistent with this perception, Thomsen (1974) reported that TBI patients interviewed one to six years following their injury acknowledged that lack of social contact and associated loneliness were the biggest problems they faced. Again, the experience of social losses was mentioned far more frequently than language, memory, or physical dysfunction. Conversely, it can be hypothesized that specific physical limitations and even cognitive disabilities such as language dysfunctions, although they may clearly impact on the family and social context, may be more easily compensated by alternative strategies. To the extent that individuals and their families are successful in adjusting their expectations related to the physical and communicative abilities of the impaired individual in the context of an otherwise rewarding relationship, feelings of burden, compromise, and, ultimately, dislike are less likely to arise.

Lezak (1978) has articulated five broad and somewhat overlapping categories of characterological alterations in persons with adult-onset brain injury that may create adjustment problems for families. Appreciation of these difficulties from a neuropsychological perspective underlines the significance of these problems for family members. These categories include (a) an impaired capacity for social perceptiveness results in self-centered behavior in which both empathy and self-reflective or self-critical attitudes are greatly diminished if not lacking altogether; (b) an impaired capacity for control and self-regulation gives rise to impulsivity, random restlessness, and impatience; (c) stimulus-bound behavior appears as social dependency, difficulty in planning and organizing activities or projects, and decreased or absent behavioral initiative that may belie the patient's verbalizations; (d) the most common specific emotional alterations are apathy, silliness, lability, irritability, and either greatly increased sexual interest or a virtual loss of the sex drive; and (e) a relative and sometimes quite complete inability to profit from experience compromises the patient's capacity for social learning even when the ability to absorb new information may be intact (p. 592).

The actual extent of disruption of family functioning, family members' distress, and changes in social roles is poorly documented in the research literature. In fact, only two studies have directly evaluated the degree of distress experienced by the relatives of TBI patients in comparison with an adequate control group.

In one study, Rosenbaum and Najenson (1976) evaluated 30 Israeli women 12 months following the Yom Kippur War. Ten women were married to brain-injured men, six were married to paraplegics, and 14 were married to uninjured veterans of the war. Each woman in the study completed a four-part questionnaire consisting of items relating to perceived change in family life, statements describing the current family and social situation, an adaptation of a marital roles inventory, and symptoms indicative of disturbances in mood. As predicted, the wives of TBI patients, relative to the wives of the paraplegic veterans, reported significantly more frequent changes in family and social activities, more frequent disruption and dissatisfaction with their current living situation, an increased "need to handle family matters outside the family," and lower mood and more frequent symptoms of depression. The authors concluded that the extreme disruption experienced by the wives of TBI patients could not be accounted for solely on the basis of physical disability. Rather, the authors suggested that the level of distress and general disruption was much more likely a function of changes in the psychological and social functioning of the TBI patient.

In contrast, Oddy, Humphrey, and Uttley (1978b) reported few significant differences between the reports of close relatives of 50 TBI patients and relatives of a comparison group of 35 individuals who had suffered traumatic limb fractures. Relatives were administered a structured interview assessing the patient's pre- and posttraumatic behavior and social adjustment, as well as a symptom checklist focusing on personality changes and somatic, cognitive, and psychiatric symptoms. Evaluations occurred at six months following the injury. The authors reported no significant changes in either pre- to posttrauma behavior or in comparing the TBI with the non-head-injured patients in relation to frequency of contact or level of friction within the family. Only one of 12 TBI patients' spouses reported that the marriage was appreciably worse. Other researchers have criticized these findings by noting that the subjects had relatively mild impairments and a high level of functioning. There appears to be a general consensus in the literature that the findings of Rosenbaum and Najenson are much more representative of the TBI population.

Studies have consistently demonstrated a significant relationship between experience of distress among family members and their perceptions of personality or behavior change among the TBI individual. Again, the study by Rosenbaum and Najenson (1976) deserves special attention. Not only did the wives of TBI patients report more frequent symptoms of depression than the wives of paraplegic patients, but from correlational analyses the authors concluded that adverse changes in family and social functioning were strongly associated with an increase in the frequency of symptoms of depression. Similarly, McKinlay and his colleagues (1981) interviewed a close family member of 55 TBI patients regarding the presence and severity of 90 possible problems (e.g., behavior problems, physical restrictions, emotional problems, and cognitive deficits). A single index of "subjective burden" rated by each family member, besides being correlated with posttraumatic amnesia (PTA) duration, was also significantly correlated with perceived subjective changes (e.g., tiredness, slowness), and emotional and disturbed behavioral changes at each follow-up period up to 12 months. Oddy and his colleagues (1978a) interviewed 54 relatives of TBI patients at one, six, and 12 months following the injury. Consistent with the above findings, the authors reported that severity of depression in the family member was significantly correlated with the number of subjective complaints about the patient at both six- and 12-month evaluation periods.

When considering the response of the family from the perspective of adjustment and coping, it has been important to evaluate changes in the families' responses over time instead of evaluating families heterogeneously with respect to time (e.g., Thomsen, 1974; Weddell et al., 1980) or at only one point in time (e.g., Rosenbaum & Najenson, 1976). Three studies evaluated family members over the course of one year at three time points (Brooks & McKinlay, 1983; McKinlay et al., 1981; Oddy, Humphrey & Uttley, 1978a). Of these studies only Oddy and his colleagues reported a significant change in reported distress over the course of one year; peak distress in that study was noted at one month post-TBI. However, all these studies consistently documented a change in the association between distress and perceived alterations in the character of the patient over the course of one year. For example, in the McKinlay et al. (1981) study, relative's reports of subjective burden were closely associated with posttraumatic amnesia (PTA) duration at three months, but by six and 12 months the association had decreased. The burden was associated with complaints of the patient's poor memory at three and six months, but not at 12 months. In contrast, burden was found to be correlated with perceptions of increased dependency at both six- and 12-month follow-ups. Oddy et al. (1978a) found that the experience of peak stress of relatives at one month post-TBI was closely associated with PTA duration and number of days hospitalized. At six and 12 months, these associations were absent. Instead, depression was associated with the number of subjective complaints at six and at 12 months, but not at three months.

In an attempt to help clarify these findings, Brooks and McKinlay (1983) reanalyzed the McKinlay et al. (1981) data and concluded that families' perceptions of patient problems rather than the objective changes among the patients likely accounted for these observed differences. When family members were asked whether or not they observed personality changes in the TBI patients, an increasing number reported "yes" by six months. However, among those changing their response from "no" at one month to "yes" at six months, as compared to those with consistent responses over time, there was not a concomitant increase in the number of perceived changes in the patient. Brooks and McKinlay suggested that distress experienced by family members may likely be associated with physical deficits early on. However, over time, the families' tolerance for other problems may decrease as manifested by increased awareness and/or appreciation of the problems. The authors concluded that "personality change is not, therefore, sufficient to cause subjective burden; other factors including personal resources and qualities of the relative are obviously important in the genesis of burden" (p. 343). Furthermore, these authors suggested that after the first six months of therapy, which should be primarily focused on the physical rehabilitation of the patient, family intervention is just as important as individual, patient-oriented intervention.

Finally, investigators have attempted to evaluate the differential impact of TBI on either spouses or parents. Although most studies have provided the opportunity to evaluate this distinction, few have done so. Evidence that has accumulated tends to support the contention that parents appear better able to withstand the stress associated with TBI than do spouses (Adler, 1945; Panting & Merry, 1972; Thomsen, 1974). Weddell, Oddy, and Jenkins (1980), however, challenged this assumption, noting the high level of distress experienced by parents of unmarried TBI patients in their sample.

Several general criticisms should be raised about the literature just reviewed before proceeding. First, the studies have relied entirely on a self-report from one individual. Although important information can be collected and hypotheses tested by evaluating the relatives' perceptions about the TBI patient, investigators should be more cautious in interpreting the validity of relatives' perceptions. This problem is exacerbated by the reliance on unvalidated and relatively subjective interview and questionnaire methods. An important advance in this literature would be a more comprehensive evaluation by incorporating a range of assessment strategies (e.g., structured observation and analogue tasks, neuropsychological evaluations, validated questionnaires, monitoring strategies) and increased attention to the psychometric properties of the instruments (cf. Turk & Kerns, in press).

Influence of the Family.   In the context of several studies just reviewed repeated allusions are made to the idea that the family may influence adaptation and recovery of the brain-injured individual. Besides providing for the increased physical needs of the TBI patient, the family may take on new roles by supporting rehabilitation efforts, increased use of the health care system and related demands (e.g., transportation), and by supporting new roles for the patient in the home. The family's ability to adapt to these changes and new demands may be expected to have an important impact on the patient.

Bicknell (1982) discussed four primary factors of potential relevance in determining the interaction between the family and the TBI patient. These factors include the age of the patient, the level and type of handicap, the coping skills within the family, and the level of external support. Romano (1974) similarly stressed the importance of the family's coping abilities in influencing the adjustment of the patient. Romano informally observed 13 patients and their families for varying lengths of time, with a few for as long as four years. She reported that the most striking observation was the persistence of denial or minimization among family members as manifested by verbal denials of disability, expectations of recovery, and other inappropriate responses to patients and staff. Based on her observation of family–patient interactions, she suggested that the family's use of denial may further reinforce the patient's own practiced minimization of deficits. More broadly speaking, Romano hypothesized that the family's characteristic manner of conceptualizing the TBI patient's deficits may be reflected in their ways of interacting with the patient and, as such, may selectively reinforce similar conceptualizations and representative behavior on the patient's part.

Unfortunately, no empirical work has thus far addressed these issues. It remains for future investigators to borrow from research implemented in other areas in order to address the potential role of the family in the rehabilitation and adjustment of the TBI patient.

Intervention.   A common complaint of TBI family members is lack of information (Oddy et al., 1978; Thomsen, 1974). Lezak (1978) emphasized that unrealistic expectations related to a lack of information and counseling about what to expect can further compound problems arising from the patient's altered character. In this regard, Lezak and others have called for family counseling in order to minimize stress and maximize satisfaction for both family members and patients. Lezak specifically mentions three immediate goals: "(1) to help family members readjust their expectations; (2) to provide practical advice for managing the patient; (3) to kindle family members' awareness of their needs and and their responsibilities to themselves and one another" (p. 595).

In addition to family counseling, several specialists have described interdisciplinary treatment programs to foster improved family adjustment (e.g., Brooks, 1980; Najenson et al., 1974; Timming et al., 1980). These authors describe programs that focus directly on the changing roles within the family through the application of contingency management strategies.

For example, Timming and his collegues (1980) report a case study of a 30-year-old male TBI patient who entered a multidisciplinary treatment program ten years following his injury. A wide range of social skills deficits leading to complaints of social isolation were readily apparent. Treatment targeted four primary social skills: (1) asking other people questions; (2) allowing others to enter conversations; (3) use of nonverbal gestures; and (4) terminating a conversation. Using a contingency management approach involving establishment of specific goals, skills training through modeling, and selective reinforcement of progress toward goals, the patient experienced dramatic improvements. Not only did he demonstrate improved social skills, but he also demonstrated improved physical (e.g., walking) and neuropsychological (e.g., memory) status. Such a program has clear implications for improving family, and more generally, social adaptation among TBI patients, even long after reasonable expectations of improvement may otherwise be minimal.

Senile Dimentia-Alzheimer's Type

Senile dementia-Alzheimer's type (SDAT) is the most prevalent form of senility in the United States, afflicting over one million individuals and about 5–10% of the population over age 65 (Katzman, 1976; National Institute on Aging Task Force, 1980). The disease is associated with a progressive and irreversible deterioration in the individual's intellectual, emotional, and perceptual–motor integrity. The average age of onset of the disease is around 75 years, but can affect individuals in their early fifties. The life expectancy in SDAT patients is reduced by about 50% (Fisk, 1979).

Influence of the Family.   Despite the often severely debilitating nature of the disorder, it is important to recognize that the majority of SDAT patients are not institutionalized (Bollerup, 1975; Kay, Beamish, & Roth, 1964). Most SDAT patients are cared for at home, and researchers have noted that families commonly refuse institutionalization despite professional advice to the contrary (Lowther & Williamson, 1966). This decision to keep the dementing patient at home may have important implications. For example, Blenkner (1967) and others have noted increased mortality rates among relocated dementia patients than among those remaining in the community. However, the decision to care for these individuals at home certainly places a stressful and demanding burden on the family. With the increasing proportion of the U.S. Census over the age of 65 and the similar increase in the diagnosis of SDAT among members of the elderly population (Benson, 1982), the importance of considering the dramatic impact of SDAT on the family is indeed timely. Fortunately, the past decade has seen increased empirical attention to a variety of issues relevant to the role of families of SDAT patients, an elaboration of transactional models, and the proliferation of support groups for family members. The following discussion will provide a brief review of some of the more salient developments in the literature.

Labeling SDAT.   Problems in understanding SDAT and its impact on the lives of affected individuals and their families begin with attempts to define and diagnose the disorder (Bensen, 1982). Although the disease involves a progressive deterioration in intellectual capacity, its clinical or subclinical presentation may vary widely from individual to individual, thus making its differential diagnosis from other forms of reversible and nonreversible dementia extremely difficult. This problem is further complicated by the complexity and confounding of the affected individuals' and family members' reports of signs and symptoms of deterioration. It is clear that the labeling of observed behaviors as "deviant" or indicative of deterioration is a function of a wide range of social and psychological variables (Blumenthal, 1979). The process of labeling the disorder apparently has important implications not only for the adjustment of the individual with SDAT, but his or her family as well.

Blumenthal (1979) discussed the potential harmful effects of labeling SDAT that are associated with increased role expectations of significant others. Once labeled as "irreversibly deteriorating" the family may come to view the individual as helplessly dependent. Attention from family members may become increasingly contingent on the SDAT individual's demonstrations of "senile" behavior, whereas more adaptive behavior is relatively ignored. Over time, the SDAT individual may increasingly emit behaviors consistent with a "sick role" regardless of their actual functional capabilities. Ultimately, early labeling of SDAT may lead to premature or unnecessary institutionalization (Blumenthal, 1979).

Several factors may be involved in delaying the labeling process. To the extent that these factors are present, the labeling process, and perhaps even the pronouncement of a significant problem, may be postponed. Of primary importance may be the availability of financial resources resulting in the ability to compensate for functional deficits through the purchase of home health services and home aides (Brody, 1974). As Blumenthal (1979) notes, "Given enough money, there is not too much difference between a wealthy young lady who does nothing because nothing is required of her, and a demented old lady of means who is equally well cared for" (p. 42).

In many ways, a supportive family can compensate for a lack of money by providing needed services. For example, Brody, Poulshock, and Masciocchi (1978) demonstrated that elderly individuals with comparable disabilities are more likely to be institutionalied if widowed, divorced, or never married. The authors concluded that this expected finding is most likely related to the unaffected partners' ability to maintain most of the functions of the household despite the limitations of their spouse. The availability of a supportive extended family can further compensate for the functional limitations of the SDAT patient (Blumenthal, 1979) as well as provide significant support for the nuclear family (Bergmann, Kay & Foster, 1973; Zarit, Reever, & Bach-Peterson, 1980).

Blumenthal (1979) further described a model for appreciating the transaction between the dementing SDAT patient and family functioning. According to the model, relatively well-functioning families, as manifested by a dynamic flexibility in accommodating change and in solving problems, may be able to make the adjustments necessary to cope with a dementing family member. The dysfunctional family, on the contrary, may respond to behavior change in the SDAT family member by increased anxiety and general disruption in family functioning. The family's anxiety may be a direct function of the inability to meet increased demands on the system. The resulting family anxiety and disorganization may be expected to increase the anxiety experienced by the SDAT patient. Completing a cycle, the patient's heightened anxiety state may be partly manifested by a further disruption of CNS functioning, exacerbation of cognitive impairments, and increased behavioral decompensation. These changes complete a positive feedback loop on the family system, resulting in further family dysfunction and anxiety, increased demands on individual family members including the SDAT patient, heightened anxiety, and so forth. The model is truly a systems model in that it incorporates transactions among individuals in an open system as well as across social, psychological, and biological levels of each transacting individual.

Elaboration of the above model may be made incorporating variables that may moderate the transactions outlined, further affecting the labeling process. As already noted, the individual's or family's financial resources may be an important moderating variable. More generally, the family's coping capacities certainly may be expected to influence the extent to which the positive feedback loop outlined becomes operational. Other specific variables have also been articulated. For example, the relative degree of social isolation experienced by the SDAT patient, even in the presence of significant family support, may be important. Blumenthal (1979) and Bennett (1973) have both discussed the likelihood that decreased social contact may exacerbate CNS deterioration as a function of lowered sensory stimulation.

Lindsley (1964) noted that specific aspects of the individual's environment may be either "prosthetic" or "demanding." Skinner (1983), in discussing issues related to the process of aging more generally, further emphasized the potential role of the physical environment in exacerbating or inhibiting deterioration and behavioral decompensation. Finally, Blumenthal (1979) notes that life stresses such as change in residence, loss of significant others, and other disruptions in the day-to-day life of the SDAT patient may have negative consequences for the individual. Many of these varibles are within the control of the family, again pointing to the family's importance in facilitating the adaptation of the SDAT patient.

It should be noted that the model just reviewed and the variables described as associated with the labeling of SDAT have not been subjected to rigorous empirical examination. The Blumenthal model is nevertheless important heuristically, not only for the investigation of SDAT but also potentially for other neurological disorders.

Impact on the Family.   Implied in the preceding section are three important hypotheses. First, the Blumenthal model suggests a reciprocal relationship between the SDAT patient and his or her family. Second, it is understood that families will respond to the presence of SDAT in a family member with varying degress of flexibility and adaptation, and will manifest widely varied levels of distress and dysfunction. Third, a range of factors will be important in mediating the transaction between the individual and the family. The literature to be reviewed in this section, although empirically derived, for the most part has failed to specifically consider the transactional model described above or its implications. The conclusions presented therefore generally mask important individual differences and only begin to investigate variables that may moderate the negative impact on the family. The literature is important, however, in addressing the problems and distress experienced by many families of SDAT patients with implications for family-oriented interventions.

There appears no doubt that the majority of families of SDAT patients experience significant problems and distress. For example, in a recent study by Rabins, Mace, and Lucas (1982), 48 of 55 family caregivers of irreversible senile dementia patients reported significant affective distress. However, demonstrations of the type, frequency, and severity of problems experienced have varied widely across studies. Problems commonly reported include the following: decreased social activities (Grad de Alarcon & Sainsbury, 1963; Sanford, 1975); increased disruption of household routines (Grad de Alarcon & Sainsbury, 1963); decreased time to themselves (Rabins et al., 1982; Sanford, 1975; Zarit et al., 1980); sleep disturbances (Rabins et al., 1982; Sanford, 1975); financial burden (Sanford, 1975); lack of information about SDAT (Aronson & Lipkowitz, 1981; Barnes, Raskind, Scott, & Murphy, 1981); lack of societal support (Rabins et al., 1982); excessive dependency of the patient (Sanford, 1975; Zarit et al., 1980); anxiety and depression (Aronson & Lipkowitz, 1981; Farkas, 1980; Grad de Alarcon & Sainsbury, 1963; Kapust, 1982; Rabins et al., 1982; Sanford, 1975); fear about patient's further deterioration (Farkas, 1980; Rabins et al., 1982; Zarit et al., 1980); and guilt (Barnes et al., 1981; Farkas, 1980; Rabins et al., 1982; Safford, 1980).

In a manner analogous to the TBI literature, researchers have attempted to evaluate the relationship between SDAT patients' disabilities and the nature and severity of problems and distress experienced by family caregivers. Interestingly, although family members' descriptions of the types of disabilities most disruptive or burdensome for the family are relatively consistent across studies, there appears to be little empirical support for a causal relationship between patient problems and experienced burden on the part of family members. Among the problems of patients most commonly reported by family caregivers are memory problems (Rabins et al., 1982; Zarit et al., 1980); catastrophic reactions (Rabins et al., 1982); sleep disturbances (Sanford, 1975); fecal and urinary incontinence (Sanford, 1975); frequent falls (Sanford, 1975); poor self-care (Zarit et al., 1980); and restlessness (Zarit et al., 1980). In the study by Zarit and his colleagues, however, the degree of burden as rated by the primary caregiver was uncorrelated with any deficit measure. A significant inverse relationship was noted between degree of burden and frequency of visits from extended family members (Zarit et al., 1980).

One other study deserves special attention. Reifler, Cox, and Hanley (1981) investigated the extent to which dementing elderly patients, family caregivers, and institutional staff agree on the presence and severity of patients' disabilities. Eighty-two patients, including a majority of SDAT patients, were interviewed by a psychiatrist to determine their appraisal to ten potential problem areas; housing and living situation, food and nutrition, self-care, physical health, emotional and mental factors, financial matters, transportation, day-to-day routine, family stress, interference with family members, and work or other activity. Family members and staff completed analogous self-administered questionnaires. Results revealed a high degree of concordance in all ten areas between the family members and staff ratings. Patients and family agreed in five of the areas, whereas patients and staff ratings were significantly correlated in only three of ten areas. Patients rated nine of the ten areas as significantly less problematic than the other two groups did. The authors concluded that this denial among dementing elderly individuals may pose a further dilemma for family members, who appear to be relatively realistic in their appraisal of problem areas. Implications for interventions with dementing individuals were also discussed in the investigation. For example, it was suggested that because physical health and mental difficulties were the most frequently acknowledged problems among patients, attention to these problems may be a way to engage the patient in a more comprehensive evaluation in spite of their denial of other problems.

Unlike the TBI literature, no investigators have attempted longitudinal investigations of the impact of SDAT on families. The few studies just reviewed have relied on a single evaluation for drawing their conclusions. Only one study, that of Zarit et al. (1980), has investigated possible mediators or moderators of the negative impact on families. Within this context, neither the characteristics of family members (e.g., demographic variables, personality, coping patterns), family structure variables (e.g., number of family members, proximity of extended family members), nor family system variables (e.g., communication patterns in the family, family coping patterns) have been investigated as to their potential role in determining the impact of SDAT on the family. It remains for future investigators to draw on relevant methodologies from other literatures in order to examine more thoroughly the complexities of the interaction between the SDAT patient and family adaptation.

Intervention. Several papers have appeared in the literature in the past four years describing support groups for SDAT family members (e.g., Barnes, Raskind, Scott, & Murphy, 1981; Farkas, 1980; Kapust, 1982; La-Vorgna, 1979; Lazarus, Stafford, Cooper, Cohler, & Dysken, 1981; Safford, 1980). The papers detail the clinical impressions of the authors regarding the problems and concerns experienced by family members, possible goals for the group, roles of the therapist, and outcomes of group participation. Most authors advocate providing opportunities for ventilation as well as discussion of specific practical problems in caring for the SDAT patients. Only one paper has incorporated an attempt to validate the efficacy of the group treatment program (Lazarus et al., 1981). However, the unanimous consensus is that such groups serve an important function in providing emotional support and solutions to many problems experienced by caregivers. The proliferation of similar support groups within hospital settings and in the community certainly speaks to the perceived need for such services.

RESEARCH AND METHODOLOGICAL ISSUES

Investigation related to the family of the neurologically impaired individual has remained largely at an exploratory level. The failure to draw upon sound theoretical models in order to develop specific testable hypotheses, and the failure to address a variety of important design and methodological issues has compromised researchers' attempts to move beyond the speculations and intuitively obvious conclusions that generally form the hallmark of article discussion sections in a journal and the current state of knowledge in this important and interesting area.

Theoretical Issues

Close reading of the majority of papers written in this area reveals a strong clinical orientation to the relative exclusion of the consideration of theoretical models, which is crucial for conceptualizing and formulating specific empirical questions (see Leventhal, Leventhal, & Van Nguyen, Chapter 5, this volume). Although the clinical significance and relevance of the problems addressed in this area cannot be minimized, the importance of investigating mechanisms that may mediate or help explain observed findings must also be undertaken. For example, it is not enough to know that the majority of families of SDAT patients experience heightened distress. It is incumbent upon researchers to begin to investigate variables that may mediate families' distress so that increasingly sound strategies for intervention may be developed.

The biopsychosocial model, discussed briefly in the introduction to this chapter, is one theoretical model that could be applied to help researchers in this area. The model draws upon systems theory (von Bertalanffy, 1968) and emphasizes the investigation of, or at least attention to, variables representing multiple dimensions or levels of the system(s) under investigation. In the present context, application of the model would include attention to biological/neurological, psychological, and social variables related to the individual under investigation and attention to the complex interaction or transaction among family members including the neurologically impaired individual at any or all of these levels. Furthermore, the model permits exploration of other social or cultural influences on the family and the impaired individual in determining the observed responses. The complexity of the model can easily become cumbersome to the investigator and thus detracts from its practical application. However, failure to attend to any one dimension of the system under investigation may compromise the validity of conclusions drawn from the study.

Models for organizing information about or understanding the transactions among members of the family, within the context of a biopsychosocial perspective, can also make an important contribution to this literature. Operant theory and family systems theory represent two conceptual schema that have begun to be applied. Only by considering these or other theoretical models can specific predictions and empirical questions be formulated about the transaction between the family and the neurologically impaired family member.

Methodological Issues

A variety of important methodological issues have already been raised in the context of the literature review. The methodological problems noted have related to the following: subject-selection criteria and population specificity; the reliance on correlational designs often without introducing multivariate analyses; the reliance on unvalidated self-report measures to the relative exclusion of other methods of data collection; the general failure to incorporate longitudinal designs; the failure to include control or comparison groups for study; and in the case of treatment outcome studies, the failure to take even rudimentary steps to ensure adequate control and experimental rigor. Until these and other methodological issues gain attention, the literature on the family of the neurologically impaired is likely to continue to rely on clinical impressions and anecdotal reports that can support almost any a priori bias of the authors.

A few of these problems deserve particular attention. First, although correlational designs may be an important means of investigation in this area, it is crucial that researchers begin to incorporate appropriate multivariate strategies for analysis and hypothesis testing. Continued reliance on primarily descriptive statistics, which is true with even recent studies appearing in the literature (e.g., McKinlay et al., 1981; Rabins et al., 1982; Weddell et al., 1980; Zarit et al., 1980) is unfortunately the rule rather than the exception.

Measurement problems also bear emphasizing. With few exceptions, investigators have relied on lengthy questionnaires and interview strategies. Most of these assessment devices were developed specifically for the study in which they were used, without attention to their psychometric properties (e.g., Reifler et al., 1981; Rosenbaum & Najenson, 1976). Besides compromising confidence in the findings of the individual studies, the continued reliance on scales that are idiosyncratic to each study precludes comparison among studies (cf. Turk & Kerns, in press).

With only a few exceptions, observational methods have not been applied in this literature. One important exception is the study by Ritchie (1981) in the childhood epilepsy literature in which videotapes of family problem-solving sessions served as the primary means of data collection. A second study (Reifler, Cox, & Hanley, 1981) included global staff ratings of SDAT patient problems in addition to patient and family member reports. Of these two observational studies, Ritchie is the only one to evaluate reliability between raters. With increasing attention to family systems variables emphasizing family interaction, the continued use of structured observation strategies appears indicated.

It is imperative that data be collected from other family members in addition to the mother or spouse. Some attention to this issue is apparent in the childhood epilepsy literature (e.g., Richardson & Friedman, 1974; Romeis, 1980), but no systematic attention is in evidence elsewhere in the literature reviewed. Related to this issue is the inclusion of spouses, parents, children, and even friends as "the primary caregiver" as the source of information in several studies (e.g., Oddy et al., 1978a). Thomsen (1974) and others have noted that parents may adjust better than spouses to TBI, thus suggesting that their inclusion as "equivalents" in investigations of family response to neurological insult is unjustified.

FUTURE DIRECTIONS

As just noted, the need to introduce contemporary psychological and social theory as well as the need to address a variety of methodological issues are perhaps the most important tasks facing investigators in this developing literature. A relatively rich clinical literature in addition to the few empirical papers available provide a basis on which to develop specific testable hypotheses. Some suggestions for further investigation are in order.

The relative neglect of the role of the family in influencing the neurologically impaired individual is readily apparent. In the childhood epilepsy literature, the role of the family in facilitating or compromising adherence to medication regimens; emotional and behavioral adjustment, cognitive development, social skills development and social maturity in addition to seizure frequency and severity are open to closer scrutiny. Similarly, in cases of resolving lesions such as TBI and stroke, the potential role of the family in influencing recovery of function and adaptation to neurological insult are attractive targets for empirical exploration, given their potential clinical importance. In cases of degenerative diseases, further attention needs to be directed toward family variables that may influence critical points in the deteriorative process such as diagnosis and institutionalization as well as the rapidity of decline. Within the context of these investigations, attention should be directed toward interactions between family-related variables and neurological, psychological, and social variables that are related to the neurologically impaired individual. Dynamic, as opposed to static, models investigating the process of these interactions and their changing relationships over time are encouraged.

More systematic investigation of family systems variables (e.g., problem-solving styles, communication patterns) that may affect the differential impact on family distress observed within each illness category appears warranted. One approach to this issue is to incorporate discriminative analytic approaches to identity variables that affect adaptation. Another approach would involve longitudinal data collection in order to follow changes over time and develop predictive models that can account for significant proportions of the variance in future adaptation. In each of these contexts, increased attention to other social variables (e.g., other social supports, health care system variables) is indicated.

Finally, in considering the application of clinical interventions, it is important to consider a variety of possible targets. The focus to date has clearly been on the development of "support" groups for family members. These groups should continue to receive attention, but need to be subjected to closer empirical scrutiny in order to improve their efficacy by examining the appropriateness of different intervention targets and strategies. Additionally, family interventions designed to improve adaptation to and/or recovery from insult for the neurologically impaired individual have yet to be systematically investigated. Strategies targeting the neurologically impaired individual's recovery and adaptation should be evaluated in terms of their impact on family functioning.

REFERENCES

Adams, R. D., & Victor, M. (1981). *Principles of neurology.* New York: McGraw-Hill.

Adler, A. (1945). Mental symptons following head injury. *Archives of Neurological Psychiatry,* 53, 34–43.

Allen, I. M. (1956). The emotional factor and the epileptic attack. *New Zealand Medical Journal*, *55*, 297–308.

Aronson, M. K., & Lipkowitz, R. (1981). Senile dementia, Alzheimer's type: The family and the health care delivery system. *Journal of the American Geriatrics Society*, *29*, 568–571.

Bagley, C. (1971). *The social psychology of the child with epilepsy*. London: Routledge & Kegan-Paul.

Barnes, R. F., Raskind, M. A., Scott, M., & Murphy, C. (1981). Problems of families caring for Alzheimer patients: Use of a support group. *Journal of the American Geriatrics Society*, *29*, 80–85.

Bennett, R. (1973). Living conditions and everyday needs of the elderly with particular reference to social isolation. *International Journal of Aging and Human Development*, *4*, 179–185.

Benson, D. F. (1982). Clinical aspects of dementia. In J. C. Beck (moderator), Dementia in the elderly: The silent epidemic *Annals of Internal Medicine*, *97*, 231–241.

Berggreen, S. M. (1971). A study of the mental health of the near relatives of 20 multihandicapped children. *Acta Paediatrica Scandinavica* (Suppl. 21), 1–24.

Bergmann, K., Kay, D. W. K., & Foster, E. (1973). A follow-up study of randomly selected community residents to assess the effects of chronic brain syndrome and cerebrovascular disease. In R. de La Fuente & M. N. Weisman (Eds.), *Psychiatry: Proceedings of the Fifth World Congress of Psychiatry* (pp. 856–865). Amsterdam: Excerpta Medica.

Bicknell, D. J. (1982). Living with a mentally handicapped member of the family. *Postgraduate Medical Journal*, *58*, 597–605.

Binger, C. M. (1973). Childhood leukemia: Emotional impact on siblings. In E. J. Anthony & C. Koupenik (Eds.), *The child in his family: The impact of disease and death*. New York: Wiley.

Blenkner, M. (1967). Environmental change and the aging individual. *Journal of Gerontology*, *7*, 101–105.

Blumenthal, M. D. (1979). Psychosocial factors in reversible and irreversible brain failure. *Journal of Clinical Experimental Gerontology*, *1*, 39–55.

Bollerup, T. R. (1975). Prevalence of mental illness among 70-year-olds domiciled in nine Copenhagen suburbs: The Grostrup survey. *Acta Psychiatrica Scandinavia*, *51*, 327–339.

Breslau, N., Weitzman, A., & Messenger, K. (1981). Psychologic functioning of siblings of disabled children. *Pediatrics*, *61*, 344–353.

Bridge, E. M. (1949). *Epilepsy and convulsive disorders in children*. New York: McGraw-Hill.

Brody, D. N. (1974). Aging and family personality: A developmental view. *Family Process*, *3*, 23–27.

Brody, S. J. Poulshock, S. W., & Masciocchi, C. F. (1978). The family caring unit: A major consideration in the long-term support system. *Gerontologist*, *18*, 556–561.

Brooks, D. N. (1979). Psychological deficits after severe blunt head injury: Their significance and rehabilitation. In D. J. Oborne, M. M. Gruneberg, & J. R. Eiser, (Eds.), *Research in psychology and medicine* (Vol. 2, pp. 469–476). London: Academic Press.

Brooks, D. N., & McKinlay, W. (1983). Personality and behavioral change after severe blunt head injury—a relative's view. *Journal of Neurology, Neurosurgery, and Psychiatry*, *46*, 336–344.

Crandell, D. L., & Dohrenwend, B. P. (1967). Some relations among psychiatric symptoms, organic illness, and social class. *American Journal of Psychiatry*, *123*, 1527–1537.

Dencker, S. J. (1958). A follow-up study of 128 closed head injuries in twins using co-twins as controls. *Acta Psychiatrica Scandanavia*, *33* (Suppl. 123), 1–125.

Denny-Brown, D. E. (1945). Disability arising from closed head injury. *Journal of the American Medical Association*, *127*, 429–436.

Diller, L. (1976). A model for cognitive retraining in rehabilitation. *Clinical Psychologist, 29*, 13–15.

Emery, R. E. (1982). Interparental conflict and the children of discord and divorce. *Psychological Bulletin, 92*, 310–330.

Engel, G. L. (1977). The need for a new medical model: A challenge for biomedicine. *Science, 196*, 129–136.

Engel, G. L. (1980). The clinical application of the biopsychosocial model. *American Journal of Psychiatry, 137*, 535–544.

Farkas, S. W. (1980). Impact of chronic illness on the patient's spouse. *Health and Social Work, 5*, 39–46.

Feibel, J. T., & Springer, C. J. (1982). Depression and failure to resume social activities after stroke. *Archives of Physical Medicine and Rehabilitation, 63*, 276–278.

Ferrari, M., Matthews, W. S., & Barabas, G. (1983). The family and the child with epilepsy. *Family Process, 22*, 53–59.

Fisk, A. A. (1979). Senile dementia, Alzheimer's type (SDAT): A review of present knowledge. *Wisconsin Medical Journal, 78*, 29–33.

Friedman, H. S. & DiMatteo, M. R. (1979). Health care as an interpersonal process. *Journal of Social Issues, 35*, 1–11.

Friedrich, W. N., & Boriskin, J. A. (1976). The role of child in abuse: A review of the literature. *American Journal of Orthopsychiatry, 46*, 580–590.

Gainotti, G. (1972). Emotional behavior and hemispheric side of lesion. *Cortex, 8*, 41–45.

Goldstein, K. (1952). The effect of brain damage on the personality. *Psychiatry, 15*, 245–260.

Grad de Alarcon, J., & Sainsbury, P. (1963). Mental illness and the family. *Lancet, 1*, 544–547.

Green, J. B. & Hartlage, L. C. (1971). Comparative performance of epileptic and nonepileptic children and adolescents. *Diseases of the Nervous System, 32*, 418–21.

Gresham, G. E., Phillips, T. F., Wolf, P. A., McNamara, P. M., Kannel, W. B., & Dawber, T. R. (1979). Epidemiologic profile of long-term stroke disability: The Framingham study. *Archives of Physical Medicine and Rehabilitation, 60*, 487–491.

Grunberg, F., & Pond, D. A. (1957). Conduct disorders in epileptic children. *Journal of Neurology, Neurosurgery and Psychiatry, 20*, 65–68.

Guttmann, E. Late effects of closed head injuries: Psychiatric observations. (1946). *Journal of Mental Sciences, 92*, 1–18.

Hauck, G. (1972). Sociological aspects of epilepsy research. *Epilepsia, 13*, 79–85.

Hauser, W. A., & Kurland, L. T. (1975). The epidemiology of epilepsy in Rochester, Minnesota, 1935 through 1967. *Epilepsia, 16*, 1–66.

Hetherington, E. G., Stouwie, R. J., & Ridberg, E. H. (1971). Patterns of family interaction and child-rearing attitudes related to three dimensions of juvenile delinquency. *Journal of Abnormal Psychology, 78*, 160–176.

Hoffman, L. (1977). Deviation amplifying process in natures groups. In J. Haley (Ed.), *Changing families*. New York: Grune & Stratton.

Horton, A. M. (1978). Behavioral neuropsychology: A tentative definition. *Behavioral Neuropsychology Newsletter, 1*, 1–2.

Hyman, M. D. (1972). Social psychological determinants of patients' performance in stroke rehabilitation. *Archives of Physical Medicine and Rehabilitation, 53*, 217–226.

Jensen, R. A. (1947). Importance of the emotional factor in the convulsive disorders of children. *American Journal of Psychiatry, 104*, 126–131.

Kapust, L. R. (1982). Living with dementia: The ongoing funeral. *Social Work in Health Care, 7*, 79–91.

Katzman, R. (1976). Editorial: The prevalence and malignancy of Alzheimer's disease. A major killer. *Archives of Neurology, 33,* 217–218.

Kay, D. W. K., Beamish, P., & Roth, M. (1964). Old age mental disorders in Newcastle-upon-Tyne. Part II. A study of possible social and medical causes. *British Journal of Psychiatry, 110,* 668–682.

Kopeloff, L. M., Chusid, J. G., & Kopeloff, N. (1945). Chronic experimental epilepsy in Macaca mulatta. *Neurology, 4,* 218–227.

Kozol, H. L. (1945). Pretraumatic personality and psychiatric sequelae of head injury. *Archives of Neurology and Psychiatry, 53,* 358–364.

Labi, M. L. C., Phillips, T. F., & Gresham, G. E. (1980). Psychosocial disability in physically restored long-term stroke survivors. *Archives of Physical Medicine and Rehabilitation, 61,* 561–565.

LaVorgna, D. (1979). Group treatment for wives of patients with Alzheimer's disease. *Social Work in Health Care, 5,* 219–221.

Lazarus, L. W., Stafford, B., Cooper, K., Cohler, B., & Dysken, M. (1981). A pilot study of an Alzheimer patients' relatives discussion group. *Gerontologist, 21,* 353–358.

Lezak, M. D. (1978). Living with the characterologically altered brain injured patient. *Journal of Clinical Psychiatry, 39,* 592–598.

Libo, S. S., Palmer, C., & Archibald, D. (1971). Family group therapy for children with self-induced seizures. *American Journal of Orthopsychiatry, 41,* 506–509.

Lindsley, O. R. (1964). Geriatric behavioral prosthetics. In R. Kastenbaum (Ed.), *New thoughts on old age.* New York: Springer.

Lipowski, Z. J. (1977). Psychosomatic medicine in the seventies: An overview. *American Journal of Psychiatry, 134,* 233–244.

Lishman, W. A. (1978). Brain damage in relation to psychiatric disability after head injury. *British Journal of Psychiatry, 114,* 373–410.

Lishman, W. A. (1978). *Organic psychiatry: The psychological consequences of cerebral disorder.* London: Blackwell Scientific Publications.

Litman, T. (1974). The family as a basic unit in health and medical care: A social behavioral overview. *Social Science and Medicine, 8,* 495–519.

Long, C. G., & Moore, J. R. (1979). Parental expectations for their epileptic children. *Journal of Child Psychology and Psychiatry, 24,* 299–312.

Lowther, C. P. & Williamson, J. (1966). Old people and their relatives. *Lancet, 2,* 1459–1460.

Lynch, M. A. (1975). Ill health and child abuse. *Lancet, 2,* 317–319.

Masland, R. I. (1982). The nature of epilepsy. In H. Sands (Ed.), *Epilepsy: A handbook for the mental health professional.* New York: Brunner/Mazel.

McKinlay, W. W., Brooks, D. N., Bond, M. R. Martinage, D. P., & Marshall, M. M. (1981). The short-term outcome of severe blunt head injury as reported by relatives of the injured persons. *Journal of Neurology, Neurosurgery, and Psychiatry, 44,* 527–533.

McMullin, G. P. (1983). A survey of epilepsy in Cheshire schoolchildren. *The British Journal of Clinical Practice* (Symposium Suppl.), *27,* 92–98.

Mellor, D. H., Lowit, I., & Hall, D. J. (1974). Are epileptic children behaviorally different from other children? In P. Harris & C. Mawdsley (Eds.), *Epilepsy: Proceedings of the Hans Breger centenary symposium* (pp. 313–316). Edinburgh: Churchill-Livingstone.

Miller, H. (1961). Accident neurosis. *British Medical Journal, 1,* 919–925; 992–998.

Mostofsky, D. I., & Balaschak, B. A. (1972). Psychobiological control of seizures. *Psychological Bulletin, 84,* 723–750.

Najenson, T., Mendelson, L., Schecter, I., David, C., Mintz, N., & Grosswasser, Z. (1974). Rehabilitation after severe injury. *Scandinavian Journal of Rehabilitation Medicine, 6,* 5–14.

National Epilepsy League. (1958). Our schools and our children with epilepsy (80 pp. mimeo) Syracuse: National Epilepsy League. (Cited in *Summaries of Articles on Juvenile Epilepsy.* The Epilepsy Foundation, 1967.)

National Institute on Aging Task Force. (1980). Senility reconsidered: Treatment possibilities for mental impairment in the elderly. *Journal of the American Medical Association, 244,* 259–263.

Nuffield, E. J. (1961). Neurophysiology and behavior disorders in epileptic children. *Journal of Mental Science, 107,* 438–457.

O'Connor, W. A. (1969). *Patterns of interaction in families with high-adjusted, low-adjusted, and retarded members.* Unpublished doctoral dissertation (cited by Ritchie, 1981), University of Kansas.

Oddy, M., Humphrey, M., & Uttley, D. (1978a). Stress upon the relatives of head injured patients. *British Journal of Psychiatry, 133,* 507–513.

Oddy, M., Humphrey, M., & Uttley, D. (1978b). Subjective impairment and social recovery after closed head injury. *Journal of Neurology, Neurosurgery and Psychiatry, 41,* 611–616.

Panting, A., & Merry, P. H. (1972). The long-term rehabilitation of severe head injuries with particular reference to to the need for social and medical support for the patient's family. *Rehabilitation, 38,* 33–37.

Piers, E. V., & Harris, D. B. (1969). The Piers-Harris Children's Self-Concept Scale. Nashville, TN: Counselor Recordings and Tests.

Pomerleau, O. F. (1957). Behavioral medicine: The contribution of the experimental analysis of behavior to medical care. *American Psychologist, 34,* 654–663.

Pond, D. A. (1952). Psychiatric aspects of epilepsy in children. *Journal of Mental Science, 98,* 404–410.

Rabins, P. V., Mace, N. L., & Lucas, M. J. (1982). The impact of dementia on the family. *Journal of the American Medical Association, 248,* 333–335.

Reifler, B. V., Cox, G. B., & Hanley, R. J. (1981). Problems of mentally ill elderly as perceived by patients, families, and clinicians. *Gerontologist, 21,* 165–170.

Reis, J. (1977). Public acceptance of the disease concept of alcoholism. *Journal of Health and Social Behavior, 18,* 338–344.

Richardson, D. W. & Friedman, S. B. (1974). Psychosocial problems of the adolescent patient with epilepsy. *Clinical Pediatrics, 13,* 121–126.

Ritchie, K. (1981). Research note: Interaction in the families of epileptic children. *Journal of Child Psychology and Psychiatry, 22,* 65–71.

Robinson, R. G., & Szetela, B. (1981). Mood change following left hemispheric brain injury. *Annals of Neurology, 9,* 447–453.

Romano, M. D. (1974). Family response to traumatic head injury. *Scandinavian Journal of Rehabilitation Medicine, 6,* 1–4.

Romeis, J. C. (1980). The role of grandparents in adjustment to epilepsy. *Social Work in Health Care, 6,* 37–43.

Rose, S. W., Penry, J. K., Markush, L. A., Radloff, L. A., & Putnam, P. L. (1973). Prevalence of epilepsy in childhood. *Epilepsia, 14,* 133–152.

Rosenbaum, M., & Najenson, T. (1976). Changes in life patterns and symptoms of low mood as reported by wives of severely brain-injured soldiers. *Journal of Consulting and Clinical Psychology, 44,* 881–888.

Rutter, M., Graham, P., & Yule, W. (1980). *A neuropsychiatric study in childhood.* Philadelphia: Lippincott.

Safford, F. (1980). A program for families of the mentally impaired elderly. *The Geronologist, 20,* 656–660.

Sanford, J. R. A. (1975). Tolerance of disability in elderly dependents by supporters at home: Its significance for hospital practice. *British Medical Journal, 3,* 471–473.

Schwartz, G. E., & Weiss, S. M. (1977). *Proceedings of the Yale Conference on Behavioral Medicine.* DHEW Publication, NIH 78–1424.

Sherwin, I. (1982). Neurobiological basis of psychopathology associated with epilepsy. In H. Sands (Ed.), *Epilepsy: A handbook for the mental health professional.* New York: Brunner/ Mazel.

Skinner, B. F. (1983). Intellectual self-management in old age. *American Psychologist, 38,* 239– 244.

Stores, G. (1981). Problems of learning and behavior in children with epilepsy. In E. H. Reynolds & M. R. Trimble (Eds.), *Epilepsy and psychiatry,* Edinburgh: Churchill-Livingston.

Thomsen, I. V. (1974). The patient with severe head injury and his family. *Scandinavian Journal of Rehabilitation Medicine, 6,* 180–183.

Timming, R. C., Cayner, J. J., Grady, S., Grafman, J., Haskin, R., Malec, J., & Thornsen, C. (1980). Multidisciplinary rehabilitation in severe head trauma. *Wisconsin Medical Journal, 79,* 49–52.

Trunkey, D. D. Trauma. (1983). *Scientific American, 249,* 28–35.

Turk, D. C., & Kerns, R. D. (in press). Assessment in health psychology: A cognitive-behavioral perspective. In P. Karoly (Ed.), *Measurement Strategies in health psychology.* New York: John Wiley & Sons.

von Bertalanffy, L. (1968). *General systems theory.* New York: Braziller.

Weddell, R., Oddy, M., & Jenkins, D. (1980). Social adjustment after rehabilitation: a two-year follow-up of patients with severe head injury. *Psychological Medicine, 10,* 257–263.

Wells, C. E. (Ed.). (1977). *Dementia.* Philadelphia: Davis.

Whitman, S., Hermann, B. P., Black, R. B., & Chhabria, S. (1982). Psychopathology and seizure type in children with epilepsy. *Psychological Medicine, 12,* 843–853.

Williams, D. T. (1982). The treatment of seizures: Special psychotherapeutic and psychobiological techniques. In H. Sands (Ed.), *Epilepsy: A handbook for the mental health professional.* New York: Brunner/Mazel.

Wolf, S. M., Carr, A., Davis, D. C., Davidson, S., Dale, E. A., Forsythe, A., Goldenberg, E. D., Hanson, R., Lulejian, G. A., Nelson, M. A., Teitman, P., & Weinstein, A. (1977). The value of phenobarbital in the child who has had a single febrile seizure: A controlled prospective study. *Pediatrics, 59,* 378–385.

Zarit, S. H., Reever, K. E., & Bach-Peterson, J. (1980). Relatives of the elderly impaired: Correlates of feelings of burden. *The Geronotologist, 20,* 649–655.

Ziegler, R. G. (1981). Impairments of control and competence in epileptic children and their families. *Epilepsia, 22,* 339–346.

7

Family Factors in Children with Acute Illness

Barbara G. Melamed

Joseph Paul Bush

The stress of medical visits for the child, particularly hospital experiences, includes fear of separation from parents, fear of strangers, the distress of unfamiliar surroundings, anxiety about painful procedures, and the actual physical discomfort of medical intervention. Recovery from even an acute illness often includes loneliness, precipitated by isolation from peers and interruption of the daily school routine. The parent also faces anxiety-producing and disruptive influences. Parents must often cope with their uncertainty about outcome, try to mitigate the child's fears, pains, and discomforts, and juggle their own expectations, past experiences, and needs, as well as maintain their continuing familial, occupational, marital, and personal roles.

The focus of this chapter is to examine the influence of parenting on children's coping when faced with acute medical stress that involves illness, elective surgery, injury, or routine pediatric or dental visits. The existing theoretical and empirical literature in both child development and actual intervention studies are critically evaluated. Both investigations providing indirect data and those specifically designed to include the parent are evaluated in an attempt to parcel out the interactive effects of parent anxiety, presence or absence, health provider-initiated or parent-initiated preparation, and child-rearing practices. Important methodological issues are identified that affect the resulting conclusions, such as individual differences, coping styles, timing and context of preparation, measurement of parenting behaviors, defining anxiety in both children and adults, and hospital policies. An illustration of future research directions is provided by our own microanalysis of parent–child interactions during outpatient medical examinations.

HISTORICAL PERSPECTIVES

The fact that the course of an illness is influenced by psychological factors has long been established. In dealing with the mind–body problem, the early psychoanalysts generated much data, albeit primarily anecdotal, relating the state of the body to unconscious motivational factors contributing to psychic stress (e.g., Alexander, 1950; Graham, 1972). Because psychosomatic symptoms were often regarded as a response to life stress, one might expect that the patterns of illness and illness behavior would be somewhat different across families. However, instead of focusing on patterns of interaction between family members, the translation of this was to define personality types likely to develop psychosomatic illness. Although it was recognized that important "others" are involved in the reaction to the stressor, there was little emphasis on the actual inclusion of family members in the primary treatment of the patient. The nature of the studies generated from these hypotheses was largely retrospective, using adult patients already suffering from disorders. Moreover, the selection of the questions asked was often biased by the nature of the theoretical expectations. Because there is little that differentiates one "type" from another, for instance, the ulcer-prone personality is overly dependent, whereas the asthmatic is crying for unfulfilled affection from the mother, the studies did not specify which disorder predominates.

More recently, Minuchin, Rosman, and Baker (1978) became interested in family structure as it affects illness manifestations in members of "psychosomatic families." However, this model has been applied more to chronic than to acute illness.

Sociologists have looked at attitudes as they affect the health care patterns of individuals. There were relatively few studies dealing with social psychological factors affecting children's patterns of health behavior; however, many myths developed. With regard to children's adjustment to acute illness, it was almost lore that the children's patterns of illness behavior were influenced by child-rearing practices, family stress, role relationships, and family definitions of health resources. However, Mechanic (1964) in a study of 350 children and their mothers failed to find support for many of the basic assumptions regarding the influence of parents' attitudes and child-rearing practices on children's attentiveness to symptoms and patterns of illness behavior. The fact that these children were older than eight years of age still leaves open the question of the importance of the earlier interactions between parents and children during periods of acute illness at a time health care behavior and anxieties may be learned.

Despite much work by Bowlby (1969, 1973), Robertson (1958, 1976), and Spitz (1950) on the dramatic effects of maternal deprivation on children's early attachment behavior and the negative effects of prolonged hospitalization on children below the age of five, there was little consideration of the quality of parental factors in the study of patterns of children's adjustment to acute medical intervention. Subsequently, theorists have employed the concept of separation to explain the effects on children when functionally deprived of parenting, such as may occur in medical environments (Brown, 1979). In addition, ill children have been found to manifest increased regression and diminished capacity to tolerate separation (Nasera, 1978). The extensive theorizing by Spitz (1950) regarding separation anxiety and the development of fear of strangers was not uniformly supported by later investigators who reported that full-blown fear reactions were far from ubiquitous even toward the first year of life, and that reactions that were positive or affiliative were often observed (Scarr & Salaptek, 1970; Schaffer, 1966; Tennes & Lampl, 1964). Bretherton and Ainsworth (1974) analyzed the behavior of young children in stranger-approach situations and found that attachment inhibited distress, thus enabling the child to engage in other coping behaviors.

With the advent of behavioral technology in the 1960s, the influence of functional analysis began to demonstrate the actual cooccurrence of symptoms in children, with the presence of the parent mediating symptom expression (Neisworth & Moore, 1972). The development of observational recording devices further allowed the simultaneous and reliable recording of interactional data. Subsequently, the development of a research literature on effects of parents' behavior on children's behavior patterns quickly led to the development of numerous therapeutic interventions in both the school and the home to alter maladaptive behavior patterns (Patterson, 1982; Sulzer-Azaroff & Meyer, 1977).

Surprisingly, the importance of early medical and dental contacts as situations through which children learn to cope with the normal stressors associated with pain and frustration has been overlooked as an arena for evaluating parental influence on children's health behaviors and concerns.

Perhaps this has not been an accident. In our society, the physician in particular is seen as an omnipotent figure who cannot be openly questioned for fear of losing access to a primary source of help. The dentist has tended to see the parent as of little help except for the very youngest children who need to be held during treatment. In fact, current policies of excluding the parent may reflect their attitude that parents pose a potentially disruptive or threatening presence. Studies have failed to support the effectiveness of parent presence versus absence in the dental operatory. Some investigators have even demonstrated a worsening of children's behavior with mothers present (Shaw & Routh, 1982; Venham, Bengstom, & Cipes, 1978). Pediatricians, although more dependent upon mothers' observations of young children's behavior during the diagnostic phase of their work, have tended to underestimate the importance of the mother as a socializing agent. There has been supporting research (Mechanic, 1964) that mothers who perceive life as stressful or experience dissatisfaction in their family relationships not only report more personal illness but also appear to recognize more illness in their children. Therefore it would seem imperative for the pediatrician to pay attention not only to the symptoms presented by the child, but also to the other stressors that may have prompted the visit. The role of the parent in determining that a child needs medical treatment is critical but poorly understood.

It would appear that policy decisions are not always based on research findings, but often result from pressures of cost-effectiveness and political interests. There is a current trend in pediatric care to include the parent in preparing children for medical procedures. In Canada the law specifies guidelines that allow parents to visit their hospitalized children at any time and to become as involved in their care as they wish. "All children have the right to specialized Child Life workers, and patients and their families should be routinely prepared for elective surgeries, before treatment, at discharge, during or after emergency care, and in clinics" (*Pediatric Mental Health*, 1983). The advent of similar legislation has also been seen in the United States. Over 75% of pediatric hospitals reportedly provide psychological preparation for children (Peterson & Ridley-Johnson, 1980). A Massachusetts Department of Public Health regulation for the licensure of pediatric facilities requires that pediatric services allow parents of hospitalized children "constant parental support of and contact with the pediatric patient throughout hospitalization" [Public Health Regulation No. 105 CMR 130.720(I)]. According to a survey by a parent advocacy group, Children in Hospitals, only 16% of the 54 hospitals surveyed in 1973 permitted open visiting; the rest had restrictions. Although 42% had rooming in, this option was often restricted to parents of nursing babies and critically ill, dying, or handicapped children. In 1982, however, 100% of the 80 hospitals surveyed had 24-hour visiting and rooming in. In addition, over 20% permitted parents in the anesthesia room during induction, and 30% permitted parents in the recovery room.

Although this practice is consistent with the literature that was developing in the early 1950s regarding the importance of the child's relationship with his or her mother during the time of hospitalization, a lag of almost three decades occurred. Noteworthy too is the fact that research demonstrated that the presence of the parent does not necessarily always have the desired outcome. Parents who are uncomfortable and anxious about their child's welfare may not be effective in mitigating their child's fears, pains, and discomforts (e.g., emotional contagion hypothesis; Escalona, 1953). Thus the time is ripe for evaluating the actual interactions that occur during the medical contact for acute illness that may affect not only the immediate adjustment of the child and family to medical interventions, but is likely to influence their future health care utilization.

There has been little research on the effects of siblings on the acutely ill child. Several authors have commented, however, on the issues of parental neglect of siblings of the chronically ill child (Breslav, Weitzman, & Messenger, 1981) and on the possible emotional consequences on other family members of behavioral disturbances in children subsequent to hospitalization (Prugh, Staub, Sands, Kirschbaum, & Lenihan, 1953). The influence of sibling interactions with the acutely ill child on his or her adjustment and recovery appears to be an underinvestigated area that could yield valuable data relating to the development of family health care attitudes and "sick-role" behaviors.

The burgeoning of current research literature in behavior pediatrics (McGrath & Firestone, 1983; Routh & Wolraich, 1982; Russo & Varni, 1982) supports the entry of the behavioral scientist as an adjunct to the delivery of health care in pediatrics. The benefits of systematically exploring theoretical positions within this context are likely to enhance our understanding of families coping with stress. Research, then, can guide us both in identifying families at risk for emotional disturbances during health care and enable us to develop appropriate skills to teach parents to be more effective allies in promoting health.

In this chapter we will focus on reviewing the theoretical and research literature relevant to posing questions for advancing knowledge about family factors in acute illness. This does not imply that we are minimizing the importance of other influences on health care learning, such as peers, teachers, and the mass media, which are beyond the scope of this chapter. In addition, the patient–physician communication influences that are crucial to the issue of anxiety reduction and adjustment to illness require a more complete account.

CURRENT STATE OF KNOWLEDGE

A substantial proportion of children suffer mild to severe traumatic psychological consequences in connection with medical treatment (Davenport

& Werry, 1970; Melamed, Robbins, & Fernandez, 1982). Hospitalization of young children has been found to be associated with in-hospital behavior problems (Brain & Maclay, 1968; Prugh, Staub, Sands, Kirschbaum, & Lenihan, 1953) and postdischarge behavioral deterioration (Wolfer & Visintainer, 1975; Danilowicz & Gabriel, 1971), and long-term psychosocial sequelae (Quinton & Rutter, 1976; Douglas 1975). A recent survey by Peterson and Ridley-Johnson (1980) indicated that a majority of American pediatric hospitals now employ some type of presurgical psychological preparation program for children.

On the other hand, some children actually seem to benefit psychologically from the medical experience. Vernon, Foley, and Schulman (1967) reported improvements in children's behavior, as rated by their mothers, subsequent to hospitalization as compared with prehospitalization ratings in 25% of their sample. Medical procedures provide children with an opportunity to learn and practice appropriate behaviors for coping with fear-arousing stimuli (Burstein & Meichenbaum, 1979; Melamed, 1981; Melamed, Dearborn, & Hermecz, 1983). Consistent with this interpretation, it has been found (Wright & Alpern, 1971) that the quality of children's previous medical experience is more predictive of cooperative behavior during medical procedures than its quantity. Thus the learning that takes place in the child's early medical experiences may be adaptive as well as dysfunctional.

Current research trends in the psychological preparation of children for medical procedures are seeking optimal prescriptive matches between various preparatory interventions and individual child characteristics of importance (Melamed, 1981; Melamed, Robbins, & Fernandez, 1982). Younger children (from three to seven years of age) in particular have been found to be more at risk for negative consequences following medical procedures (Belmont, 1970; Shade-Zeldow, 1977; Brain & Maclay, 1968; Prugh et al., 1953; Sides, 1977). A related trend places increasing emphasis on the role of parents in determining children's handling of medical procedures (Wolfer & Visintainer, 1975). Concurrently, hospital practice is involving parents to an increasing extent in psychological aspects of their children's treatment (Roskies, Mongeon, & Gagnon-Lefebvre, 1978).

Unfortunately, the current state of knowledge has lagged behind, with sparse attention being paid to the collection of empirical data on critical aspects of the task of parenting the acutely ill child. Existing reserch has measured parents' responses to various questionnaires, parental anxiety in the medical setting, and parental presence versus absence as variables relating to children's adjustment to medical and dental procedures. However, the content of the parents' interactions with the child has been neglected, despite the theoretical importance of its impact on children's behavior. An extensive review of the research literature with respect to dental and medical settings has found few studies utilizing direct observation of parent behaviors.

Preparatory Intervention Programs: Focus on the Child

Much of the existing data relating to the issue of parenting acutely ill children are derived from research studies that evaluate procedures preparing children for medical or dental treatments. Studies often include a treatment group and one or more control groups in which the elements of an intervention program are successively eliminated in order to identify the effective component. Manipulated components have included level of parental involvement, information provision, and provision of supportive relationships/interactions with caregiving personnel. This research will be reviewed, focusing first on information provision and then looking at modeling, coping skills training, systematic desensitization, and preparatory play. Although this portion of the review is organized by technique, the reader's attention is directed to the influences of information and support as well as of parental involvement. Whatever the primary modality of any particular preparatory program may be, it is unrealistic to consider any element in isolation. The importance of individual child characteristics mediating the effects of preparatory programs will next be explicitly considered, followed by a review of studies focusing on parental involvement in preparing children for medical procedures. Theoretical models for understanding parent influences on children's adjustment to stressful medical situations will then be evaluated and pertinent research reviewed, including the factors of parental presence, anxiety, preparatory efforts, and child-rearing practices. Methodological issues raised by these studies will be discussed. Finally, we will share our own systematic approach to research on actual parenting during outpatient clinic visits.

Information Provision and Modeling.   Programs based upon providing information to the child patient are reviewed in several sources (e.g., Melamed & Siegel, 1980; Kendall & Watson, 1981). Clough (1979) argues that information provision serves the dual function of supplying reassurance through the fostering of a trusting relationship between the child and the informing agent as well as reducing the child's anxiety by decreasing uncertainty about what is going to happen and thereby checking the child's tendency toward negative distortions and fantasies (Becker, 1972). Thus, although the research literature is generally favorable as to the effects of information provision (Kendall, 1982), it is indeed difficult to isolate those effects attributable to information alone.

In a study attempting to quantify how hospital-relevant information influences cooperation, four- to 17-year-old children hospitalized for elective surgery were evaluated (Melamed, Dearborn, & Hermecz, 1983). The study found that the subjects who scored higher on a hospital information test, regardless of whether they had previously been shown a hospital information film, were rated by their mothers four weeks after surgery as having adjusted better to the hospital experience and as manifesting fewer posthospitalization behavior problems than lower-scoring subjects. It was also found that children over eight years of age and those with previous surgery experience retained significantly more hospital information after viewing the hospital-relevant film than if they had seen an unrelated control film. Younger children (four to eight years of age) and children without previous experience did not get a significantly higher percent of the hospital–knowledge test questions correct after seeing the hospital-relevant film. In fact, children who were under eight and had previous surgery experience were shown to be initially more upset behaviorally, and they reported an increase in medical concerns after viewing a hospital-relevant slide tape than those shown a distracting film. Knowledge by itself can perhaps have a detrimental effect.

The supportive context in which information is imparted may be critical. Fernald and Corry (1981) found that empathic preparation was superior to directive information in preparing three- to nine-year olds to have blood drawn.

The use of peer models may provide one example of the supportive context for preparation. However, presurgical preparation programs using modeling, typically with filmed or videotaped models, have also been found to be differentially effective according to children's individual characteristics. Melamed and Siegel (1975) found more favorable postoperative recovery indices (amount of pain medication, cooperativeness ratings, etc.) in children who had been shown a peer-modeling film than in those who had not. The authors attempted to replicate this finding (Melamed & Siegel, 1980) with children having their second surgery. The Palmar Sweating Index measures suggested that some experienced children's autonomic arousal levels were too high to allow them to benefi from the preparation.

Kendall and Watson (1981), reviewing the resea :h literature, concluded that filmed modeling has been the most successful preparatory program for young children. However, not all modeling films are identical, and several authors have found the coping-mastery distinction to be important. Kendall (1982) reviewed research showing that the coping model, who demonstrates fear and stress at the outset and then achieves successful coping, is generally more effective than the mastery model, who demonstrates successful coping only. Klorman, Hilpert, Michael, LaGana, and Sveen (1980), observing children's cooperativeness during dental procedures, found significantly better effects using a coping rather than a mastery model. They found, however, that once children had previous dental experience, exposure to models was not as important because there was already a low level of disruptiveness. Children with previous experience who are afraid need to practice what to do to control their fears. Klingman, Melamed, Cuthbert, and Hermecz (1984) compared children who viewed a modeling film showing coping skills prior to dental treatment with children who saw the same film but were encouraged to practice the modeled skills during the film. Children receiving "active participant modeling" were found to have acquired more information relevant to dental treatment, showed decreased anxiety and disruptiveness during treatment, and reported using the coping skills more during treatment than did the nonparticipant group. Children who had reported higher self-mastery showed more benefit from the practice condition. Thus practice in skills needs to be assessed both in terms of what the situation demands and what capacities the child has.

Coping Skills Training. Preparing children for medical procedures by means of coping skills training has taken numerous forms. In a study, Kendall and Watson (1981) conclude that coping training has thus far been more clearly shown to have an effect on postsurgical recovery than on presurgical anxiety and subjective distress. In an earlier study of adults undergoing cardiac catheterization (Kendall et al., 1979), it was found that patients who received coping training showed better adjustment to the procedure, less anxiety, and reported fewer negative self-statements than subjects prepared with information only. The latter subjects in turn were rated more favorably on these indices than an unprepared control group.

These authors argued that timeliness and repeated preparatory contact with the stressing stimuli were the critical elements in their intervention, and that it would be important to take into consideration the patient's own preferred coping style before attempting to train the patient in a coping technique. A similar conclusion regarding the importance of matching coping training with individual styles was reached by Pickett and Clum (in press) after reviewing research on coping training for pain tolerance and individual differences in responses to psychotherapeutic approaches. The work on children needs to assess the actual repertoire of the children's coping skills and rely more heavily on the use of parents and peers to teach these skills. There is very little research on children's individual coping styles.

Systematic Desensitization. Systematic desensitization has also been used to prepare children for dental treatment, and has been found to be as effective as filmed modeling for reducing disruptiveness in this setting (Machen & Johnson, 1974). Using a similar population, Sawtell, Simon, and Simeonsson (1974) found that children going to the dentist for the first time and who were highly aroused prior to dental procedures were equally prepared by modeling and systematic desensitization. However, they also found that interaction with a friendly receptionist was as beneficial as these behavioral procedures. Thus the effects may be due to exposure to feared stimuli within a supportive context. Relaxation training alone, without the anxiety hierarchy, has also shown some effectiveness with children (Kendall & Watson, 1981).

Preparatory Play.   Exposure to hospital-related toys prior to contact with the actual stressing situation has been investigated under the assumption (Janis, 1958) that children who accomplish the "work of worrying" will adjust better to hospitalization (Burstein & Meichenbaum, 1979). Children who did in fact play with the stress-related toys prior to hospitalization reported lower anxiety levels subsequent to hospitalization. However, not all children chose to play. Children high in defensiveness scores avoided playing with stress-relevant toys. High-defensive children also had more posthospital anxiety. Their results, although correlational, shed some light on characteristics of children who apparently do cope well with hospitalization, and raise the question of whether other children who are presumably less likely to spontaneously engage in preparatory play might be profitably induced to do so. In fact, the refusal to play with dental toys in the play area of a clinic discriminated those children who had previously behaved negatively during restorative treatment from those who were very cooperative (McTigue & Pinkham, 1978).

Importance of Individual Child Characteristics

Preparatory intervention programs are not uniformly beneficial for all children. Current research efforts are beginning to build a data base upon which to make optimal prescriptive matches between particular types of children and specific preparatory techniques. Becker (1972) warns that presurgical preparation is not inevitably benign, and may in fact break down adaptive defenses in children. Knight, Atkins, Eagle, Evans, Finkelstein, Fukushima, Katz, and Weiner (1979) found that children who used certain types of defenses, such as intellectualization, and had flexible defenses coped more successfully than children who used denial, displacement, or projection in a rigid defense structure when told about impending medical procedures. This suggests that careful attention be paid to the way a child copes with information in the environment before he or she is given "threatening" information. Unger (1982) found that children high in defensiveness tend not to retain as much information from film modeling prior to impending dental injections. However, the children high in denial tended to be younger in age and lower in intellectual capability. Those defensive children who received information from a model expressing affective concern were actually more disruptive during dental treatment.

Furthermore, age is an important consideration for both the type and the appropriate timing of preparation. Melamed, Meyer, Gee, and Soule (1976) found that children younger than seven shown a modeling film one week prior to hospitalization were sensitized by this exposure and emitted more disruptive behaviors postoperatively than those viewing the film at the time of hospital admission. Melamed, Dearborn, and Hermecz (1983) found that whereas slide-tape hospital information preparation was beneficial for most children hospitalized for elective surgery, children under eight years of age who had previous surgery experience were actually sensitized by exposure to the preparatory film relative to a control group. Clearly, the importance of systematically examining individual child characteristics in determining the if, when, and how of presurgical intervention has been amply demonstrated. Surprisingly, there were few studies in the literature that have looked at developmental trends.

In a cross-sectional study of 48 children from six to 60 months of age observed during routine outpatient medical visits, Hyson (1983) examined developmental trends in emotional responses and coping mechanisms before, during, and after examination. Negative emotional responses were found to decrease in frequency with age and to be greater during the examination than before or after. Information seeking was the most commonly observed coping behavior, particularly during the preexamination period, whereas autonomy seeking was found to increase during and after the exam. Older children engaged in less autonomy seeking during the exam, which was generally more instrumental before the exam, and expressive (e.g., crying, verbal protesting) during the exam. The ratio of instrumental to expressive autonomy seeking was also found to increase with age. Younger children were more threatened by concrete (e.g., actual touch with instruments) events and older children by symbolic (e.g., verbal) events. Thus with increasing age, fear responses and coping behaviors were found to be more realistic and more anticipatory and goal directed. These results provide evidence for the importance of providing developmentally appropriate assistance to children in coping with stressful medical events.

These results are not surprising, in view of research on children's developing concepts of illness (Melamed, Robbins, & Fernandez, 1982). Wright (1982) found increasingly sophisticated concepts of illness with increasing age in children over six years old. Specifically, it has been shown that older children retain more information (Perlmutter & Myers, 1976; Melamed, Dearborn, & Hermecz, 1983) and have a more realistic grasp of illness causation (Nagy, 1951).

Preparatory Programs: Focus on the Parent

Research has also been conducted on the impact of parent-focused preparatory intervention programs for children about to undergo medical or dental procedures. Mahaffey (1965) provided mothers of two- to ten-year-old children hospitalized for tonsillectomy or adenoidectomy with extensive attention, information, and support, whereas control group children and their mothers underwent standard hospital procedures. Experimental group children showed greater ease of fluid intake, less crying and calls for help, earlier voiding, less emesis, less fever, and less worrisome behavior postoperatively than control group children. Because children were also present during the preparatory periods, this study leaves unanswered questions as to what it was that mothers did if anything that was differentially associated with the children's postoperative recovery, as well as to what extent results were attributable to direct effects of experimental nursing on the children. These studies suggest the efficacy of preprocedure support and information as ways of reducing the mother's anxiety when her child is to undergo dental or other medical treatment. They do not, however, uniformly establish that reductions in maternal anxiety lead to reductions in children's anxiety nor to other desirable changes in the child's medical experience.

An experiment conducted by Skipper, Leonard, and Rhymes (1968) also explored the effects of nurses' interactions and information provision to mothers on children's hospital adjustment. Mothers of children hospitalized for tonsillectomy were given preparatory information by nurses who were instructed to avoid paying any more attention to these children than was received by those in the control group. As predicted, mothers receiving "supportive information" reported less stress, and their children received more favorable ratings on several postoperative indices (both behavioral and somatic) than control group subjects. The authors inferred that the intervention allowed mothers to more effectively assist their children in coping with the stress of hospitalization. They did not, however, document any differences between the behavior of experimental and control group mothers to clarify this inference.

Using a more temporally extended model of medical treatment, Wolfer and Visintainer (1975) identified five "stresspoints" in hospitalization: admission, blood test, preoperative medication, transport to the operating room, and return from the recovery room. Nurses provided child–parent units with information and reassurance just prior to each stresspoint. Children and parents were also encouraged to ask questions and to rehearse behavioral prescriptions provided for coping at stresspoints. Children receiving stresspoint nursing care were rated as more cooperative and less upset during the stresspoint procedures, as well as showing more favorable postoperative indices, than control group children. Similarly, parents in the stresspoint nursing group self-reported less anxiety than control group parents. The authors later replicated these findings (Visintainer & Wolfer, 1975), with the addition of a relationship/supportive care control group, in which a nurse spent as much time with the mother-child dyad as in the experimental group, but did not provide stresspoint preparation. A second experimental group was also added, in which stresspoint preparation was provided in a single initial session rather than just before each stresspoint. Children in both experimental groups received more favorable upset, cooperativeness, and postoperative ease of fluid intake ratings than those in either control group. Parents in the stresspoint preparation group reported less anxiety, more satisfaction with care, and feeling better informed than those in the single-session preparation or in the control groups.

Pinkham and Fields (1976) provided mothers of 3- to 5-year-old children with visits to the dentist's reception room 1 week prior to the child's treatment. In addition, some of the children were shown a modeling videotape which mothers were told had been found to improve children's behavior in the operatory. A control group received no pretreatment preparation. Only those mothers in the visit-plus-positively-suggested-videotape group reported significantly lower Taylor Manifest Anxiety scores at the time of the child's appointment. This difference was not accompanied, however, by any significant differences in observer ratings of children's cooperativeness during treatment. Similar results were obtained by Wright, Alpern, and Leake (1973), who found reduced self-reported anxiety scores in mothers sent a supportive letter prior to their 3- to 6-year-old children's dental visits without obtaining any effect on children's cooperativeness in the operatory.

More recently, in the area of surgery preparation, researchers have been increasingly explicit in defining the behaviors parents have been taught and instructed to use in their preparation of children before and during hospitalization. For example, a variety of preparatory procedures presented conjointly to hospitalized children and their parents was also the experimental variable in an important study by Peterson and Shigetomi (1981). Two- to ten-year-old children and their parents were provided either with information alone, coping skills training (deep muscle relaxation, distracting mental imagery, comforting self-talk), filmed modeling, or the coping skills and modeling film treatments combined. Children in both coping skills training groups were rated by both their parents and by observers as superior on a combination of measures of anxiety and cooperativeness. The most consistent effects on parents' self-ratings showed coping groups parents to be more confident and less anxious than the information and modeling groups. The authors suggested that the coping groups' preparation involved procedures that involved the parent to a greater degree in influencing the child's response to stress, for example, by cueing and guiding the child's use of the coping techniques.

In a replication of this study, Peterson, Schultheis, Ridley-Johnson, Miller, and Tracy (1984) found that children in the parent–child groups receiving modeling were rated calmer and more cooperative before and during surgery than those receiving routine preparation by the hospital staff. These findings suggested that the formal presentation of information to both the parent and the child by using a coping model who demonstrates adaptive behavior was much more important to the successful preparation of children than either the similarity of the model to the child, the actual medical setting, or the order in which the medical procedures were shown. In addition, the cost effectiveness of using a modeling procedure was demonstrated in a comparative analysis in which the addition of modeling and coping skills led to fewer maladaptive behaviors than a hospital tour alone (Peterson, Ridley-Johnson, Tracy, & Mullins, in press).

Peterson et al. (in press) and Zastowney, Kirschenbaum, & Meng (in press) extended the findings of Peterson and Shigetomi (1981) by manipulating parents' activity more explicitly in terms of the parents' role in helping their children cope. Six- to ten-year-old children hospitalized for elective surgery were included in one of three treatment groups. In the control group, parents and children viewed a coping model videotape two weeks before admission. Anxiety reduction group subjects also viewed the modeling videotape in the same context, and parents were then trained in relaxation. Finally, subjects in the coping skills group also saw the modeling tape. These parents were then given a rationale and training in the use of deep breathing and physical relaxation, and viewed a videotape that modeled parental use of these techniques to facilitate a child's coping at hospitalization stresspoints. They were then given a booklet to help them structure and individualize their use of these techniques with their own children. Children in the coping skills group were rated by parents as behaving less problematically at home both during the preadmission week and during the second postdischarge week, and these parents rated themselves as less stressed during the prehospitalization period than the control group. Coping skills children were also rated by observers as engaging in fewer maladaptive behaviors than control group children during six hospital stresspoints. Although providing some of the strongest evidence currently available that preparatory interventions can differentially increase parental enhancement of children's positive coping with medical stress, this study does not specifically assess whether the actual use of parental behaviors taught was related to children's coping.

To summarize, the effects of pretreatment preparatory intervention programs have been found to vary according to several factors. Research results have been highly consistent in showing such programs to be more effective with older (usually over seven years) than with younger (usually two to seven years) children (Brain & Maclay, 1968; Melamed, Robbins, & Fernandez, 1982; Prugh et al., 1953; Siegel & Peterson, 1980; Vernon, Foley, & Schulman, 1967). Other patient characteristics have also been found to be of significance, including cognitive style variables (Kendall, 1982; Kendall & Watson, 1981; Wilson, 1981); prior experience with medical procedures (Klorman et al., 1980; Melamed et al., 1983; Melamed & Siegel, 1980); the child's fear or anxiety level (Klorman et al., 1980; Melamed, 1981; Melamed, Robbins, & Fernandez, 1982; Burstein & Meichenbaum, 1979; Wilson, 1981); locus of control (Auerbach, Kendall, Cuttler, & Levitt, 1976; Kendall & Watson, 1981; Pickett & Clum, 1982); arousal (Faust & Melamed, 1984; Sawtell et al., 1974); intelligence (Melamed, 1981); coping style (Melamed, Robbins, & Fernandez, 1982; Siegel, 1981; Wilson, 1981); and defensiveness (Burstein & Meichenbaum, 1979; Knight et al., 1979; Unger, 1982).

Parental factors have also been shown to enhance the effectiveness of preparatory intervention programs. Programs focusing on the parent–

child unit have been shown to be effective (Wolfer & Visintainer, 1975; Skipper, Leonard & Rhymes, 1968; Mahaffey, 1965; Peterson & Shigetomi, 1981; Zastowney et al., in press), but have not pinpointed the parental behaviors of importance. The next section will identify theoretically meaningful predictions regarding the content of these critical parent–child interactions.

Theoretical Importance of Parent Influences on Children's Adjustment

Models accounting for parental influences on children's coping with stressful medical situations include the emotional contagion and crisis-parenting hypotheses. The emotional contagion hypothesis (Escalona, 1953; Visintainer & Wolfer, 1975; Heffernan & Azarnoff, 1971; Vernon et al., 1967; Skipper et al., 1968; Robinson, 1968) states that parental anxiety is communicated to the child by nonverbal as well as verbal means, and that this in turn increases the child's anxiety level. The hypothesis is nonspecific as to exactly how and why parental anxiety elicits child anxiety, as well as with respect to possible interacting variables such as situation, but as a general model the hypothesis enjoys empirical support in studies correlating parental and child state anxiety in medical situations (Bailey, Talbot, & Taylor, 1973; Sides, 1977).

A second model to account for parents' effects on children's handling of stressful medical procedures might be called the "crisis-parenting hypothesis." This model emphasizes the increased importance of parenting when children face stressors (Kaplan, Smith, Grobstein, & Fischman, 1973). Support for this model was obtained by Vernon et al. (1967) in their study of two- to six-year-old children hospitalized for elective surgery. They compared the effect of maternal presence on children's behavior during a relatively nonstressful hospital procedure (admission) to a more highly stressful procedure (anesthesia induction). During the less stressful procedure the children evidenced little upset, and maternal presence or absence had no significant effect. During the highly stressful procedure, however, maternal presence was negatively related to children's distress levels. High parental anxiety at such times is thought to lead to impaired parental functioning (Skipper et al., 1968; Duffy, 1972), and consequently to less adequate parental support for the child's coping efforts. Supportive of this hypothesis, Robinson (1968) found that more fearful mothers of hospitalized children were likely to spend less time visiting, entered less frequently into conversations with the child's surgeon, and were less likely to complain about or criticize aspects of their children's hospitalizations.

Parental Anxiety.   Relevant to both models, the generality of this problem is evidenced by studies that have shown that parents of hospitalized children often experience considerable anxiety. Gofman, Buckman, and

Schade (1957) interviewed 100 parents at the time of their children's admission to the hospital. They report that all of the parents described themselves as anxious, with 57 of them calling it overwhelming. They describe over half of the parents as having been plainly upset and unable to provide adequate support to the child during his or her time of stress. Similar results were obtained by Skipper et al. (1968) using a self-report measure of maternal anxiety before, during, and after the child's surgery.

The emotional contagion hypothesis differs the most critically from the crisis-parenting model in that the latter places greater emphasis on the importance of parenting behaviors, whereas the former is nonspecific with regard to this. The models are compatible to the extent that parental anxiety is positively correlated with disruption of parenting competence, and (by extension) to the degree that parental calmness is positively correlated with effective parenting in the medical situation.

It has been widely assumed (Becker, 1972; Mellish, 1969; Glaser, 1960; Belmont, 1970) that parental anxiety has a negative effect on the child's adjustment to medical procedures. Correlational studies have been generally supportive, although not unanimously, of this assumption.

Johnson and Baldwin (1969), looking at three- to seven-year-old children undergoing dental extractions, found a significant negative relationship between mothers' scores on the Taylor Manifest Anxiety Scale and observer ratings of children's cooperativeness during treatment. These results were replicated by Wright and Alpern (1971) with three- to four-year-olds, and by Wright, Alpern, & Leake (1973) using three- to six-year-olds. These authors also found this relationship to be stronger in preschool than in older children.

Children's Manifest Anxiety Scale scores were found by Bailey, Talbot, and Taylor (1973) to correlate positively with mothers' Taylor Manifest Anxiety Scale scores, when the children were taken to a dental clinic, for nine- and ten- but not for eleven- and twelve-year-olds. These correlations were also higher among children who were experiencing their first visit to the dentist. Similarly, Koenigsburg and Johnson (1972) found a positive association between maternal and child anxiety levels during the child's first dental visit. Hawley, McCorkel, Wittemann, and Van Ostenberg (1974) also found a direct relationship between mothers' anxiety and children's uncooperative behavior in the dental operatory. Brown (1979) found that highly anxious mothers were more likely to have children who showed distress and withdrawal during a short hospital stay. On the other hand, several studies have failed to show an association between maternal anxiety and children's noncooperative behavior during dental treatment (Klorman, Ratner, King, & Sveen, 1977, 1978; Pinkham & Fields, 1976).

Parental Presence. To the extent that parental anxiety is not positively correlated with children's fear and noncooperativeness during medical procedures, the crisis-parenting hypothesis may account for much of this variance in terms of parental competence in coping with the fearful child in the setting. It is not surprising, according to either model, that studies of the effect of parental absence or presence that do not take into account parental anxiety or parenting behaviors have at times failed to show main effects (Allen & Evans, 1968; Venham, 1979).

In one of the earliest experimental studies examining young children's anxiety, when parents were asked to wait outside the dental operatory, it was demonstrated that considerable crying and negative behavior occurred in three- to four-year-olds during the first dental visit (Frankl, Shiere, & Fogels, 1962). Because these youngsters are most presumably vulnerable to separation anxiety, it is difficult to interpret this as protest behavior or anxiety about the actual medical procedures.

Supporting the notion that parental influences are enhanced during stressful procedures, Vernon et al. (1967) found that maternal presence showed a significantly more pacifying effect during highly stressful than during slightly stressful hospital procedures.

Ziegler and King (1980), evaluating the effects of a foster grandparent program for hospitalized 6-month to five-year-olds, observed significantly more tranquil, happy, and responsive behavior in parented children (whether by their own parent or a foster grandparent) only while the parenting figure was actually present. While unattended by a parenting figure, the behavior of the children in all three groups did not differ significantly in terms of observed tranquility, happiness, or responsivity.

Shaw and Routh (1982), however, found the opposite results. They systematically compared parent presence or absence in studying groups of children across two age groups (18 months and five years) during well-child examinations. They randomly assigned mothers to be present or absent during parts of the physical examination involving immunizations. Mothers remained in the room initially, and in the mother-absent-group children were held by the rater at points where mothers were asked to assist. The behavioral observations revealed a greater degree of crying in the younger group of children whose mothers were excluded. However, during the actual injections, those children in the mother-present group received the most negative ratings. Older children, with parents present, also showed negative behavior and fussed more during the tetanus injection and tuberculin tine test. They concluded that although protest may occur with separation, the presence of the mother serves to disinhibit or reinforce the overt expression of anxiety.

In another study of four- to six-year-old versus seven- to ten-year-old children receiving venipunctures, similar findings were reported (Gross, Stern, Levin, Dale, & Wojnilower, 1983). The presence of the mothers in both age groups immediately prior to the initiation of the blood test resulted in more frequent crying than when the mothers remained in the waiting room. However, this effect was not significant at other points. The younger group of children exhibited more aggression, resistance, and crying regardless of whether the mothers were present or absent. The investigators interpret the data as providing evidence that a mother serves as a discriminative cue for crying behavior and suggest that if she is instructed in a specific set of comforting procedures, the reduction of crying may be accomplished.

Venham and his colleagues (1978) published one of the only studies in which the actual parenting behaviors during children's dental appointments were studied. Parents were given a choice as to whether or not they wished to accompany their children in the operatory. No main differences were found in how well children adjusted during the procedures between groups whose parents were or were not present. They found that the quality of the interaction between child and mother varied with the intensity of the child's response during treatment and that parents demonstrated a variety of operatory behaviors including ignoring, coercing, reassuring, and instructing their children.

In a study with preschool children (aged one to five) having outpatient surgery (Hannallah & Rosales, 1983), it was found that when mothers or fathers elected to stay with their children during the induction of anesthesia, there was a significant decrease in the number of very upset or turbulent children in this group relative to a group unaccompanied by their parent. Thus the relationship between parents electing to stay may indicate something about their relationship.

Studies of the significance of parental presence frequently suffer from a potentially significant confound, as pointed out by Prugh et al. (1953). These authors found that parents who visited their hospitalized children less fequently were more likely than frequently visiting parents to have nonsatisfactory relationships with these children. Several authors (Dimock, 1960; Gofman, Buckman, & Schade, 1957; Prugh et al., 1953) have contended that the quality of this relationship is a crucial variable influencing the child's hospital adjustment. In fact, there are data (Brown, 1979) that demonstrate that a child's response to hospitalization varies with the child's ongoing relationship to the family at home, as well as what the mother actually does during the hospital stay. It was found that three- to six-year-old children who had close proximity to their families at home were most likely to withdraw and show distress during a short stay in the hospital. Mothers who were themselves anxious and accepted hospital authority had children who were distressed and withdrawn.

Couture (1976) attempted to control for this variable by randomly assigning parents of three- to six-year-old hospitalized children to a limited visiting, unlimited visiting, or rooming-in conditions. Although his prediction that parental presence would be more significant for younger children was not supported, he did find a main effect for these conditions. Significantly less problematic behavior was observed in children of parents who roomed in. This replicated an earlier finding (Brain & Maclay, 1968), who found better in-hospital and posthospitalization adjustment in young children whose mothers roomed in.

These results, then, indicate that parental presence may be helpful to children in medical situations (e.g., Frankl et al., 1962), but that any benefits may be limited to times of high stress when the parent is actually with the child. The overall unclarity of the results of studies of parent presence, particularly in conjunction with previously reported findings regarding the correlates of parental anxiety levels, suggests the need for further investigation into differential effects associated with differences in how the parent interacts with the ill child. The age of the child and developmental differences in competence must also be considered.

Parent-Initiated Efforts to Prepare Children. Research has generally supported the commonsense assumption that a child's illness and/or hospitalization is stressful to parents (Mahaffey, 1965; Skipper, et al., 1968; Mechanic, 1964; Gofman et al., 1957; Prugh et al., 1953). Researchers found that many parents attempt to cope with this stress by providing psychological preparation for medical procedures to their children themselves, independently of professional involvement. Forty-seven out of 100 parents of hospitalized children interviewed by Gofman et al. (1957) reported attempting to do this. Bailey, Talbot, and Taylor (1973) found that children whose mothers reported providing them with preparatory information and trying to reduce the children's fears received higher observer ratings of cooperativeness during dental treatment than those whose parents did not report attempting such preparation.

Similar results were found by Heffernan and Azarnoff (1971) with a sample of children receiving outpatient medical examinations if the child had initiated the preprocedural discussion with the mother. The authors propose a desensitization paradigm to account for this finding, arguing that preprocedural information constitutes a form of exposure to the feared stimulus situation, and that the child's initiation of information seeking indicates a readiness to handle this degree of exposure.

Child-Rearing Variables. The task facing parents in helping their children cope with stressful medical procedures is apparently more complex than simply being present or providing the child with information about what to expect. In addition to coping with his or her own anxiety, the parent must respond to the individual child's needs. Several researchers have accordingly looked at child-rearing variables in an attempt to explore the relationship of parental behaviors toward the child in other stressful situations with the child's coping in the medical situation. Levy (1959) tested the hypothesis that parents' previous training of the child in how to respond in stress situations would predict the child's adjustment to hospitalization. Results failed to support this hypothesis, but a significant relationship was found between observer ratings of hospitalized children's behavior at several stresspoints and parents' prior provision of stress-response training specific to hospitalization. A low but significant positive correlation was obtained between parents' provision of general training and of hospital-specific stress-response training. Studies have also suggested that parents' child-rearing behaviors may be related to children's attitudes toward illness, medical practitioners, and the sick role (Mechanic, 1964). Support for this hypothesis is apparent in research findings associating parent and child attitudes toward dental treatment (Forgione & Clark, 1974; Johnson & Baldwin, 1969; Venham, Murray, & Gaulin-Kremer, 1979; Skipper et al., 1968; Wright, Alpern, & Leake, 1973), or child anxiety during medical examination with mother's self-report of anxiety when she undergoes such examination (Heffernan & Azarnoff, 1971).

Venham et al. (1979) found significant associations between observational and physiological measures between the parents' and three- to five-year-old children's anxiety during dental treatment and observational and self-report measures of home child-rearing practices. In general, children who were more anxious during treatment had parents who tended to avoid the use of reward and punishment, whereas low child anxiety during treatment was related to maternal responsivity and the organization of the home environment. The authors conclude that children's ability to tolerate a stressful dental treatment situation was related to socialization practices and with parents' noninterference with the child's daily stresses. These findings suggest that the learning of appropriate behaviors as well as how to cope with potentially fear-arousing stimuli are involved in determining the children's adjustment to medical procedures.

Several other studies have focused on relationships between parental discipline and other parenting behaviors during children's stress experiences with children's behavior during medical procedures, but findings were inconsistent. Shade-Zeldow (1977) failed to find a significant correlation between parent scores on measures of dependency-fostering behaviors and attitudes with nurses' ratings of the in-hospital behavior of three- to 15-year-olds.

Zabin and Melamed (1980) mailed the Child Development Questionnaire, a self-report measure of disciplinary steps used in connection with children's approach to fearful situations, to parents of four- to 12-year-old children within one year of their children's hospitalization for elective surgery. Previously acquired self-report, observational, and physiological measures of children's in-hospital anxiety showed significant correlations with several disciplinary categories. Use of punishment by the father was found to be associated with high self-reported state of anxiety in the hospitalized children. High preoperative anxiety was observed in children whose parents reported using disciplinary approaches scored as reinforcing of dependency. On the other hand, lower pre- and postoperative anxiety was found in children whose parents used more modeling. Although the Child Development Questionnaire has not been validated in terms of correspondence between self-report and actual parental disciplinary behaviors, these findings are consistent with the other studies discussed above and suggest a relationship between parenting variables and children's handling of stressful medical situations.

Heffernan and Azarnoff (1971) looked at mothers' self-reported attitudes toward their children's expressing fear along with children's self-reported anxiety about an imminent medical examination. They found a significant interaction between a child's previous anxiety about such examinations (as rated retrospectively by the mother) and the mother's suppressiveness of the child's crying when frightened. Among children rated by their mothers as previously nonfearful, children with suppressive mothers reported high anxiety, whereas children with nonsuppressive mothers reported low anxiety about the impending examination. In addition, a main effect for maternal suppressiveness was significant, with children of suppressive mothers reporting greater anticipatory anxiety regardless of maternally reported anxiety on previous clinic visits.

Summary

Research has shown that pediatric medical intervention often results in negative psychosocial sequelae and that children's contacts with medical practitioners are frequently highly stressful for themselves as well as their parents. On the other hand, such experiences provide an opportunity for beneficial learning in terms of the development of positive health care attitudes and abilities to cope with stressful situations. Current health care trends reflect these research findings in emphasizing the importance of psychologically preparing young children for medical intervention. Increasingly, such preparatory programs are including a role for the child's parents.

Research on parents' influence on children's adjustment to medical procedures has implicated the importance of child-rearing styles, parent-initiated preparation, parental anxiety, and interventions to reduce this anxiety and to train situation-specific parenting skills have been evaluated. However, there is a lack of empirical data relating what parents actually do with their children in medical situations and how this influences their children's adjustment.

Models for conceptualizing parent influences include the emotional contagion hypothesis, which states that parents communicate their anxiety to their children primarily by nonverbal means, and the crisis-parenting hypothesis, which states that although parenting becomes critical during crisis situations, parental anxiety at such times may have a disorganizing influence on effective parenting behaviors.

RESEARCH AND METHODOLOGICAL ISSUES

The critical literature reviews in the area of parental involvement in preparing children for medical intervention have revealed an interesting paradox. There has long been recognition that parental factors can positively influence or exacerbate children's stress responses. This information has come largely from anecdotal reports of large field studies. However, the result of this recognition has been largely ignored by the medical community, who prefer not to add to the complexity of their medical goals by including the parents in the process. The psychologists who have become involved have largely ignored the developmental literature and have instituted large-scale intervention studies to demonstrate the effectiveness of various procedures, such as stresspoint preparation and using parents to cue the children's use of coping techniques. There have been several studies in which parent presence or absence has been related to the child's anxiety as if the nature of this interaction were insignificant. The intention of our review was to remind the psychologists that we do have a data base from which to construct interventions that may be age appropriate, and to specify what new baseline information may be useful in identifying family patterns of interaction that may lead to problematic behaviors with respect to health care.

Neglect of Individual Differences

The studies we have reviewed have suggested that individual factors, including intellectual and developmental factors, previous experiences with medical stressors, and the nature of the parent–child interaction, must all be considered in determining if children should be prepared and if parental involvement facilitates or impairs adjustment.

The age of the children will also have an influence on how important the parent can be in modifying the children's behavior. As children grow older, they develop a more diverse repertoire of coping behaviors. They have had experience in many other situations that may have led them to expect more pain and discomfort than a younger child. The peer group may have a more important influence upon the expression of their fears than parents' presence has. Behaviors such as attachment may have different implications regarding adaptability, depending upon the children's age. Whereas this may be appropriate and facilitative of cooperation in the very young child, older children may have problems complying with invasive procedures if they show an excess of attachment responses toward their parent.

Lack of Focus on Parents' Affect

The success of using parents as agents to promote children's adjustment cannot be viewed without understanding their own strategies for coping with stress, their level of anxiety, and the expectations they have for their children's abilities to cope. Our recent studies of dyadic patterns of interaction between children and their mothers (presented in the next section) suggested that the same parenting strategies may have different results depending upon contextual factors such as parental anxiety. The previous level of support that the parent has shown the child is likely to affect the probability that the child will look toward the parent for support in the current situation.

Failure to Consider Timing of Preparation

Several of the studies reviewed have looked at the timing of preparation as a factor in the success of children's readiness for hospitalization. Those studies that have intervened at home prior to the admission of a child to the hospital have relied on the parents as part of the treatment package (Ferguson, 1979; Wolfer & Visintainer, 1975). Different outcomes have been found to be attributable to the timing of the preparation, with those parents who were instructed in stresspoint preparation appearing to have greater impact than those who were provided with general strategy teaching at a time removed from the stressful medical event. Our previous research investigated the openness of children for processing hospital-relevant information at the time of the crisis, and supported the better effectiveness of crisis timing within the context of the stressor (Faust & Melamed, 1984). Younger children who were prepared too far in advance were in fact more aroused at the time of admission to the hospital (Melamed et al., 1976). Furthermore, it was found that if the children were prepared immediately prior to the stress event, and were too young or had previous surgery experience, then relevant preparation might even sensitize them and impair their adjustment (Melamed et al., 1983).

Overlooking Longitudinal Data Base

Although many investigators have loosely used the concept of coping, few studies have actually examined the behaviors of respondents over repeated instances with the stressors. The ability to learn from experience is unquestioned, yet most studies focused on a unique experience or single-stress exposure. The definition of a taxonomy of events that arouse medical concerns with a recognition of the demands upon both the children and the parents can allow us to observe the adjustment across many seemingly different situations. Thus repeated experience can be viewed as a learning opportunity, and changes in coping behaviors over time and the generalization to different events should be assessed.

Absence of Integration of Theory with Measurement

In our quest for knowledge regarding the reduction of fears, we have overlooked many psychological theories that postulate that the ability to cope effectively may be related to reassurance or to orienting the individuals to the information to be presented. Thus measures that are related to theoretical postulates need to be developed. For instance, we postulated a crisis-parenting conception in which parents' ability to support their children during crises may be negatively related to the demands or anxieties these situations have for the parents. Yet few studies have done more than assess parents' verbal reports about anxiety. In a study to be described on dyadic interactions, we were able to see that the same parenting behaviors—informing and distraction—might have quite different effects, depending upon whether the parent is concurrently agitated or ignoring the child. The use of reassurance may also backfire if threatening events are communicated within the same message. Highly anxious parents are more likely to feel that they cannot get the needed information from physicians. Thus the arousal and information-processing theories should be applied in making predictions regarding the usefulness of information for decreasing children's and parents' anxiety.

Importance of Health Care Provider

To some extent, the lack of studies that focus on the influence of physician and nursing personnel on facilitating the communication process and asssisting the parent and child in adjustment to the stressor is either chauvinistic, naive, or based on a self-consciousness that fears criticism. The lack of interactive measures may also hamper research regarding the health care provider's role. The interesting field study of nurses reported by Jacobs (1979) may be useful in shedding light on these phenomena. Her findings clearly implicated the nursing staff in fostering a closed system that excluded the parent from daily participation in their child's inpatient hospital care. The issue of role usurption by the parent who desires to assist in his or her child's treatment and recovery is an interesting paradox, given the greater knowledge most parents possess regarding their particular child's individual coping style.

Measurement of Constructs

The measurement of constructs of both the parents' behavior and the children's distress responses are biased evaluatively. The use of terms such as *reassurance* and *distress* have typically been associated with good or bad evaluative dimensions. However, our current data base revealed the necessity of using functional relationships without presupposing their presumed effect. Thus the patterns of interaction that predict future success in receiving necessary medical treatment should be examined empirically, with reference to well-specified outcome criteria.

Policy Issues

To some extent, the advent of natural childbirth and Lamaze techniques has changed the course of hospital policies regarding the use of anesthesia and the presence of the husband in the labor and delivery rooms. This policy change has allowed for the realization that many more healthy babies could be born without the heavy medication to reduce excruciating pain that the obstetricians and anesthesiologists were attempting to spare the mother.

As more and more hospitals begin to allow rooming in of a parent with an ill child, the benefits of speedier recoveries and relieving burn-out among nursing staff may reinforce these policies prior to actual evaluations from an accumulating data base and thereby provide an increased opportunity for naturalistic observation regarding actual parenting effects.

FUTURE DIRECTIONS: MICROANALYSIS OF PARENT–CHILD DYADS

Thus the questions we are asking are very complex. The need to sort out how information provided by the parent to the child may be contributing supportive effects above and beyond what they could read in a book requires more microlevel analysis of what occurs in this interaction. The advent of more sophisticated data analysis schemes such as Gottman's (1979) sequential analysis will allow for greater precision in attempting to answer questions posed about causality in examining dyadic interactions.

Our own recent research attempts to deal with some of the gaps in the literature by (a)providing an observational measure of dyadic interaction between parent and child, specific to acute medical intervention; and (b) obtaining normative data on this family interaction with regard to parent and children's health concerns and behaviors. The identification of families at risk for dysfunction in the face of acute illness is a planned by-product of our investigations.

Fifty children between four and ten years of age who were seen as outpatients in the Pediatric Clinic at Shands Teaching Hospital at the University of Florida were videotaped along with their mothers while waiting for the physician in clinic examining rooms. These children were referred to Shands for routine diagnostic or specialized medical attention and post-surgical follow-up. Children with severe chronic disabilities were excluded from this study.

Prior to entering the examining room, self-report measures of anxiety were administered to both mothers and children. Mothers were given the State-Trait Anxiety Inventory (Spielberger, Gorusch, & Lushene, 1976), and both mothers and children indicated current medical concerns on the Hospital Fears Rating Scale (Melamed & Siegel, 1975). Mothers also rated their own and their children's current anxiety on 4-point scales, along with their assessment of their children's past reaction to medical visits and expected reaction to the current visit. Mothers also completed the Coping Questionnaire (Billings & Moos, 1981), which yields scores for the extent to which they reported using coping behaviors focused on their own emotional reactions to their child's current health crisis and the extent to which they reported seeing coping behaviors focused on the problems constituting that crisis. Background information was obtained from mothers by means of a short, structured interview, including demographic data and detail about the child's previous medical experiences. After the examination, the physician rated the child's diagnosis on a 10-point severity scale, along with the mother's cooperativeness during the examination procedures. Observers rated mothers' effectiveness in helping their children cope with examination procedures and their anxiety during the examination, also on 10-point scales. Finally, mothers were asked whether they had been able to ask the doctor all of their questions.

An observational scale of parent–child interactions was used to rate the videotapes. The Dyadic Prestressor Interaction Scale (DPIS) was constructed after review of related literature and extensive narrative–descriptive clinic observation (Bush, 1983). Four classes of child behaviors and six of parent behaviors were selected, and four specific behaviors operationally defined within each class (see Table 7.1).

TABLE 7.1   DYADIC PRESTRESSOR INTERACTION SCALE: FUNCTIONAL DEFINITIONS

Child Behavior Categories

Attachment
    Look at parent: Child looking at parent
    Approach parent: Child motorically approaching parent
    Touch parent: Child physically touching parent
    Verbal concern: Child verbalizing concern with the parent's continuing presence throughout the procedures
Distress
    Crying: Child's eyes watering and/or he or she is making crying sounds
    Diffuse motor: Child running around, pacing, flailing arms, kicking, arching, engaging in repetitive fine motor activity, etc.
    Verbal unease: Child verbalizing fear, distress, anger, anxiety, etc.
    Withdrawal: Child silent and immobile, no eye contact with parent, in curled-up position
Exploration
    Motoric exploration: Child locomoting around room, visually examining
    Physical manipulation: Child handling objects in room
    Questions parent: Child asking parent a question related to doctors, hospitals, etc.
    Interaction with observer: Child attempting to engage in verbal or other interaction with observer
Social-Affiliative
    Looking at book: Child is quietly reading a book or magazine unrelated to medicine or looking at its pictures

TABLE 7.1 (Continued)

Other verbal interaction: Child is verbally interacting with parent on topic unrelated to medicine

Other play: Child playing with parent, not involving medical objects or topics

Solitary play: Child playing alone with object brought into room, unrelated to
medicine

Parent Behavior Categories

Ignoring

Eyes shut: Parent sleeping or has eyes shut

Reads to self: Parent reading quietly

Sitting quietly: Parent sitting quietly, not making eye contact with child

Other noninteractive: Parent engaging in other medically unrelated solitary activity

Reassurance

Verbal reassurance: Parent telling child not to worry, that he or she can tolerate
the procedures, that it will not be so bad, etc.

Verbal empathy: Parent telling child he or she understands his or her feelings,
thoughts, situation; questions child for feelings

Verbal praise: Parent telling child he or she is mature, strong, brave, capable,
doing fine, etc.

Physical stroking: Parent petting, stroking, rubbing, hugging, kissing child

Distraction

Nonrelated conversation: Parent engaging in conversation with child on unrelated topic

Nonrelated play: Parent engaging in play interaction with child unrelated to
medicine

Visual redirection: Parent attempting to attract child's attention away from medically related object(s) in the room

Verbal exhortation: Parent telling child not to think about or pay attention to
medically related concerns or objects

Restraint

Physical pulling: Parent physically pulling child away from an object in the room

Verbal order: Parent verbally ordering child to change his or her current activity

Reprimand, glare, swat: Parent verbally chastising, glaring at, and/or physically
striking child

Physically holds: Parent physically holding child in place, despite resistance

Agitation

Gross motor: Parent pacing, flailing arms, pounding fists, stomping feet, etc.

Fine motor: Parent drumming fingers, tapping foot, chewing fingers, etc.

Verbal anger: Parent verbally expressing anger, dismay, fear, unease, etc.

Crying: Parent's eyes watering, verbal whimpering, sobbing, wailing

Informing

Answers questions: Parent attempting to answer child's medically relevant/sit-
uationally relevant questions

Joint exploration: Parent joining with child in exploring the room

Gives information: Parent attempting to impart information, unsolicited by
child, relevant to medicine/the current situation, to the child

Prescribes behavior: Parent attempting to describe to the child appropriate behaviors for the examination session

Child behavior categories were adapted from Bretherton and Ainsworth's (1974) functional systems of behavior in stranger approach situations. Parent behaviors correspond to dimensions of parent behavior indicated by past research as relevant to children's adjustment to stressful medical procedures. Specific constituent behaviors were defined according to criteria of face validity, observed occurrence in the clinics during narrative-descriptive observation, and inclusion of verbal and motoric behaviors across the age span.

Ratings were made on all dyads for which at least 5 minutes of uninterrupted videotaped interaction was obtained while waiting for the physician up to a maximum of 10 minutes. Instantaneous scan ratings (Altmann, 1974) were made every 5 seconds to ascertain which of the ten behavior classes were being engaged in at that moment.

Interobserver reliability for each of the ten behavior classes was evaluated by comparing ratings made by three independent observers on each of the 50 videotapes. Reliability coefficients, presented in Table 7.2, were obtained by means of the repeated-measures analysis of variance procedure described by Winer (1962).

The behavior of mothers in the waiting rooms was expected to influence the anxiety level and behaviors of their children. From the emotional contagion hypothesis, it was predicted that mothers who showed agitation would have children high in distress. Younger children were expected to show more distress in this condition, as they tend to seek attachment to mothers. From the crisis-parenting hypothesis, it was predicted that mothers who showed more agitation and used more ignoring and distracting would have children high in distress who would engage in few exploratory behaviors, whereas the use of information provision or distraction in the absence of maternal agitation would be accompanied by less distress in the children.

The four child behavior categories were found to measure reasonably independent functional systems. Only two significant correlations were

TABLE 7.2   DYADIC PRESTRESSOR INTERACTION SCALE
Interrater Reliability of Behavior Categories $n = 50$

Child behaviors	Attachment	.94
	Distress	.80
	Exploration	.92
	Socializing	.94
Parent behaviors	Ignoring	.97
	Reassuring	.96
	Distracting	.96
	Restraining	.52[a]
	Informing	.96
	Agitation	.98

[a]Scored dichotomously for presence or absence in entire session.

found among child categories: Distress was negatively related to socializing ($r = -.43$, $p < .01$) with distressed children engaging in fewer social-affiliative behaviors. Distressed children also engaged in fewer exploratory behaviors ($r = -.28$, $p < .05$). Parent behavior categories were also highly independent, with the exception of ignoring. Ignoring, defined as the active nonresponding of a mother who occupied herself to the exclusion of the child was negatively correlated with each of these four behavior systems with which it could not, by definition, simultaneously cooccur: (a) reassurance ($r = -.30$, $p < .05$); (b) distraction ($r = -.59$, $p < .0001$); (c) restraining ($r = -.39$, $p < .01$); and (d) informing ($r = -.34$, $p < .05$). Ignoring and agitation were positively associated ($r = .31$, $p < .05$). In addition, mothers who were more agitated provided less information to their children ($r = -.28$, $p < .05$).

A number of significant correlations were found between mother and child behaviors. Attachment in children was associated with maternal reassurance ($r = .56$, $p < .0001$). This frequently represented reciprocal interactions. Although free to vary independently, attachment behaviors (e.g., reaching for mother) were often reciprocally consequated by reassurance behaviors (e.g., picking the child up) and vice versa. Another strong pattern of reciprocal interaction was evident in the strong correlation between maternal use of distraction and child socializing behaviors ($r = .77$, $p < .0001$). Yet another was seen between maternal information provision and child exploration ($r = .57$, $p < .0001$).

As predicted according to the emotional contagion hypothesis, children of agitated mothers showed more distress ($r = .32$, $p < .05$). Child distress was also associated with maternal use of reassurance ($r = .39$, $p < .01$). On the other hand, low distress in the child was correlated with mothers' use of distraction ($r = -.31$, $p < .05$). While it might be inferred that maternal agitation elicited children's distress and distraction reduced or inhibited it, and that maternal reassurance was responsive to the child's distress, these data are inconclusive as to causal direction. Further research is currently underway employing sequential analyses by means of which such causal hypotheses may, at least in part, be evaluated.

The remaining mother-child correlations consisted of tendencies for maternal ignoring to be associated with less exploration by children of their current situation ($r = -.30$, $p < .05$) and with children's engaging in less social-affiliative behavior ($r = -.46$, $p < .001$).

To understand the contextual effects of using various techniques while looking at maternal affect (ignoring, agitation), patterns of relationship between combinations of parent behaviors with combinations of child behaviors were examined by canonical correlation analysis. All of the possible canonical functions were significant. The first canonical function yielded an R^2 of .67 ($p < .0001$). Mothers who used much distraction and little reassurance had children who showed more social-affiliative behavior. This relationship did not significantly differ with children of different ages.

The second canonical function, orthogonal to the first, showed that mothers who provided more information and little reassurance had children who engaged in more exploration (R^2 = .48, p < .0001). This effect was partly age-related [$F(1, 42)$ = 4.40, p < .05], with informing contributing more strongly to exploration in the youngest group of children (under five years, nine months).

The third canonical function showed that mothers who used a great deal of reassurance had children who were high in distress and showed a lot of exploratory, social-affiliative, and attachment behaviors (R^2 = .43, p < .0001). In particular, highly reassuring mothers had children high in both attachment and distress [$F(1, 28)$ = 6.11, p < .05]. This effect was most pronounced among the youngest children [$F(1, 28)$ = 5.15, p < .05].

The last significant canonical function supported the prediction drawn from the crisis-parenting hypothesis. It showed that mothers who were highly agitated and who made use of distraction or ignored their children had children who were high in distress and showed little attachment (R^2 = .26, p < .01). This function was not age mediated.

Redundancy analysis of the canonical functions (Thorndike, 1978) indicated that maternal behaviors measured on the DPIS accounted for 49% of the variance in observed children's behaviors, whereas children's behaviors accounted for 36% of the variance in maternal behaviors. This implies that knowing either child or parent behaviors relates meaningfully to behaviors in medical contexts.

Younger children showed fewer social-affiliative behaviors (r = $-.35$, p < .05), and their mothers used less distraction (r = $-.38$, p < .01) and ignored them more (r = .30, p < .05). Neither children's sex, rated severity of diagnosis, nor children's previous medical experience was found to be related to any interactive behaviors that occurred while awaiting the physician. However, children who were expected by their mothers to have worse reactions to the examination engaged in more exploratory behavior (r = .32, p < .05), and mothers who reported using more problem-focused coping were observed using more reassurance with their children (r = .37, p < .01). Few questionnaire measures of mother or child anxiety were predictive of either mother or child behaviors.

Self-reported maternal anxiety was, however, related to mothers' self-reported perceptions of the task of parenting their ill children and with maternal functioning during the medical examination itself. Self-reported trait anxiety was correlated with maternal ratings of children's difficulties with previous medical visits (r = .48, p < .001), with their ratings of the stressfulness of dealing with their children's current health problems (r = .35, p < .05), and with their predictions of their children having difficulty with the upcoming examination (r = .32, p < .05). The same pattern of correlations was found with maternal state anxiety. Children with hospitalization experience were expected by their mothers to handle the examination better (r = .31, p < .05), but mothers whose children had been to the clinic before had higher self-rated anxiety (r = .30, p < .05). Parents with higher medical concerns were rated by observers as less effective in helping their children cope with examination procedures ($r = .25$, $p < .05$). Mothers high in state anxiety were not as effective during the exam, reporting that they were not getting to ask the doctor all their questions ($r = .30$, $p < .001$), whereas mothers rated by observers as less anxious were rated as more cooperative with the examining physician ($r = .27$, $p < .05$).

The results of our analysis of parenting behaviors while awaiting clinic examinations supported the emotional contagion hypothesis that predicts that children are responsive to maternal anxiety. This was found, however, with respect to maternal behavioral manifestations of anxiety while interacting with children in the clinic waiting rooms and not by questionnaire measures of anxiety. Those mothers, who also ignored their children more and provided less information, had children who showed few exploratory behaviors and remained more attached to them. On the positive side, we found that less behaviorally anxious mothers were more likely to use distraction effectively to keep the children from becoming distressed. However, the effectiveness of distraction as well as information was found to depend upon the interactive context in which they occurred. Thus if mothers who are agitated use distraction, children remain high in distress. The use of maternal reassurance can also be associated with more distress when the mother is agitated, whereas informing and distraction were associated with more exploring and social-affiliative behaviors in children of mothers who used little reassurance.

The implications of this research are exciting. They suggest that parents can be identified according to their skills in helping their acutely ill children cope with a stressful medical situation. The next step, of course, is to develop ways to modify parenting through teaching more effective strategies. Rather than use standard behavioral packages (e.g., teach relaxation or coach parents to simply provide information or reassurance), it is important to do a functional analysis of relevant dyadic patterns of interaction.

SUMMARY

The critique of literature on family factors in acute illness has identified some of the shortcomings in research designs. The need to carefully assess the individual differences between children of different ages and capabilities is a major factor in determining the appropriateness of a given psychological preparation. The well-accepted assumption that all children can benefit from parental support during medical interventions needs to be reexamined from the data base. The anxiety of the parent may contribute to the maladaptive coping of children involved in acute health care. The investigations thus far conducted do not answer some of the primary questions that concern both psychologists and health care practitioners. Who needs to be prepared, how, at what time, and by whom? The current policies of involving parents in medical settings provide a unique opportunity for the advent of naturalistic studies in which the interactions of children and their parents during stressful events can be studied. The advantage of a theory-based rather than a technique-oriented approach to improving family functioning during stressful events was discussed. The opportunity for collaboraton of psychologists and health care providers should lead to enrichment both in a research literature and the practices upon which to base recommendations for enhancing utilization of health care systems.

REFERENCES

Alexander, F. (1950). *Psychosomatic medicine: Its principles and applications*. New York: Norton.

Allen, B. P., & Evans, R. I. (1968). Videotape recording in social psychological research: An illustrative study in pedodontia. *Psychological Reports, 23*, 1115–1119.

Altmann, J. (1974). Observational study of behavior: Sampling methods. *Behaviour, 49*, 227–267.

Auerbach, S. M., Kendall, P. C., Cuttler, H. F., & Levitt, W. R. (1976). Anxiety, locus of control, type of preparatory information, and adjustment to dental surgery. *Journal of Consulting and Clinical Psychology, 44*(5), 809–818.

Bailey, P. M., Talbot, A., & Taylor, P. P. (1973). A comparison of maternal anxiety levels with anxiety levels manifested in the child dental patient. *Journal of Dentistry for Children, 40*, 277–284.

Becker, R. D. (1972). Therapeutic approaches to psychopathological reactions to hospitalization. *International Journal of Child Psychotherapy, 2*, 64–97.

Belmont, H. S. (1970). Hospitalization and its effect upon the total child. *Clinical Pediatrics, 9*(8), 472–483.

Billings, A. G., & Moos, R. H. (1981). The role of coping responses and social resources in attenuating the stress of life events. *Journal of Behavioral Medicine, 4*(2), 139–157.

Bowlby, J. (1969). *Attachment and loss. Vol. 1. Attachment*. New York: Basic Books.

Bowlby, J. (1973). *Attachment and loss. Vol. 2. Separation and Anger*. New York: Basic Books.

Brain, D. J., & Maclay, I. (1968). Controlled study of mothers and children in hospital. *British Medical Journal, 1*, 278–280.

Breslav, N., Weitzman, M., & Messenger, K. (1981). Psychological functioning of siblings of disabled children. *Pediatrics, 67*(3), 344–353.

Bretherton, I., & Ainsworth, M. (1974). Responses of one-year-olds to a stranger in a strange situation. In M. Lewis and L. A. Rosenblum (Eds.), *The origins of fear*. New York: Wiley.

Brown, B. (1979). Beyond separation. In D. Hall and M. Stacey (Eds.), *Beyond separation*. London: Routledge and Kegan-Paul.

Burstein, S., & Meichenbaum, D. (1979). The work of worrying in children undergoing surgery. *Journal of Abnormal Child Psychology, 7*(2), 121–132.

Bush, J. (1983). An observational measure of parent-child interactions in the pediatric medical clinic: Relationship with anxiety and coping style. Unpublished doctoral dissertation proposal, University of Virginia.

Clough, F. (1979). The validation of meaning in illness-treatment situations. In D. Hall and M. Stacey (Eds.), *Beyond separation*. London: Routledge and Kegan-Paul.

Couture, C. J. (1976). The psychological responses of young children to brief hospitalization and surgery: The role of parent-child contact and age. *Dissertation Abstracts International, 37*(B), 1427B.

Danilowicz, D. A., & Gabriel, H. P. (1971). Postoperative reactions in children: "Normal" and abnormal responses after cardiac surgery. *American Journal of Psychiatry, 128*(2), 185–188.

Davenport, H. T., & Werry, J. S. (1970). The effect of general anesthesia, surgery and hospitalization upon behavior of children. *American Journal of Orthopsychiatry, 40*(5), 806–824.

Dimock, H. G. (1960). *The child in hospital: A study of his emotional and social well-being.* Philadelphia: Davis.

Douglas, J. W. B. (1975). Early hospital admissions and later disturbances of behavior and learning. *Developmental Medicine and Child Neurology, 17,* 458–480.

Duffy, J. C. (1972). Emotional reactions of children to hospitalization. *Minnesota Medicine, 55,* 1168–1170.

Escalona, S. (1953). Emotional development in the first year of life. In M.J. Senn (Ed.), *Problems of infancy and childhood.* NJ: Foundation Press.

Faust, J., & Melamed, B. G. (1984). The influence of arousal, previous experience, and age on surgery preparation of same day surgery and in-hospital pediatric patients. *Journal of Consulting and Clinical Psychology, 52,* 359–365.

Ferguson, B. F. (1979). Preparing young children for hospitalization: A comparison of two methods. *Pediatrics, 64,* 656–664.

Fernald, C. D., & Corry, J. J. (1981). Empathic versus directive preparation of children for needles. *Children's Health Care, 10*(2), 44–47.

Forgione, A. G., & Clark, R. E. (1974). Comments on an empirical study of the causes of dental fear. *Journal of Dental Research, 53*(2), 496.

Frankl, S. N., Shiere, F. R., & Fogels, H. R. (1962). Should the parent remain with the child in the dental operatory? *Journal of Dentistry for Children, 29,* 150–163.

Glaser, K. (1960). Group discussions with mothers of hospitalized children. *Pediatrics, 26,* 132–140.

Gofman, H., Buckman, W., & Schade, G. (1957). Parents' emotional responses to children's hospitalization. *American Journal of Diseases of Children, 93,* 157–164.

Gottman, J. M. (1979). Time-series analysis of continuous data in dyads. In M. E. Lamb, S. J. Suomi, & G. R. Stephenson (Eds.), *Social interaction analysis.* University of Wisconsin, Madison.

Graham, D. T. (1972). Psychosometric medicine. In N. S. Greenfield and R. A. Sternbach (Eds.), *Handbook of psychophysiology.* New York: Holt, Rineholt and Winston.

Gross, A. M., Stern, R. M., Levin, R. B., Dale, J., & Wojnilower, D. A. (1983). The effect of mother-child separation on the behavior of children experiencing a diagnostic medical procedure. *Journal of Consulting and Clinical Psychology, 51,* 783–785.

Hannallah, R. S., & Rosales, J. K. (1983). Experience with parents' presence during anesthesia induction in children. *Canadian Anesthesiology Society Journal, 30,* 286–289.

Hawley, B. P., McCorkel, A. D., Wittemann, J. K., & Van Ostenberg, P. (1974). The first dental visit for children from low socioeconomic families. *Journal of Dentistry for Children, 41,* 376–381.

Heffernan, M., & Azarnoff, P. (1971). Factors in reducing children's anxiety about clinical visits. *HSMHA Health Reports, 86*(12), 1131–1135.

Hyson, M. C. (1983). Going to the doctor: A developmental study of stress and coping. *Journal of Child Psychology and Psychiatry, 24*(2), 247–259.

Jacobs, R. (1979) The meaning of hospital: Denial of emotions. In D. Hall & M. Stacey (Eds.), *Beyond Separation.* London: Routledge and Kegan-Paul.

Janis, I. L. (1958). *Psychological stress*. New York: Wiley.

Johnson, R., & Baldwin, D. C. (1969). Maternal anxiety and child behavior. *Journal of Dentistry for Children, 36*, 87–92.

Kaplan, D. M., Smith, A., Grobstein, R., & Fischman, S. E. (1973). Family mediation of stress. *Social Work, 18*, 60–69.

Kendall, P. C. (1982). Stressful medical procedures: Cognitive-behavioral strategies for stress-management and prevention. In D. Meichenbaum and M. Jaremko (Eds.), *Stress reduction and prevention: A cognitive-behavioral perspective*. New York: Plenum Press.

Kendall, P. C., & Watson, D. (1981). Psychological preparation for stressful medical procedures. In C. A. Prokop and L. A. Bradley (Eds.), *Medical psychology*. New York: Academic Press.

Kendall, P. C., Williams, L., Pechacek, T. F., Graham, L. E., Shisslak, C., & Herzoff, N. (1979). Cognitive-behavioral and patient education interventions in cardiac catheterization procedures: The Palo Alto medical psychology project. *Journal of Consulting and Clinical Psychology, 47*(1), 49–58.

Klingman, A., Melamed, B., Cuthbert, M., & Hermecz, D. (1984). Effects of participant modeling on information acquisition and skill utilization. *Journal of Consulting and Clinical Psychology, 52*, 414–422.

Klorman, R., Hilpert, P. L., Michael, R., LaGana, C., & Sveen, O. B. (1980). Effects of coping and mastery modeling on experienced and inexperienced pedodontic patients. *Behavior Therapy, 11*, 156–169.

Klorman, R., Ratner, J., Arata, C. L. G., King, J. B., & Sveen, O. B. (1978). Predicting the child's noncooperativeness in dental treatment from maternal trait, state, and dental anxiety. *Journal of Dentistry for Children, 45*, 62–67.

Klorman, R., Ratner, J., King, J. B., & Sveen, O. B. (1977). Pedodontic patients' noncooperativeness and maternal anxiety. *Journal of Dental Research, 56*, B160.

Knight, R. B., Atkins, A., Eagle, C. J., Evans, N., Finkelstein, J. W., Fukushima, D., Katz, J., & Weiner, H. (1979). Psychological stress, ego defenses, and cortisol production in children hospitalized for elective surgery. *Psychosomatic Medicine, 41*, 40–49.

Koenigsburg, S. R., & Johnson, R. (1972). Child behavior during sequential dental visits. *Journal of the American Dental Association, 85*, 128–132.

Levy, E. (1959). Children's behavior under stress and its relation to training by parents to respond to stress situations. *Child Development, 30*, 307–324.

Machen, J., & Johnson, R. (1974). Desensitization, model learning, and the dental behavior of children. *Journal of Dental Research, 53*, 83–89.

Mahaffey, P. R. (1965). The effects of hospitalization on children admitted for tonsillectomy and adenoidectomy. *Nursing Research, 14*(1), 12–19.

McGrath, P. J., & Firestone, P. (Eds.). (1983). *Pediatric and adolescent behavioral medicine: Issues in treatment* (Vol. 10). New York: Springer.

McTigue, D. J., & Pinkham, J. (1978). Association between children's dental behavior and play behavior. *Journal of Dentistry for Children, 8*, 42–46.

Mechanic, D. (1964). The influence of mothers on their children's health attitudes and behavior. *Pediatrics, 3*, 444–453.

Melamed, B. G. (1981). Effects of preparatory information on the adjustment of children to medical procedures. In M. Rosenbaum and C. M. Franks (Eds.), *Perspectives on behavior therapy in the eighties*. New York: Springer.

Melamed, B. G., Dearborn, M. J., & Hermecz, D. (1983). Necessary considerations for surgery preparation: Age and prevous experience. *Psychosomatic Medicine*.

Melamed, B. G., Klingman, A., & Siegel, L. J. (1983). Anxiety disorders in children: Individualizing cognitive behavioral strategies in the reduction of medical and dental stress. In A. Meyers and N. E. Craighead (Eds.), *Cognitive behavior therapy in children*. New York: Plenum Press.

Melamed, B. G., Meyer, R., Gee, C., & Soule, L. (1976). The influence of time and type of preparation on children's adjustment to hospitalization. *Journal of Pediatric Psychology, 1*(4), 31–37.

Melamed, B. G., Robbins, R. L., and Fernandez, J. (1982). Factors to be considered in psychological preparation for surgery. In D. Routh and M. Woolraich (Eds.), *Advances in developmental and behavioral pediatrics* (Vol. 3). New York: JAI Press.

Melamed, B. G., Robbins, R. L., & Graves, S. (1982). Preparation for surgery and medical procedures. In D. Russo and J. Varni (Eds.), *Behavioral pediatrics: Research and practice*. New York: Plenum Press.

Melamed, B. G., & Siegel, L. J. (1975). Reduction of anxiety in children facing hospitalization and surgery by use of filmed modeling. *Journal of Consulting and Clinical Psychology, 43*(4), 511–521.

Melamed, B. G., & Siegel, L. J. (1980). *Behavioral Medicine: Practical Applications in Health Care*. New York: Springer.

Mellish, R. W. P. (1969). Preparation of a child for hospitalization and surgery. *Pediatric Clinics of North America, 16*(3), 543–553.

Minuchin, S., Rosman, B., & Baker, L. (1978). *Psychosomatic families*. Cambridge, MA: Harvard University Press.

Nagy, M. (1951). Children's ideas of the origin of illness. *Health Education Journal, 9*, 6–12.

Nasera, H. (1978). Children's reactions to hospitalization and illness. *Child Psychiatry and Human Development, 9*, 3–19.

Neisworth, J. T., & Moore, F. (1972). Operant treatment of asthmatic responding with the parent as therapist. *Behavior Therapy, 3*, 95–99.

Patterson, G. (1982). *Coercive family process*. Eugene, OR: Castalia.

Pediatric Mental Health. (1983). Psychosocial care of hospitalized Canadian children. 2(4), 3.

Perlmutter, M., & Myers, N. A. (1976). A developmental study of semantic effects on recognition memory. *Journal of Experimental Child Psychology, 22*, 438–453.

Peterson, L., & Ridley-Johnson, R. (1980). Pediatric hospital response to a survey on prehospitalization preparation for children. *Journal of Pediatric Psychology, 5*(1), 1–7.

Peterson, L., Ridley-Johnson, R., Tracy, K., & Mullins, L. J. (1984). Developing cost-effective presurgical preparation. *Journal of Pediatric Psychology*.

Peterson, L., Schultheis, K., Ridley-Johnson, R., Miller, D. J., & Tracy, K. (1984). Comparison of three modeling procedures on the presurgical and postsurgical reactions of children. *Behavior Therapy, 15*, 79–83.

Perterson, L., & Shigetomi, C. (1981). Use of coping techniques to reduce anxiety in hospitalized children. *Behavior Therapy, 12*, 1–14.

Peterson, L., & Shigetomi, C. (1983). Psychosocial care of hospitalized Canadian children. *Pediatric Mental Health, 2*(4), 3.

Pickett, C., & Clum, G. A. (1982). Comparative treatment strategies and interaction with locus of control in the reduction of post-surgical pain and anxiety. *Journal of Consulting and Clinical Psychology, 50*, 439–441.

Pinkham, J., & Fields, H. W. (1976). The effects of preappointment procedures on maternal manifest anxiety. *Journal of Dentistry for Children, 43*, 180–183.

Prugh, D. G., Staub, E. M., Sands, H. H., Kirschbaum, R. M., & Lenihan, E. A. (1953). A study of the emotional reactions of children and families to hospitalization and illness. *American Journal of Orthopsychiatry, 23*, 70–106.

Quinton, D., & Rutter, M. (1976). Early hospital admissions and later disturbances of behavior: An attempted replication of Douglas' findings. *Developmental Medicine and Child Neurology, 18,* 447–459.

Robertson, J. (1958). *Young children in hospitals.* New York: Basic Books.

Robertson, J. (1976). The children in hospitals. *South African Medical Journal, 50,* 749–752.

Robinson, D. (1968). Mothers' fear, their children's well-being in hospital, and the study of illness behavior. *British Journal of Preventive Social Medicine, 22,* 228–233.

Roskies, E., Mongeon, M., & Gagnon-Lefebvre, B. (1978). Increasing parental participation in the hospitalization of young children. *Medical Care, 16*(9), 767–777.

Routh, D. K., & Wolraich, M. (Eds.). (1982). *Advances in developmental and behavioral pediatrics* (Vol. 3). NJ: JAI Press.

Russo, D. C., & Varni, J. W. (Eds.). (1982). *Behavioral pediatrics: research and practice.* New York: Plenum Press.

Sawtell, R. O., Simon, J. F., & Simeonsson, R. J. (1974). The effects of five preparatory methods upon child behavior during the first dental visit. *Journal of Dentistry for Children, 41,* 367–365.

Scarr, S., & Salapatek, P. (1970). Patterns of fear development during infancy. *Merrill Palmer Quarterly, 16,* 53–90.

Schaffer, H. R. (1966). The onset of fear of strangers and the incongruity hypothesis. *Journal of Child Psychology and Psychiatry, 1,* 95–106.

Seidl, F. W., & Pillitteri, A. (1967). Development of an attitude scale on parent participation. *Nursing Research, 16*(1), 71–73.

Shade-Zeldow, Y. (1977). Attachment and separation: Effects of hospitalization on pediatric patients. *Dissertation Abstracts International, 37B,* 5376-B.

Shaw, E. G., & Routh, D. K. (1982). Effect of mothers' presence on children's reaction to aversive procedures. *Journal of Pediatric Psychology, 7,* 33–42.

Sides, J. P. (1977). Emotional responses of children to physical illness and hospitalization. *Dissertation Abstracts International, 38B,* 917-B.

Siegel, L. J. (1981). *Naturalistic study of coping strategies in children facing medical procedures.* Paper presented at Southeastern Psychological Association, Atlanta Convention.

Siegel, L. J., & Peterson, L. (1980). Stress reduction in young dental patients through coping skills and sensory information. *Journal of Consulting and Clinical Psychology, 48*(6), 785–787.

Skipper, J. K., Jr., Leonard, R. C., & Rhymes, J. (1968). Child hospitalization and social interaction: An experimental study of mothers' feelings of stress, adaptation, and satisfaction. *Medical Care, 6*(6), 496–506.

Spielberger, C. D., Gorusch, R. L., & Lushene, R. (1970). *State-Trait Anxiety Inventory.* Palo Alto, CA: Consulting Psychologists Press.

Spitz, R. A. (1950). Anxiety in infancy: A study of manifestations in the first year of life. *International Journal of Psychoanalysis, 31,* 138–143.

Sulzer-Azaroff, B., and Meyer, G. R. (1977). *Applying behavior analysis procedures with children and youth.* New York: Holt, Rinehart and Winston.

Tennes, K. H., & Lampl, E. E. (1964). Stranger and separation anxiety in infancy. *Journal of Nervous and Mental Diseases, 139,* 247–254.

Thorndike, R. (1978). *Correlational procedures for research.* New York: Gardner Press.

Unger, M. (1982). *Defensiveness in children as it influences acquisition of fear-relevant information.* Unpublished masters thesis, University of Florida.

Venham, L. L. (1979). The effect of the mother's presence on the child's response to a stressful situation. *Journal of Dentistry for Children, 46,* 219–225.

Venham, L. L., Bengston, D., & Cipes, M. (1978). Parents' presence and the child's response to dental stress. *Journal of Dentistry for Children, 45,* 213–217.

Venham, L. L., Murray, P., & Gaulin-Kremer, E. (1979). Child-rearing variables affecting the preschool child's response to dental stress. *Journal of Dental Research, 58,* 2042–2045.

Vernon, D. T. A., Foley, J., & Schulman, J. (1967). Effect of mother-child separation and birth order on young children's responses to two potentially stressful experiences. *Journal of Personality and Social Psychology, 5*(2), 162–174.

Visintainer, M. A., & Wolfer, J. A. (1975). Psychological preparation for surgical pediatric patients: The effect on children's and parents' stress responses and adjustment. *Pediatrics, 64*(5), 646–655.

Wilson, J. F. (1981). Behavioral preparation for surgery: Benefit or harm? *Journal of Behavioral Medicine, 4*(1), 79–102.

Winer, B. J. (1962). *Statistical principles in experimental design.* New York: McGraw-Hill.

Wolfer, J. A., & Visintainer, M. A. (1975). Pediatric surgical patients' and parents' stress responses and adjustment. *Nursing Research, 24*(4), 244–255.

Wright, F. (1982). Children's concepts of dental illness. *Journal of Dentistry for Children, 49*(1), 25–29.

Wright, G. Z., & Alpern, G. D. (1971). Variables influencing children's cooperative behavior at the first dental visit. *Journal of Dentistry for Children, 38,* 124–128.

Wright, G. Z., Alpern, G. D., & Leake, J. L. (1973). The modifiability of maternal anxiety as it relates to children's cooperative dental behavior. *Journal of Dentistry for Children, 40,* 265–271.

Zabin, M. A., & Melamed, B. G. (1980). Relationship between parental discipline and children's ability to cope with stress. *Journal of Behavior Assessment, 2*(1), 17–38.

Zastowney, T. R., Kirschenbaum, D. S., & Meng, A. L. (in press). Coping skills training for children: Effects on distress before, during and after hospitalization for surgery. *Journal of Consulting and Clinical Psychology.*

Ziegler, S., & King, J. (1980, September). *Evaluating a foster-grandparent program in a pediatric hospital.* Paper presented at the American Psychological Association, Montreal.

8

The Family and the Child with Chronic Illness

Suzanne Bennett Johnson

Advances in medical treatment have reduced acute illness in children and permitted youngsters with more chronic physical conditions to live longer. For example, the discovery of insulin in 1922 enabled children with insulin-dependent diabetes to have more reasonable life expectancies. Similarly, before the advent of antibiotics few children with cystic fibrosis lived beyond infancy. Today many live into young adulthood. These changes in childhood morbidity have resulted in increasing the number of chronically ill youngsters. It is estimated that 7–10% of children are affected with a serious chronic illness and that these patients currently comprise almost 50% of pediatric practice (Magrab & Calcagno, 1978). Be-

Supported by Grant #R01HD12820 from the National Institute of Child Health and Human Development.

cause youngsters with diabetes, cancer, cystic fibrosis, and end-stage renal failure are living longer, they must face new problems as adolescents and adults. Frequently, physical treatments for these conditions have been developed with little consideration given to the psychological and social support necessary to enhance the quality as well as the length of the child's life (Drotar, 1981).

Chronic illness differs from acute physical conditions in several important respects. First, a chronic illness is usually treatable but not curable. This means the disease must be "managed" in some way for long periods of time, usually until the patient's death. Typically, there is transfer of medical responsibility from the physician to the patient. Although the doctor remains involved, it is the patient who must manage the illness on a day-to-day basis. For many youngsters, this means a lifelong commitment to often complex, expensive, and sometimes painful procedures for manageing their disease.

For the child with a chronic illness, the situation is further complicated by the necessity of involving parents and family. Frequently, the patient is too young to be responsible for all aspects of his or her medical management. Parents must therefore assume this responsibility and the family as a whole must adapt to the demands of the child's illness. However, this adaptation often requires constant change and readaptation as the child grows older and becomes capable of playing different roles within the family and as the disease itself changes, thus placing more or less stress on the patient and the parents. Unlike acute illness, chronic illness places ongoing demands upon the family. Consequently, adaptation by both patient and family is best viewed as a process that changes over time.

How a child with chronic illness adjusts to or copes with his illness can be viewed as the product of three variables: (1) the disease itself; (2) individual characteristics of the child; and (3) environmental factors within the child's life.

Although there is a tendency to refer to "chronic illness" as a single entity, there are numerous chronic illnesses with very different characteristics. Certainly, for the purposes of communication it makes sense to discuss the "family and the child with chronic illness." It is a class of illness that differs in some important respects from acute illness. Nevertheless, while discussing the class "chronic illness," it is important that we do not lose sight of the impact of specific illness characteristics on the patient or family. For example, chronic illnesses differ in their visibility and prognosis. Different illnesses place varying limitations on the patient's functioning. Treatment requirements differ in difficulty, complexity, frequency, discomfort, and resultant side effects. And some diseases are associated with other disorders or "complications" that place additional demands upon the patient and family. Not only does each disease have its own special characteristics, but the illness itself can change over time, becoming more or less severe with resultant changes in treatment, prognosis, and the patient's functional capabilities. Although the purpose of this chapter is to focus on the family of a child with chronic illness, both the clinician and the researcher would do well to recognize the importance of disease variables on both the patient's and the family's adjustment.

Historically, the psychosocial literature has not taken an interactive view of patients' adjustment to chronic illness. Instead of studying disease variables, patient variables, and environmental variables in combination, it has generally focused exclusively on patient variables. The most popular approaches have been attempts to identify specific personality types associated with specific diseases or to compare a chronic illness group with a "normal," physically healthy group on one or more measures of psychopathology or adjustment. Although this literature suffers from numerous methodological flaws, it does suggest that (a) specific personality patterns are not associated with specific illnesses; and (b) most children facing chronic disease cope reasonably well (Drotar, 1981; Johnson, 1980). Fortunately, there has been a recent trend toward the study of patient variables associated with good or poor functioning *within* a specific illness. Clearly, this approach has greater practical application than prior efforts to delineate specific illness personalities or to compare ill children with healthy ones.

Understanding what child or patient variables are related to successful coping have obvious implications for the management of any disorder. However, many child or patient variables should be considered in addition to the more traditional approach of studying a youngster's personality. As one example, the child's age or cognitive developmental level is probably an important contributor to what he or she is capable of understanding about the disease, how the child communicates concerns to the parents and doctor, and what aspects of the management of the disease should be the youngster's responsibility. Yet this particular patient variable has often been ignored both in the research literature and in educational program development. Of course, other patient variables are equally worthy of consideration. Many of these will be discussed in subsequent portions of this chapter.

As investigators and clinicians have turned away from the study of the patient in isolation, the role of the environment and particularly the family has become paramount. The publication of this volume is an example of this changing perspective. The patient is viewed as coping with illness within an environmental context that is necessarily affected by the patient's illness, which in turn influences the patient's ability to cope and adjust. It is the purpose of this chapter to take a closer look at the family and its interaction with the child who has a chronic illness.

Children, of course, are highly dependent upon their parents for much of their growth and development. Consequently, the family should play a major role in a child's adjustment to a chronic disease. Similarly, the child's disease should impact on the family's functioning. Although these assumptions seem reasonable, it is important to recognize that research in this area is in its infancy. Our conceptualizations have changed, but the methodology to test these assumptions is only now being developed. This chapter will raise more questions than provide answers, but hopefully it will serve as a guide to both the interested clinician and the researcher.

Yancy (1972) suggested that pediatricians who care for children with chronic disease should have three major goals. First, they must attempt to treat the disease itself. This involves correcting any specific defects as much as is feasible, controlling any illness symptoms as they arise, and arresting the progress of the disease as much as possible. Second, they must prevent the disease and its treatment from interfering with the child's development. Third, they must prevent the illness and its management from disrupting the family unit. Parents of children with chronic illness have essentially the same goals. First, they must manage or help the child manage his or her illness. Second, they must help the child cope with the realities of the illness while encouraging the youngster to develop as normally as possible. Third, they must accomplish the first two goals without totally disrupting the family's normal functioning. Families' inability to meet one or more of these goals is typically what brings them to the attention of a mental health professional.

MANAGING THE CHILD'S ILLNESS

The day-to-day management of any chronic illness rests with the patient and family. Many illnesses require relatively complex treatment procedures. The child with diabetes must take daily insulin injections, test his urine or blood for its sugar content, and maintain certain dietary restrictions. Youngsters with cystic fibrosis must have physiotherapy two or three times a day to rid their lungs of excess mucus, and are usually on special diets and regular medication. These management programs are not only time consuming, but often involve discomfort on the child's part. Rarely can the child be given total responsibility for disease management. The treatment regimen may be beyond the child's cognitive capabilities. Motivating the youngster to participate may be difficult because management tasks can be uncomfortable; they may take the child away from more pleasant activities and can make the youngster feel different from peers. Often, compliance with daily management tasks results in no immediate, pleasurable experience for the child. Rather, treatments are designed to prevent illness that may take days or weeks to develop. Similarly, there are rarely immediate, negative consequences for noncompliance. Because there are few rewards inherently associated with the child's adherence to management prescriptions and few punishments associated with noncompliance, it is usually the parent's task to motivate the child to perform these daily routines.

Managing a child's chronic illness usually requires that the parent (a) be well educated about the disease and its treatment; (b) communicate with the child's physician about the child's management; (c) determine which aspects of the child's daily management should be the child's responsibility and which aspects should be the parent's responsibility; and (d) teach and supervise the child's efforts at managing his or her own illness. Parents are variable as to how adequately they meet these demands. Unfortunately, there has been little research addressing any of these issues.

Learning About the Illness

Although parents are often given extensive education about their child's illness, few studies have addressed the success of these educational efforts or the best methods for teaching this information. Patient instructional efforts have been given much closer attention, although research on educational programing for the patient and various family members is generally lacking. There is some evidence that mothers, fathers, and patients all differ in what they know about and how they perceive the illness. Mothers of youngsters with diabetes, for example, know more about managing this disease than fathers or young children with the illness. However, some adolescents are as knowledgeable as their mothers and more knowledgeable than their fathers (Etzwiler & Sines, 1962; Johnson et al., 1982; La Greca, Follansbee, & Skyler, 1982). Mothers and fathers of diabetic youngsters also differ in their perception of and involvement in various management tasks (Etzwiler & Sines, 1962).

Factor analytic studies suggest that the mother's perceptions of observant or supervisory behaviors in which the parent watches the child closely for signs of illness are distinct from her perceptions of how disruptive the illness is on the family's functioning. In contrast, fathers often view the necessity of closely monitoring a child as evidence that the illness is generally disruptive of the parents' and family's efforts to live normally (Johnson, 1982). Although mothers may take greater responsibility for their child's management and consequently may be better educated about the disease than are fathers, it is unclear whether this is an ideal arrangement. The role of the father as well as that of the mother in the child's management needs to be more carefully assessed. In fact, methods for successfully educating all family members about a child's chronic condition have received remarkably little attention.

Communicating with the Child's Physician

In addition to learning about the child's illness, the parent is usually a primary source of information for the physician. The parent describes ongoing management behaviors, personal observations, and the results of daily tests relevant to the child's condition. The mother or father usually alerts the physician in times of crisis and is often the first to implement the physician's recommendations. Yet little is known about the best methods of ensuring adequate physician–parent, as well as physician–patient, communication. Mothers and fathers often have highly positive or negative attitudes toward their child's physician, but variables associated with these attitudes are often unclear (Johnson, 1982). There is some evidence that compliance with prescribed treatment increases when parents' expectations about parent–physician encounters are met and when the physician interacts with the parent in a friendly manner (Frances, Korsch, & Morris, 1969; Freemon, Negrete, Davis, & Korsch, 1971). However, these studies were conducted with acute rather than chronically ill children and employed unvalidated measures of compliance. It is clear that this is a critical area in need of further research.

Defining Patient and Parent Responsibilities

It is unrealistic to expect a child with a chronic illness to manage his or her disease completely. Some tasks may be beyond the child's ability, whereas others may be left undone because they are time consuming, boring, or even uncomfortable. Children are simply too immature, both cognitively and emotionally, to be given complete responsibility for managing their own illness. Yet parents are offered few guidelines as to who should handle which aspects of the treatment program and often have age-inappropriate expectations for their children (Hill & Hynes, 1980). Only recently have we begun to explore the relationship of children's cognitive developmental level to the understanding of illness and its treatment. In our own work, we have found that youngsters' knowledge about diabetes and skills at various management tasks increase in age-related stages (Gilbert et al., 1982; Harkavy et al., 1983; Johnson et al., 1982). Most youngsters, for example, seem to be capable of self-injection around nine years of age. However, nine-year-old youngsters cannot be expected to accurately test their urine for sugar. It is best to wait until children are around 12 years of age before expecting them to independently perform this task.

The importance of realistically defining a child's illness management responsibilities is highlighted in a recent study by La Greca (1982). She found that in preadolescent diabetic patients, the degree of responsibility the child assumed for his or her care and the level of the mother's knowledge were both predictive of how well or poorly the diabetes was controlled. Although good maternal knowledge was associated with good diabetic control, greater child responsibility was associated with poorer control. In contrast, among adolescent patients their compliance with treatment regimen and their knowledge about diabetes were both positively related to their level of diabetic control. This study suggests that for younger patients, parents may need to assume the primary responsibility for managing the child's illness. Giving the youngster too much responsibility too early may prove disasterous.

Because the child's abilities and emotional maturity change over time, patient and parent responsibilities for managing the child's illness should change as well. As the child grows older, he or she should perform more and more of the necessary treatment procedures. Helping the child through this transition from relative dependence to independence is primarily the parent's responsibility. Adolescence is sometimes particularly problematic because the youngster expects and often should have increased control over disease management. Yet it can be difficult for the parent to relinquish this control because the youngster's failure to manage the illness properly can have such serious health consequences (Johnson & Rosenbloom, 1982). In the absence of data-based research, health professionals can do little more than offer parents well-meaning advice.

Teaching and Supervising the Patient

Because chronically ill children's self-management skills are expected to improve and expand over time, the parent must teach and supervise the youngster through the various stages of this process. Not only must the parent define patient versus parent responsibilities, but also must remain observant of the child's performance on various treatment tasks. Even if a child is capable of carrying out a particular management task, this does not mean the child will consistently and accurately perform the task without any parental supervision. This places additional demands upon the parent and can be a source of parent–child conflict. Parents and children often have very different perceptions about the illness and its management. In one study, mothers and children were asked what the child disliked most about diabetes. Although the youngsters focused on injections and social restrictions, their mothers emphasized dietary regimens. The mothers of these particular children seemed to have inaccurate perceptions of how their own children viewed the daily demands placed upon them by diabetes (Kronenfeld & Ory, 1981).

HELPING THE CHILD COPE

Much is expected of the child with a chronic illness. He or she may experience pain, discomfort, and physical limitations from the illness itself or from its prescribed treatments. Both the disease and its management may interfere with the child's social and emotional development. Necessary hospitalizations mean repeated separations from the family. Frequent illness episodes mean school absences. The affected child may feel jealous of others who are healthy and who can lead a less constricted existence. Feelings of being different from peers and siblings may result in a sense of isolation and loneliness. The future may be viewed with little optimism and the spector of death may be quite real.

Each disease places its own special demands upon the child. A severely burned child must initially endure great pain and then must cope with the effects of disfigurement. A diabetic youngster must lead a life of daily injections, urine tests, and dietary constraints. A child with leukemia must face painful spinal taps, hair loss, and the imminence of death.

Youngsters' reactions to these different demands may depend upon their cognitive and emotional developmental levels. Young children may be primarily stressed by mother–child separations and the discomfort of medical procedures. They may feel angry at day-to-day restrictions placed upon them but show little concern for their future. In contrast, adolescents may be particularly sensitive to how the demands of their illness separate them from their peers. Their ability to live independently, marry, work and support themselves become important foci of concern as they develop the capability of considering and planning for their future.

Through all of this, the parent and family must help the child cope. Yet we are just beginning to study the relationship of parent or family variables to good versus poor adaptation in this population. A number of studies have focused on (a) the relationship between child adjustment and physical health; (b) the relationship between family factors and the child's adjustment; and (c) the relationship between characteristics of the family and the child's health.

Child Adjustment and Physical Health

All parents hope that their children will be well adjusted emotionally. However, the stresses and special demands of a chronic illness may impede this process. Adequate adaptation to the disease is critical if the child is to develop normally. In addition, there is some evidence that the child's psychological status may be related to the youngster's physical condition. Simonds (1976, 1977), for example, reported that the frequency of psychiatric diagnosis among a group of insulin-dependent diabetic children was no higher than that found in the normal, nondiabetic population. However, patients in poor diabetic control had more interpersonal conflicts than those in good control. Other investigators have also reported more emotional and behavioral problems in patients in poorer diabetic control compared with their well-controlled counterparts (Anderson, Miller, Auslander, & Santiago, 1981; Gath, Smith, & Baum, 1980; Grey, Genel, & Taborlane, 1980). Although chronic illness is not always associated with poor adaptation in the child, those youngsters in the poorest health do seem to have more adjustment problems.

The mechanisms by which the child's psychological status is related to his or her physical condition are not entirely clear. In some cases, the severity of the illness and the child's generally poor health may so severely limit functioning that the child is deprived of critical experiences, resulting in less than adequate social skills, poor self-esteem, and excessive dependency on parents and family. It is also possible that maladaptive patient attitudes may negatively influence the course of the disease itself. For instance, negative attitudes may result in noncompliance with recommended treatment with resultant effects on the child's health. In some cases, emotional stress may affect the child's condition more directly. In diabetes, for example, emotional upset may lead to an increase in the stress hormones, which in turn may result in an increase in glucose and free fatty acids, thus placing the child in poor metabolic control (Tarnow and Silverman, 1981–1982).

Childhood asthma is a prototypical example of how emotions and health may interrelate. There is some evidence that asthmatic patients may have more difficulty expressing their emotions overtly compared with persons with other respiratory conditions (Rubenstein, King, & London, 1979). There is also some evidence that anger and fear may actually reduce pulmonary flow rates in asthmatic youngsters (Tal & Miklich, 1976). Emotionally inhibited youngsters seem to be more difficult to treat (Kapotes, 1977). Patients with fearful response styles seem to ask for and receive more medication (Dahlem, Kinsman, & Horton, 1977; Dirks, Jones & Kinsman, 1977), and are often hospitalized for longer periods of time (Kaptein, 1982). In one published report, patients who were more difficult to treat also had experienced more stressful life events (Zlatich, Kenny, Sila, & Huang, 1982). These studies suggest that certain emotional response styles may be an important determinant of whether a child has many or very few asthmatic attacks.

Matus (1981) has proposed that psychological variables may influence asthma in several ways. First, a psychological stimulant may actually elicit respiratory distress, serving as a precipitant of an attack. Second, when a patient detects a change in respiration, this may result in an emotional response, which may in turn heighten the respiratory change. In this case, the patient's emotions are actually exacerbating the condition. Finally, psychological factors may be important influences in the maintenance of the condition. For example, the secondary gain the child receives while ill may be sufficiently rewarding that he or she fails to take medication as prescribed or actually deliberately induces an attack by engaging in a behavior that is known to precipitate attacks.

Although there is theoretical and some empirical support for the view that patient attitudes or emotions may be causally linked to health, the hypothetical nature of the relationship must be emphasized. In our own work we have found that youngsters in poor diabetic control often view their disease as a disruptive force in their lives, whereas youngsters in good diabetic control perceive the disease and its impact quite differently (Johnson, 1982). However, it is unclear whether patients' perceptions of the disease as disruptive result in deteriorated health or whether the patients' perceptions are a consequence of the limitations and frustrations associated with repeated illness episodes.

A recent study by Staudenmayer (1982) makes a similar point. The amount of debilitation experienced by children with asthma was significantly correlated with a number of patient perceptions including despair over social limitations due to the illness, dread of the illness, judgments of quality of life, and attitudes about compliance with medications. Pre- and posttreatment assessment of these perceptions indicated that as the child's medical condition improved, the child's perceptions of the disease changed as well. In this particular study, it appeared that negative patient attitudes and perceptions were a consequence of poor medical management rather than an antecedent condition that undermined good medical care. Clearly, the relationship between child adjustment and physical health is not unidirectional.

Child Adjustment and the Family

Few would argue with the proposition that family functioning is closely related to psychopathology or psychological health in the child. Only recently has this relationship been examined within chronically ill childhood populations. In a now classic study, Pless, Roghmann, and Haggerty (1972) examined the relationship between child adjustment, family functioning, and chronic illness in a large sample of youngsters living in Monroe County, New York. Two hundred nine children with documented chronic illness were compared to 113 healthy controls. Using semistructured household interviews, symptom checklists of child behavior completed by the parent, information obtained from the child's teacher, and the child's self-report on a self-esteem inventory, each youngster was rated on a mental-health adjustment index and each family was rated on a family-functioning index. Both family functioning and physical health seemed to contribute to a child's psychological adjustment, with ill youngsters and those from poorly functioning families showing more adjustment problems. Youngsters who were ill and lived in dysfunctional families showed the highest incidence of psychological disturbance. This was particularly true for older youngsters, thus suggesting that there may be a cumulative effect over time of poor health and an unfavorable family situation.

The results of the Pless et al. (1972) survey suggested that chronically ill youngsters who live in poorly functioning families may be particularly at risk for developing social/emotional problems. In their attempts to address this relationship more specifically, different investigators have focused on various child and family characteristics. Some have studied family variables related to the child's general emotional development. Others have been concerned with child behaviors that are more directly tied to the youngster's illness.

Marital discord is considered by some to be an important negative influence on a chronically ill youngster's psychological adjustment (Kupst et al., 1982; Lawler, Nakielny, & Wright, 1966). Others point to parental self-esteem (Grey, Genel, & Taborlane, 1980); overprotective or overcontrolling parental behavior (Meijer, 1981; Rubenstein, King, & London, 1979); and closed family communication (Spinetta & Maloney, 1978) as critical parameters leading to behavioral or emotional problems in the chronically ill child.

One study attempted to use home observation techniques to assess the family interaction patterns of well-adjusted children versus maladjusted children with cystic fibrosis (Kucia et al., 1979). Both groups of families were observed in their own homes where they were asked to work together to discover the rules of a game presented by the experimenter and to obtain the highest possible score. (The observers were unaware of the patients' adjustment status.) During the game, the families were given feedback; a green light indicated a rule had been observed, whereas a red light meant a rule had been broken. Observers recorded the percentage of green lights the families obtained (family successes), the number of different ways of playing the game originated by each person (creativity), and whether each person offered positive or negative support. The results suggested that the two groups of families did not differ in terms of total communication and support. However, the families of the well-adjusted children offered more creative problem solutions. Fathers were particularly creative and supportive in the well-adjusted group. The authors conclude that family creativity (i.e., the ability to generate many different solutions to a problem) may be very helpful in the management of certain chronic illnesses. A child's adjustment to the illness may be enhanced if maternal care for the child is balanced by paternal support.

Perhaps the most interesting studies focus on parental variables that relate to children's ability to cope specifically with their illness. At least two studies have assessed children's perceptions of their disease and related these perceptions to other family members' attitudes toward the child's illness. Among diabetic youngsters, patients who view their illness as highly disruptive often have mothers who share these negative attitudes. Similarly, children with very authoritarian attitudes toward diabetes management frequently mimic attitudes held by their mothers (Johnson, 1982). Studying a different chronically ill population, Susman et al. (1982) found that patient and parent conceptions of cancer were similar, particularly in the areas of knowledge about the illness, realistic perceptions of the future, feelings associated with discussions about the future, and the extent to which the patient planned to participate in or withdraw from his or her environment.

Family variables associated with patient compliance were assessed by Korsch, Fine, and Negrete (1977). Fourteen patients who interrupted immunosuppressive treatment following renal transplantation were compared with their more compliant peers. Nonadherent youngsters came from lower socioeconomic backgrounds and usually lived in fatherless households. Based on a semistructured parental interview, these youngsters' families evidenced greater communication difficulties both within the family and with their medical caretakers. For example, noncompliant patients were described as being closest to persons outside the family. Their parents reported increased quarreling, angry outbursts, and difficulty communicating with the child, and their mothers perceived someone other than the child's physician as the most helpful during the youngster's illness.

Evaluating pediatric cancer patients reactions to painful medical procedures, Jay and her colleagues (Jay, Ozolins, Elliot, & Caldwell, 1983) found both child and parent variables to be important predictors of child behavior. Younger children and those with less experience with bone marrow aspiration showed greater distress. In addition, parental anxiety was associated with increased patient distress. Of course, heightened parental anxiety could be the result as well as the cause of the patient's anxious behaviors.

Although few in number, these studies point to the importance of parental or family variables as possible determinants of good versus poor coping in a chronically ill child.

Child Health and the Family

Family disturbance has been linked to childhood psychopathology in both physically healthy and chronically ill populations. However, when a child has a chronic illness, family problems are often linked to health problems in the child. Reviews of the literature suggest that youngsters in poor diabetic control often live in less than ideal family circumstances (Anderson & Auslander, 1980; Johnson, 1980). In one of the few longitudinal studies available, Koski and Kumento (1975) followed a sample of diabetic youngsters over a five-year period. A high incidence of family disruption was found among youngsters whose health deteriorated. Family adversity in poorly controlled diabetic children has also been reported by Gath, Smith, and Baum (1980). Simonds (1977) noted an unusually low rate of divorce in families of well-controlled patients as compared to those with unstable diabetes or nondiabetic comparison groups. The Simonds (1977) study suggests the interesting hypothesis that good control may be associated with unusually healthy or well-integrated families. Even "normal" family conflicts may be related to poor control in some youngsters.

Clinicians who treat diabetic children have pointed to specific family patterns as particularly detrimental to the patient's health. The most common include (a) overanxious patterns; (b) overindulgent patterns; (c) overcontrolling patterns; (d) patterns of resentment and rejection; and (e) disinterest and neglect (Johnson, 1980). Minuchin and his colleagues have done the most extensive theorizing regarding the relationship between parental or family patterns and the child's diabetic condition. They suggest that psychological factors may influence diabetes in two ways. First, emotional disturbance may result in behavior problems (e.g., refusing to take insulin and eating inappropriately), which can have metabolic consequences. Second, emotional disturbance may cause metabolic derangements directly through psychophysiological mechanisms. It is this latter relationship that the authors have termed "psychosomatic" and that has been the focus of their research. In particular, they have studied the role the family may play in producing "psychosomatic" diabetes.

Their psychosomatic family is defined by four characteristics: (1) enmeshment to such an extent that individual identities and roles are unclear; (2) overprotectiveness toward all family members; (3) rigidity in maintaining the status quo; and (4) lack of conflict resolution. The sick child plays an important role in the family's attempts at conflict avoidance. However, some family conflict unavoidably occurs, leading to emotional and physiological arousal, described as the "turn-on" phase. In the psychosomatic family the turn off phase (or return to normal levels of physiological responding) is handicapped by the family's attempts to avoid conflict with a consequent lack of conflict resolution (Baker, Minuchin, Milman, Leibman, & Todd, 1975; Minuchin, Rosman, & Baker, 1978). In order to test this model, stress was induced in several individuals within the context of a family interview and physiological responding was monitored. The model seemed to aptly describe some children with diabetes; stress led to an increase in arousal and free fatty acid production that did not "turn off" once the interview was terminated (Baker et al., 1975; Minuchin et al., 1978).

Research findings by Anderson et al. (1981) also offer some support for this model. Parents of well-controlled compared to poorly controlled youngsters encouraged greater independence and direct expression of feelings within the context of a relatively cohesive, conflict-free environment. Family therapy has been reported to be helpful when managing poorly controlled diabetic children (Minuchin et al., 1975), although no appropriate control groups have been used. Although these studies are supportive of the psychosomatic family hypothesis, it is unclear how many children with unstable diabetes come from such families.

Little is known as to how physiologically reactive psychosomatic diabetic youngsters are to most any stress, including family conflict. Certainly, specific family patterns (e.g., conflict avoidance) might develop in response to heightened somatic reactivity rather than being a unique cause of it. It is also unclear how applicable Minuchin et al.'s (1975) model is to other chronic illness groups (Burbeck, 1979; Loader, Kinston, & Stratford, 1980). Minuchin and his colleagues should be commended for providing a specific model of how particular family interaction patterns might result in health or illness in a chronically ill child. However, more empirical work needs to be done to confirm or disconfirm this model.

It is likely that no one model will be descriptive of all chronically ill families or even all families within one chronic illness group. Wikran, Faleide, and Blakar (1978), for example, pointed out that parents of asthmatic children are a heterogeneous group. In their study, two thirds of both parents studied showed communication patterns that were as efficient as those of controls. However, one third of the sample demonstrated extremely inefficient communication. It is this subgroup that might have particular problems managing a child with asthma. There is little doubt that some chronically ill children are negatively affected by exposure to certain family environmental conditions. Specifying which children will be affected by what family characteristics remains a difficult, but important topic for further inquiry.

IMPACT OF THE CHILD'S ILLNESS ON THE FAMILY

A family with a chronically ill child must exert a great deal of effort to manage effectively the child's disease while encouraging normal psychological development in the child. At the same time, the youngster's illness may seriously impact on the family. Preventing the illness from disrupting normal family functioning is an important goal that often receives too little attention. Our focus is usually on the patient and how the family hinders or helps with the management of the child's disease and general adjustment. Stein and Riessman (1980) have suggested that chronic illness may negatively impact upon the family financially. It may influence the quality and quantity of interactions outside of and within the family unit. It may cause considerable personal strain and distress for one or both parents. Siblings of the affected child may receive less parental attention. However, it is also possible that the illness may impact positively as well as negatively on the family's functioning. There may be increased sharing, support, and heightened self-esteem gained by the family's efforts to cope with and master the stress of the illness. Although such positive effects are certainly possible, the available literature has focused exclusively on negative consequences of the child's illness.

Financial Effects

There is no doubt that a child's chronic illness may be a serious financial burden. In survey studies, approximately 60% of parents with severely disabled children feel they have financial problems (Satterwhite, 1978). One or both parents often take on supplementary employment, leaving less time for the children and for each other (McCollum, 1971). How well the child's illness is controlled often has a direct bearing on the family's finances, with more seriously ill children requiring more frequent and more expensive medical intervention (McCollum, 1971; Vance & Taylor, 1971). In addition to the costs of medicines, special equipment, and hospitalizations, there are other less obvious expenses. These include the need for special diets, custom clothing, special living arrangements, travel expenses to see the doctor, time off from work for medical visits, and increased insurance premiums.

Effects upon Interactions Within the Family

A youngster's chronic illness can potentially affect parent–child relationships, sibling–child relationships, sibling–parent relationships, and marital relationships.

Although divorce rates do not appear to be unusually high among parents of chronically ill youngsters, there is some evidence of increased marital disharmony (Begleiter, Burry, & Harris, 1976; Lansky, Cairns, Hassanein, Wehr, & Lowman, 1978; Satterwhite, 1978). Parents often report that there is insufficient time to devote to their spouse (Turk, 1964). It is doubtful that all chronic illnesses affect marital relationships in the same way. Some illnesses may be more stressful than others (Lansky et al., 1978).

Many parents struggle with disciplinary issues particularly in regard to the sick child (Driscoll & Lubin, 1958). They frequently view themselves as more dominant and strict when dealing with their ill son or daughter (Long & Moore, 1979). Siblings tend to see parents as overindulgent and overprotective of the sick child (Cairns, Clark, Smith, & Lansky, 1979). However, not all authors report differences in patient versus sibling disciplinary practices (King, 1981; Steinhausen, 1976). Peterson (1972) interviewed adolescents regarding how controlling they perceived their parents to be (i.e., how strongly the parent attempted to direct the youngster to behave according to parent determined standards of conduct). A similar evaluation was made as to how interested the adolescents perceived their parents to be in the adolescents' activities, concerns, problems, and so forth. Compared with healthy youngsters, the chronically ill adolescents interviewed did not view their parents as more controlling or concerned. However, when ill, they did perceive changes in both parent–patient and patient–sibling relationships. Both parents and siblings were viewed as being "friendlier" and "nicer" during illness episodes. Parents were also seen as exerting greater control over the patient when sick. The chronically ill adolescents also admitted to pretending to be ill more often than their healthy peers. This suggests that some patients may use their illness to get things they want and to avoid experiences or responsibilities they dislike. In one study of parental attitudes toward diabetes, the child's use of illness to manipulate others was a concern expressed by both mothers and fathers (Johnson, 1982).

Not only do parents sometimes feel that there is insufficient time to devote to each other, but siblings are often ignored or given less than ideal amounts of attention. Some studies suggest that physically healthy brothers and sisters of sick children often feel isolated, deprived, outside of family relationships, and have difficulty openly discussing their feelings with other family members (Cairns et al., 1979; Taylor, 1980; Turk, 1964). Other studies report that very few mothers feel that their ill child's presence has seriously interfered with their care of siblings (Breslau, Weitzman, & Messenger, 1981). There is, however, very little empirical data addressing this issue.

Effects on Relationships Outside the Family

Several authors have commented that a child's chronic illness may limit or interfere with family members' experiences outside the family (Anderson, Miller, Auslander, & Santiago, 1981; Turk, 1964) although very few studies have tested the validity of this assumption. A factor analysis of a measure developed by Stein and Riessman (1980) called the Impact-on-Family Scale suggested that interference with relationships outside the family was highly related to interference with relationships within the family. In other words, if a family member felt that a child's chronic illness had disrupted interactions between family members, they usually felt that the illness had been problematic for their relationships with persons outside the family as well.

Personal Distress

In previous sections we have discussed the interplay between the child's psychological adjustment and his or her physical health. In this section, the personal distress of parents and siblings of the child is emphasized.

A number of studies suggest that mothers in particular may experience significant strain when coping with a child's chronic illness or serious burns. Wright and Fulwiler (1974) reported that although burned children did not differ from healthy controls on several psychological variables, their mothers experienced significantly more distress than mothers of healthy children. Other investigators have described similar findings. Mothers are often more neurotic, depressed, introverted, lacking in self-confidence, and generally more distressed than either fathers of chronically ill youngsters or mothers of healthy controls (Borner & Steinhausen, 1977; Breslau, Staruch, & Mortimer, 1982; Gayton, Friedman, Tavormina, & Tucker, 1977; Tavormina, Boll, Dunn, Luscomb, & Taylor, 1981; Tew & Laurence, 1976). Although experiencing increased personal strain, mothers' general parenting attitudes often do not differ from comparison groups (Boll, Dimino, & Mattsson, 1978; Tavormina et al., 1981). Because mothers are usually the primary caretakers of chronically ill children (King, 1981; Tavormina et al., 1981), they may experience greater demands upon their personal resources and consequently feel more distressed. The fact that most children with chronic illness appear to cope reasonably well is a tribute to their parents' (and most frequently their mothers') efforts at managing the child's disease and helping the child cope. However, mothers in their efforts to assist the child with his or her illness may suffer significant distress. The literature on this topic, although limited, is highly consistent. A greater focus on maternal adjustment to the child's illness seems warranted.

Even less appears to be known about paternal adjustment. The few existing studies present somewhat inconsistent findings. Borner and Steinhausen (1977) and Tavormina et al. (1981) reported that fathers of chronically ill children were similar to fathers of healthy controls on a number of personality indices. However, Tavormina et al. did suggest that fathers' attitudes toward child rearing and parenting seemed to have been negatively influenced by the presence of a chronically ill child. The investigation of Gayton et al. (1977) indicated that both mothers and fathers of children with cystic fibrosis had similar perceptions about their family and both believed that the family would be more satisfied and better adjusted if it did not have to cope with a seriously ill child. Almost a third of the fathers studied showed evidence of significant psychopathology, scoring at least two standard deviations above the mean on one or more clinical scales of the Minnesota Multiphasic Personality Inventory. Cummings (1976) also reported that fathers of chronically ill youngsters were more depressed and felt less competent than fathers of a healthy child comparison group.

Like maternal and paternal adjustment, sibling reactions have received only limited investigation. Some studies find little evidence of psychological problems among brothers and sisters of chronically ill children (Gath, 1972; Gayton et al., 1977). Others report that although overall indices of adjustment suggest that siblings are quite normal, more specific indices suggest some impairment (Breslau, Weitzman, & Messenger, 1981; Cairns, Clark, Smith, & Lansky, 1979; Lavigne & Ryan, 1979). However, the nature of this impairment differs from study to study, with some authors pointing to increased social withdrawal and feelings of isolation (Cairns et al., 1977; Lavigne & Ryan, 1979) and others describing increases in aggressive or acting-out behaviors (Breslau et al., 1981).

The inconsistencies found in this literature are probably the result of several factors. Studies vary in the measures used and the populations assessed. Although the population of parents or siblings as a whole may not be experiencing serious distress as a consequence of living with a chronically ill child, a substantial minority of these individuals may indeed have problems coping with the added demands or stresses placed upon them. In some studies, this minority may be sufficiently large to yield significant group differences. In other studies, this may not be the case. Parents and siblings of chronically ill children, like the patients themselves, may be a group that is "high risk" for developing social and emotional problems. Our task is to define what factors or variables are associated with good versus poor adaptation.

TREATMENT

This chapter has focused on the family and the child with chronic illness. Consequently, only those treatments specifically addressing family problems or treatment designed to assist the child within the family context will be discussed. There are, of course, treatment or educational programs aimed at helping individual children cope with one or more aspects of their medical management. For example, preparation programs using peer-modeling techniques have sometimes been helpful for children facing unpleasant medical procedures (Melamed & Siegel, 1975). Because these programs are aimed at the individual patient and do not typically involve the family, they will not be reviewed here. Also, most of these programs are aimed at children with acute illness, which makes their application to chronically ill populations questionable (Gilbert et al., 1982).

Family-oriented programs for chronically ill children can be conceptualized along a continuum from educational supportive approaches that might be appropriate for many or all families to more intense, psychotherapeutic strategies aimed at particularly problematic patients and their families. However, there are little empirical data addressing the usefulness of any of these approaches.

Parent-Inclusive Pediatric Units

Because chronically ill youngsters are typically hospitalized during the course of their diagnosis and treatment, the role of the family in the child's hospitalization is an important consideration. Parental support for the child in times of distress is now considered so important that most hospitals offer liberal visiting privileges. However, the extent of these privileges and the use hospital personnel make of family members vary from hospital to hospital. A survey study by Hardgrove and Kermoian (1978) indicated that two thirds of the hospitals responding to their questionnaire provided sleeping arrangements for parents but only one half of the hospitals allowed well siblings to visit. One third of the hospitals provided parent education either prior to or after the child's hospitalization. An even smaller percentage provided parental support groups; parents were often barred from medical tests and procedures administered to their child. As the authors point out, institutional support for family members' presence is usually limited to providing sleeping arrangements for the child's parents. Although parental visiting privileges are often liberal, hospitals do not seem to make optimal use of parents.

There are, of course, exceptions. A few hospitals have developed "parent care units" in which parents are trained to take a primary role in the care of the hospitalized child. These programs seem to be ideal for parents who need to develop expertise in managing their child's illness or who have fears of being able to handle their youngster's medical problems once the child returns home. These programs appear to be cost effective—costing less than routine hospital care (Tonkin, 1979; Vermilion, Ballantine, & Grosfeld, 1979).

Supportive Approaches

In an effort to provide support to families with a chronically ill child, Pless and Satterwhite (1972) trained six laypersons to serve as family counselors. All six were women and four of the six had a child with a chronic disease in their own family. They served as listeners, educators, and advisors to 48 families, helping to provide and coordinate relevant services. They worked an average of 4.6 hours per month per family, which included home visits and telephone contacts. Mothers who received this assistance appeared to be very pleased with the program and saw their children as better adjusted psychologically compared with control families who were not assigned a family counselor. The program appeared to be less effective with families who had multiple problems, thus suggesting that supportive approaches may be best for relatively normal families facing an abnormal situation (i.e., a chronically ill child).

Support groups have also been advocated for this population. However, the literature on this topic has been generally limited to program descriptions (Hill & Hynes, 1980; Johnson, 1982; Kartha & Ertel, 1976; Mattsson & Agle, 1972). These programs differ in terms of group membership (parents only versus children only versus families), number of sessions (limited versus open ended), and session content (specific topics or tasks versus unstructured discussion). However, they have a number of characteristics in common. They are aimed at normal families facing chronic illness in a child. They assume that interactions with other families facing a similar dilemma are therapeutic. Their goals are to help the family successfully cope with the consequences of the child's illness and to educate the family as to the best methods for managing the youngster's disease.

One of the few empirical studies using group therapy was described by Hock (1977). This study differs from others not only in its attempt to evaluate program effectiveness, but also in its focus on families with asthmatic boys who had distinct psychological problems. Youngsters were seen in groups separate from their parents and were given relaxation training and assertiveness exercises. They were encouraged to openly discuss their emotions, feelings of anger, and ways of expressing anger. Parents in separate groups discussed child management problems, feelings toward their children, and other interpersonal concerns. After one year, treated children had significantly improved pulmonary function as compared to controls. Unfortunately, this study did not use random assignment to treatment/control groups and does not permit any assessment of the importance of the group process. No follow-up data were collected and the study's use of Forced Expiratory Volume/First Second (a measure of pulmonary function) as the sole outcome variable can be criticized. Forced expiratory volume measures show only a weak correlation with other measures of airway resistance and depend on the patient's willingness to cooperate. Thus they reflect motivational factors as well as pulmonary function (Richter & Dahme, 1982). Although certainly useful, the study could have been improved by using multiple outcome measures.

Behavioral Interventions

In a number of studies, parents have been taught to use reinforcement programs to increase compliance with medical management programs. Lowe and Lutzker (1979) used written instruction and a reward system to increase foot care, urine testing, and appropriate dietary intake in a nine-year-old girl with diabetes. Nineteen diabetic youngsters were studied by Epstein and his colleagues (1981). In the context of an intensive educational program, parents were taught to use praise and points to reward children not only for conducting urine tests, but also for getting "good" results (i.e., urine glucose readings of less than 1%). This study and a subsequent report (Carney, Schechter, & Davis, 1983) suggest that behavioral methods may be effectively used by families to improve patient adherence, and improved adherence may result in improved health. Although few in number, these studies indicate that behavioral interventions may be powerful methods to help families with daily management aspects of the child's disease (King, 1980).

Family Therapy

Family therapy is based on the assumption that the patient's problems are a function of a maladaptive family structure. When this is the case, individually oriented psychotherapy will be unsuccessful because it does not address the role of the patient's problems within the family constellation. Minuchin and his colleagues (1975) have been the primary proponents of this form of treatment. Because chronically ill children are physiologically vulnerable, the child's illness may encourage overinvolvement by one parent. This parent, usually the mother, then neglects other family members. Her neglect places strain on the marital relationship and also results in feelings of hostility toward the patient by siblings. However, these feelings of resentment are not expressed openly because the patient is not to be "upset." The parents' focus on the child's symptoms permit them to avoid their own marital conflicts and consequently the patient's symptoms are reinforced. In order to help the patient, these maladaptive family patterns must be identified and changed. Efforts are first directed at alleviating the child's symptoms so as to decrease the family's use of the patient's illness as a means of avoiding or detouring family conflict. This then gives the family more freedom to identify family patterns that seem to exacerbate the child's illness. Thus the structure and the functioning of the family are changed in order to develop and promote more healthy family interactions (Liebman, Minuchin, and Baker, 1974).

Although Minuchin et al.'s conceptualizations have intuitive appeal and enjoy widespread clinical application, little empirical data are available as to their effectiveness with chronically ill populations. The authors have provided evidence that family therapy has been useful for children with intractable asthma, superlabile diabetes, and anorexia nervosa (Minuchin et al., 1975; Liebman, Minuchin, & Baker, 1974). However, controlled studies are needed.

Residential Treatment

When all efforts to treat a child on an outpatient basis have failed, residential treatment is often suggested. The treatment of intractable asthma has the longest history utilizing this approach. Dr. Murray Peshkin was the earliest advocate of convalescent care in which asthmatic children were removed from their own homes and successfully treated in different environments, separate from their families. As early as 1930, he made a plea for the development of such homes after working with asthmatic youngsters. About 10% of his patients maintained their illness despite all attempts to manage them medically and to remove any allergens from their home environments. Yet most of these youngsters became symptom free when hospitalized. It was not until 1935, however, that Peshkin began to suspect a psychological component to these children's illness. Prior to that time, he believed that hospitalization was effective because it removed the child from some unknown allergen in the child's usual living environment. In 1935, when reviewing his patients' records, he noted that many hospitalized children would have asthma attacks that coincided with maternal visits. Thereafter he began to focus on the mother–child relationship as a possible exacerbating influence on the child's asthmatic condition. He coined the term "parentectomy," and recommended separating the child from his or her parents for as long as two years (Robinson, 1972).

Additional support for separating the child and family as a treatment modality came from the work of Long et al. (1958) who reported that children with intractable asthma remained symptom free while hospitalized even when their rooms were sprayed with dust collected from the children's homes. Purcell et al. (1969) took the interesting approach of removing the family from the child's home and studying asthmatic symptomatology in the child while cared for by a parent substitute. Predictions were made as to which of 25 children studied would beenfit from this approach and which would not. Youngsters with a history of asthma attacks that were precipitated by emotional upset were predicted to do best The data supported the authors' hypothesis. Those children with emotional precipitants improved when the family left home and worsened when they returned.

Residential treatment programs for intractable asthmatic patients have been developed in both the United States and Europe. Youngsters usually reside in these programs for a year or more. Most programs report good success while the child is in the residential facility, but problems often reappear when the child returns home (Kapotes, 1977; Kellock, 1970; Peshkin, 1968; Purcell et al., 1969; Sadler, 1975). As Sadler has pointed out, providing residential treatment for a child may give a family a much needed rest. However, when the child's problems are a function of the family's maladaptive interactions, the child's hospitalization may only defer any resolution of the family's pathology. The child may get better while in residential treatment but become difficult to treat effectively when returned home.

Residential treatment facilities aimed at chronically ill children are much more common in Europe than in the United States (Peshkin, 1968; Rosenbloom, 1983). However, physicians who treat childhood diabetes in the United States report that they need such facilities for 5–12% of their patients. Rarely are there appropriate facilities available (Rosenbloom, 1982).

During the past three years we have developed a residential treatment program for youngsters with insulin-dependent diabetes. Youngsters admitted have a history of repeated hospitalizations and school absences. Their diabetes has remained in poor control despite intensive efforts to manage the child on an outpatient basis. The facility consists of an apartment with three bedrooms, a living room, kitchen, several baths, and two staff offices. Up to four youngsters can be housed at any one time. Because the program is physically situated in a University Hospital, the children are medically managed by the hospital's pediatric endocrinologists. Yet their life is more "normal" than would be the case in a hospital pediatric ward. The youngsters are supervised by child care workers with expertise in juvenile diabetes and they attend public school in the local community.

Treatment is focused on the psychological as well as the medical management of the child. Separating the child and family permits the child's diabetes to be stabilized in a controlled environment. At the same time, the demands of school, parent substitutes, and fellow patients normalize the child's environment, making it more "homelike" than is possible in a pediatric hospital setting. The purpose of the program is not to provide long-term residential treatment. Rather, methods of successfully managing the children and their diabetes are developed and then communicated to the youngsters' families. Parents must agree to participate in family therapy on a weekly basis during the child's residence and every effort is made to follow these families once the child is discharged.

When the child is first admitted to the program, a thorough assessment is made of the patient's and parents' knowledge about diabetes and their management skills. The youngster's food preferences and usual activity level is monitored. The parents' eating habits and activity level are discussed as well. The parents' role in the management of the child's illness at both an active and a supervisory level is evaluated. These data serve as the basis of educational sessions for both the patient and parent. Beyond this type of information exchange, family sessions are aimed at dealing with the patient's and parents' affect about one or more aspects of their relationship. One or both parents may be angry at the child for repeated dietary (or other) indiscretions. A mother may be angry or hurt that her husband offers so little help with managing the child's illness. The patient may be responding to perceived parental disinterest except when the patient is in crisis. Siblings may blame the ill child for everything that goes wrong in the family. These problems are approached in several ways. The child's manipulative behaviors, misconceptions, and disciplinary problems usually become apparent to the residential treatment staff within two to three weeks of the youngster's admission. Plans are made to encourage and reward more appropriate attention-seeking behaviors.

Once the youngster is functioning well in the residential setting, home visits are initiated so that treatment gains can be "practiced" at home. These visits provide an opportunity for the family to identify specific problem areas and to try different ways of dealing with these difficulties. At least once during the child's stay, we encourage the family to move into our residential setting for a weekend. This provides us with an opportunity to do a more complete assessment of the family's usual style of interaction and provides the family with an intense educational experience that they have found to be very useful.

One measure of the program's success is change in the child's total glycosolated hemoglobin (HbA_1) levels, a widely accepted and objective indicator of diabetic control. Although children without diabetes have HbA_1 levels in the 7–10% range, youngsters with diabetes have generally higher values (8–23%). Youngsters in poor control have high HbA_1 levels, whereas patients in good control have values closer to nondiabetic youngsters (Williams & Savage, 1979).

Figures 8.1 and 8.2 describe the HbA_1 levels of 13 children admitted to our facility. Values prior to treatment, during residence, and at follow-up are provided. Children varied in length of stay from two to six months and available follow-up data ranged from two to 24 months. Note that all 13 children show decreases in HbA_1 levels within the first two months of inpatient treatment. Some of these patients (Figure 8.1) seemed to maintain these gains throughout their stay with us. These youngsters were referred to as "stable responders" because their diabetes, once stabilized, remained in relatively good control as long as the child was in residence. Other youngsters showed initial improvement in diabetic control, but began to deteriorate prior to discharge (see Figure 8.2). A review of this second group of children's case histories suggests that their deterioration was associated with increased therapeutic efforts aimed at discharging the child back to the home environment.

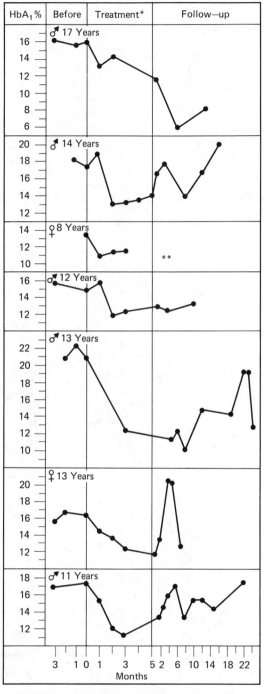

* Treatment varied from two to five months
** HbA$_1$ values unavailable. Repeated hospitalizations

FIGURE 8.1 Pretreatment, treatment, and follow-up HbA$_1$ values for stable responders.

243

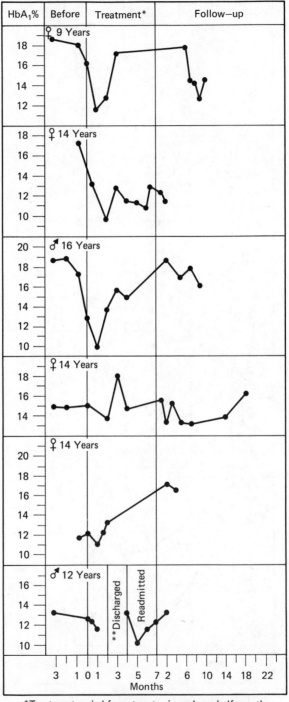

*Treatment varied from two to six and one half months
**HbA, values unavailable. Repeated hospitalizations.

FIGURE 8.2 Pretreatment, treatment, and follow-up HbA₁ values for stress responders.

244

Soon after a child is admitted to our facility, work with the family begins. However, this work intensifies and plans for discharge become more explicit over the course of the child's residential treatment. For some youngsters, deterioration in diabetes control seemed to be a direct result of the stress engendered by therapeutic activities focused on the patient's ultimate discharge. We have labeled these patients "stress responders" because initial improvements in diabetic control were not maintained once the patient was faced with discharge. The idea that there are two types of patients—stable responders and stress responders—who respond to our program quite differently is, of course, a working hypothesis in need of further validation. Also of note is the high relapse rate found in both stable and stress responders. Most of the youngsters returned to pretreatment levels of HbA$_1$ once discharged, although the length of time it took for this to occur varied considerably from individual to individual.

Our experiences suggest that so-called brittle diabetes is clearly treatable. Youngsters with difficult to control diabetes improved when removed from their families and placed in a residential program. However, some of these youngsters appeared to be more "stress-sensitive" than others. For them, planning their return to their home environment seemed to induce deterioration in diabetes control even prior to discharge. In our small sample, whether or not the patient was stress-sensitive appeared to be unrelated to relapse rates once discharged. Patients who regularly participated in outpatient therapy seemed to do better at follow-up. Although outpatient therapy is regularly recommended for all patients, many families either refuse to participate or participate irregularly. Many of our patients come from lower socioeconomic backgrounds and feel they lack the financial resources to pay the transportation costs of regularly scheduled outpatient visits. Many parents' inability to give their child's diabetes priority attention except when the patient is in crisis is characteristic of the family's pathology. For some families, relatively short-term residential placement for the patient with intensive family therapy and regular outpatient care may be a successful approach to help the family cope with the child's diabetes. For other families, the parents' unwillingness to make any significant changes and their inability to successfully manage the child's diabetes demand that an alternative approach be considered. Perhaps in this very small subgroup of chronically ill youngsters, more permanent residential placement should be a viable option. European countries have considerable experience with this approach although empirical data are lacking (Rosenbloom, 1983).

METHODOLOGICAL ISSUES

Our knowledge about the family and the child with chronic illness is necessarily limited by our methodological sophistication. Unfortunately, a number of methodological problems exist in the current literature.

Measurement

First and foremost is the general lack of reliable and valid methods of measuring families. This is a difficult task, but one that must be given serious attention if advances are to be made in this field. Of course, measurement problems are not limited to the assessment of families. Other variables presumed to be related to family functioning are often measured inadequately. For example, child adjustment is frequently assessed by clinician ratings and the health of the child is often determined by physician judgments. Such global measures are potentially unreliable and may be particularly subject to bias.

Construct Independence

When studying the relationship between family functioning, child adjustment, and child health, it is important that each of these variables be clearly defined and measured independently. Often the same individual (e.g., the physician) rates the child's and the family's ability to "cope" and provides some estimate of the child's health. This introduces the possibility of spurious relationships between variables. A related problem is the lack of clear differentiation between constructs. For example, compliance with recommended treatment is sometimes confused with more metabolic parameters in studies assessing diabetic control (Keiding, Root, & Marble, 1952; Lowery & Ducette, 1976; Stone, 1961). Although compliance or adherent behaviors are presumed to be related to the health status of the child, these two constructs must be defined and assessed separately if their interrelationship is to be understood.

Specificity

Global terms such as "compliance," "health," "adjustment," "family functioning," and even "chronic illness" are commonly used. However, they offer too little information as to what the child did or did not do that affected what specific aspects of his or her health or psychological adjustment. Research in this area demands greater attention to specifics that can be reliably measured. Investigations that focus on one chronic illness and the particular behaviors that are necessry to manage that illness may be more productive than studies that attempt to study "chronic illness" and "compliance" in general.

Theoretical Clarity

Although it is reasonable to assume that family functioning influences child health and adjustment (and vice versa), the mechanisms by which this occurs are often left unclear. For example, family variables are frequently correlated with child health variables, but the intervening variables (e.g., patient or parent knowledge about the disease, compliance with treatment tasks) are left unmeasured. Methods need to be developed to measure these intervening variables, and the nature of the relationships between specific family characteristics and child variables needs to be more clearly hypothesized.

Correlational/Longitudinal Approaches

Most of the available research in this area has been correlational in nature. Several parameters are studied at a single point in time and relationships between variables are noted. Cause and effect cannot be determined. Nevertheless, correlational methods permit the identification of relationships in need of further study without the expense incurred by longitudinal approaches. When sufficient evidence is accumulated using correlational methods, longitudinal studies should be designed and undertaken. Particularly in an area like childhood chronic illness, much of what needs to be known is not a static event but a process. Children grow and change, diseases get better or worse, parent–child relationships differ depending upon the youngster's maturity. Both correlational and longitudinal approaches have their advantages and limitations. Both should be appropriately used to better understand this process.

Who Is Studied

When studying the family and the child with chronic illness, there has been a tendency to focus on the patient and the mother. Fathers and siblings are often ignored. Yet there is evidence that each member of the family (patient, mother, father, and sibling) may differ in terms of knowledge, attitudes, emotions, and behaviors relevant to the child's condition. To properly understand the role of the family, greater consideration needs to be given to which family members are studied. Probably of equal importance is the relationship between different family members' perceptions. Similarities and differences between family members' views may be as important as the perceptions themselves.

Other Environmental Variables

The importance of studying the chronically ill child within an environmental context has gained widespread acceptance in the past few years. Previously, the emphasis was on the patient and particular patient characteristics that were indicative of good or poor adjustment. The child's family has now become a primary focus of attention. Although this is a laudable change in both our conceptual and practical approaches to this population, the family is not the only environmental variable of potential influence. Family support systems and physician or health provider behaviors are other environmental factors in need of further research scrutiny.

SUMMARY

It is estimated that chronically ill children now comprise nearly 50% of pediatric practice. Historically, the psychosocial literature has focused primarily on personality traits or other indices of emotional adjustment in this population. However, because children are highly dependent upon their parents, the family should play a primary role in the child's adaptation to his or her disease. Similarly, the child's illness should impact upon the family. Although these assumptions seem reasonable, it is important to recognize that research in this area is in its infancy. Nevertheless, certain significant areas have emerged that seem to warrant further investigation.

First, there are issues related to the family's managing or helping the child manage the illness. These include family educational programs, parent–physician as well as patient–physician communication, and developing data-based guidelines for defining parent versus child responsibilities. The child's cognitive developmental level should be given greater consideration in all these areas (i.e., educating the child, communicating with the patient about the disease, and assigning disease management tasks to the youngster).

Second, there are issues related to helping the child cope with the disease. It is remarkable that most chronically ill youngsters appear to cope reasonably well. However, those youngsters in poorer health do seem to have more adjustment problems. The mechanisms by which the child's psychological status is related to his or her physical condition are not entirely clear. In some cases, the severity of the illness may negatively impact on the child's psychological adjustment. In other cases, negative attitudes may result in poor adherence with recommended treatment. Or emotional upset may negatively influence certain conditions such as diabetes and asthma through the direct and indirect effects of the stress hormones.

Although family functioning is presumed to relate to children's psychological adjustment, there is little agreement as to what family characteristics are most critical to what aspects of adjustment in the child. One fruitful approach may be to study specific demands placed upon the child (e.g., taking medication, cooperating with painful medical procedures) and the relationship of parental or family variables to the child's success at coping with these demands.

Just as family functioning is presumed to be related to a child's psychological adjustment, it is also presumed to relate to the child's health. In support of this hypothesis, there is some evidence that youngsters in poorer health come from less than ideal family circumstances. How certain family characteristics result in good or poor health in the child is often left unspecified. Certain family constellations may result in poor adherence with treatment regimens. In other cases, the stress of the family's maladaptive functioning may result in metabolic derangements in the child with resultant negative health effects. It is unlikely that one family pattern will be characteristic of all families of children with chronic illness. Rather, our goal should be to identify subgroups of children that appear to be negatively or positively affected by certain family characteristics.

Of course, evidence of maladaptive family functioning could be the result of as well as a cause of a child's poor health. In fact, the impact of the child's illness on the family has received relatively little attention and is a third area in need of further investigation. We do know that mothers usually serve as the primary caretakers for the chronically ill child. There are limited data suggesting that mothers of these children may be particularly subject to personal distress. There are also very few published studies addressing the impact of the child's disease on the father and siblings. Parents and siblings of chronically ill children, like the patients themselves, may be at "high risk" for developing social and emotional problems. Our task is to define what factors are associated with good versus poor adaptation.

Treatment research assessing the effectiveness of family-oriented intervention programs is also needed. Such programs include parent-inclusive pediatric units, individual and group supportive therapies, behavioral interventions, family therapy, and residential treatment. The nature and content of family problems and pathology seem to be particularly important parameters in selecting particular intervention strategies. The fact that some families are unwilling to change in spite of the child's deteriorating health raises an ethical and moral dilemma. For some, permanent separation of the child from the family may be necessary if the child is to survive.

Our knowledge about the family and the child with chronic illness is necessarily limited by our methodological sophistication. Reliable and valid methods of measuring families and other relevant constructs (e.g., health status) are needed. Variables selected for study should be clearly defined and measured independently. Where possible, global terms such as "compliance," "health," and "family functioning" should be avoided and replaced by more specific terminology. Investigations that focus on one chronic illness and the particular behaviors that are necessary to manage that illness may be more productive than studies that attempt to study chronic illness or compliance in general. Specific mechanisms by which two or more variables (e.g., family functioning and child health) are presumed to relate need to be hypothesized and tested. Based upon data obtained from our initial correlational investigations, longitudinal studies need to be designed and conducted so that the changing nature of the child, the disease, and the family may be given greater appreciation.

REFERENCES

Anderson, B., & Auslander, W. (1980). Research on diabetes management and the family: A critique. *Diabetes Care, 3*, 696–671.

Anderson, B., Miller, J., Auslander, W., & Santiago, J. (1981). Family characteristics of diabetic adolescents: Relationship to metabolic control. *Diabetes Care, 4*, 586–594.

Baker, L., Minuchin, S., Milman, L., Leibman, R., & Todd, T. (1975). Psychosomatic aspects of juvenile diabetes melitus: A progress report. In Z. Laron (Ed.), *Diabetes in juveniles: Medical and rehabilitation aspects: Vol. 12. Modern problems in pediatrics.* New York: Karger

Begleiter, M., Burry, V., & Harris, D. (1976). Prevalence of divorce among parents of children with cystic fibrosis and other chronic diseases. *Social Biology, 23*, 260–264.

Boll. T., Dimino, E., & Mattsson, A. (1978). Parenting attitudes: The role of personality style and childhood long-term illness. *Journal of Psychosomatic Research, 22*, 209–213.

Borner, A., Steinhausen, H. C. (1977). A psychological study of family characteristics in juvenile diabetes. *Pediatric and Adolescent Endocrinology, 3*, 46–51.

Breslau, N., Staruch, K., & Mortimer, E. (1982). Psychological distress in mothers of disabled children. *American Journal of Diseases of Childhood, 136*, 682–686.

Breslau, N., Weitzman, M., & Messenger, K. (1981). Psychologic functioning of siblings of disabled children. *Pediatrics, 67*(3), 344–353.

Burbek, T. (1979). An empirical investigation of the psychosomatogenic family model. *Journal of Psychosomatic Research, 23*, 327–337.

Cairns, N., Clark, G., Smith, S., & Lansky, S. (1979). Adaptation of siblings to childhood malignancy. *The Journal of Pediatrics, 95*, 484–487.

Carney, M., Schechter, K., & Davis, S. (1983). Improving adherence to blood glucose testing in insulin-dependent diabetic children. *Behavior Therapy, 14*, 247–254.

Cummings, S. (1976). The impact of the child's deficiency on the father: A study of fathers of mentally retarded and of chronically ill children. *American Journal of Orthopsychiatry, 46*(2), 246–255.

Dahlem, N. W., Kinsman, R. A., & Horton, D. J. (1977). Panic-fear in asthma: Requests for as-needed medications in relation to pulmonary function measurements. *Journal of Allergy and Clinical Immunology, 60*, 295–300.

Dirks, J. F., Jones, N. F., & Kinsman, R. A (1977) Panic-fear: A personality dimension related to intractability in asthma. *Psychosomatic Medicine, 39*, 120–126.

Driscoll, C., & Lubin, A. (1972). Conferences with parents of children with cystic fibrosis. *Social Work*, 140–146.

Drotar, D. (1981). Psychological perspectives of chronic childhood illness. *Journal of Pediatric Psychology, 6*(3), 211–228.

Epstein, L. H., Beck, S., Figueroa, J., Farkas, G., Kazdin, A. E., Kaneman, D., & Becker, D. (1981). The effects of targeting improvements in urine glucose on metabolic control in children with insulin-dependent diabetes. *Journal of Applied Behavior Analysis, 14*, 365–375.

Etzweiler, D. D., & Sines, L. K. (1962). Juvenile diabetes and its management: Family, social and academic implications. *Journal of the American Medical Association, 181*, 94–98.

Francis, V., Korsch, B. M., & Morris, M. J. (1969). Gaps in doctor-patient communication: Patients' response to medical advice. *New England Journal of Medicine, 280*, 535–540.

Freemon, B., Negrete, V. F., Davis, M., & Korsch, B. M. (1971). Gaps in doctor-patient communication: Doctor-patient interaction analysis. *Pediatric Research, 5*, 298–311.

Gath, A. (1972). The mental health of siblings of congenitally abnormal children. *Journal of Child Psychology and Psychiatry, 13,* 211–218.

Gath, A., Smith, M., & Baum, J. (1980). Emotional, behavioral, and educational disorders in diabetic children. *Archives of Disease in Childhood, 55,* 371–375.

Gayton, W., Friedman, S., Tavormina, J., & Tucker, F. (1977). Children with cystic fibrosis: Psychological test findings of patients, siblings, and parents. *Pediatrics, 59,* 888–894.

Gilbert, B. O., Johnson, S. B., Spillar, R., McCallum, M., Silverstein, J., & Rosenbloom, A. (1982). The effects of a peer modeling film on children learning to self-inject insulin. *Behavior Therapy, 13,* 186–193.

Grey, M., Genel, M., & Taborlane, W. (1980). Psychosocial adjustment of latency-aged diabetics: Determinants and relationship to control. *Pediatrics, 65,* 69–73.

Hardgrove, C., & Kermoian, R. (1978). Parent-inclusive pediatric units: A survey of policies and practices. *American Journal of Public Health, 68,* 847–850.

Harkavy, J., Johnson, S. B., Silverstein, J., Spillar, R., McCallum, M., & Rosenbloom, A. (1983). Who learns what at diabetes camp? *Journal of Pediatric Psychology, 8*(2), 143–154.

Hill, E., & Hynes, J. (1980). Fostering self-esteem in families with diabetic children. *Child Welfare, LIX,* 576–582.

Hock, R. (1977). A model for conjoint group therapy for asthmatic children and their parents. *Group Psychotherapy, Psychodrama, and Sociometry, XXX,* 108–113.

Jay, S. M., Ozolins, M., & Elliott, C. H. (1983). Assessment of children's distress during painful medical procedures. *Journal of Health Psychology, 2,* 133–147.

Johnson, M. (1982). Support groups for parents of chronically ill children. *Pediatric Nursing, 8,* 160–163.

Johnson, S. B. (1980). Psychosocial factors in juvenile diabetes: A review. *Journal of Behavioral Medicine, 3,* 95–116.

Johnson, S. B. (1982). *Coping with childhood diabetes.* Presented at the annual meeting of the American Psychological Association, Washington, D.C.

Johnson, S. B., Pollak, R. T., Silverstein, J., Rosenbloom, A., Spillar, R., McCallum, M., & Harkavy, J. (1982). Cognitive and behavioral knowledge about insulin-dependent diabetes among children and parents. *Pediatrics, 69,* 708–713.

Johnson, S. B., & Rosenbloom, A. (1982). Behavioral aspects of diabetes mellitus in childhood and adolescence. *Psychiatric Clinics of North America, 5,* 357–369.

Kapotes, C. (1977). Emotional factors in chronic asthma. *The Journal of Asthma Research, 15*(1), 5–14.

Kaptein, A. A. (1982). Psychological correlates of length of hospitalization and rehospitalization in patients with acute, severe asthma. *Social Science Medicine, 16,* 725–729.

Kartha, M., & Ertel, I. (1976). Short-term therapy for mothers of leukemic children. *Clinical Pediatrics, 15,* 803–808.

Keiding, N., Root, H., & Marble, A. (1952). Importance of control of diabetes in prevention of vascular complications. *Journal of the American Medical Association, 150,* 964.

Kellock, T. D. (1970). Residential care of the diabetic child. *Postgraduate Medical Journal, 46,* 629–630.

King, E. (1981). Child-rearing practices: Child with chronic illness and well sibling. *Issues in Comprehensive Pediatric Nursing, 5,* 185–194.

King, N. (1980). The behavioral management of asthma and asthma-related problems in children: A critical review of the literature. *Journal of Behavioral Medicine, 3,* 169–189.

Korsch, B., Fine, R., & Negrete, V. (1977). Noncompliance in children with renal transplants. *Pediatrics, 61,* 872–876.

Koski, M., & Kumento, A. (1975). Adolescent development and behavior: A psychosomatic follow-up study of childhood diabetics. *Modern Problems in Pediatrics, 12,* 348–353.

Kronenfeld, J., & Ory, M. (1981). Familial perceptions of juvenile diabetes. *Diabetes, 70,* 83–90.

Kucia, C., Drotar, D., Doershuk, C., Stern, R., Boat, T., & Matthews, L. (1979). Home observation of family interaction and childhood adjustment to cystic fibrosis. *Journal of Pediatric Psychology, 4,* 189–195.

Kupst, M., Schulman, J., Honig, G., Maurer, H., Morgan, E., & Fochtman, D. (1982). Family coping with childhood leukemia: One year after diagnosis. *Journal of Pediatric Psychology, 7,* 157–174.

La Greca, A. M., Follansbee, D., & Skyler, J. S. (1982). *Behavioral aspects of diabetes management in children and adolescents.* Presented at the annual meeting of the American Psychological Association, Washington, D.C.

Lansky, S., Cairns, N., Hassanein, R., Wehr, J., & Lowman, J. (1978). Childhood cancer: Parental discord and divorce. *Pediatrics, 62,* 184–188.

Lavigne, T. & Ryan, M. (1979). Psychological adjustment of siblings of children with chronic illness. *Pediatrics, 63,* 616–627.

Lawler, R., Nakielny, W., & Wright, N. (1966). Psychological implications of cystic fibrosis. *Canadian Medical Association Journal, 94,* 1043–1946.

Liebman, R., Minuchin, S., & Baker, L. (1974). The use of structural family therapy in the treatment of intractable asthma. *American Journal of Psychiatry, 131,* 535–540.

Loader, P., Kinston, W., & Stratford, J. (1980). Is there a "psychosomatogenic" family? *Journal of Family Therapy, 2,* 311–326.

Long, C., & Moore, J. (1979). Parental expectations for their epileptic children. *Journal of Child Psychology, 20,* 299–312.

Long, R. T., Lamont, J. H., Whipple, B., Bandler, L., Blom, G. E., Burgin, L., & Jessner, L. (1958). A psychosomatic study of allergic and emotional factors in children with asthma. *American Journal of Psychiatry, 114,* 890–899.

Lowe, K., & Lutzker, J. R. (1979). Increasing compliance to a medical regimen with a juvenile diabetic. *Behavior Therapy, 10,* 57–64.

Lowery, B., & DuCette, J. (1976). Disease-related learning and disease control in diabetes as a function of locus of control. *Nursing Research, 25,* 358.

Magrab, P., & Calcagno, P. (1978). Psychological impact of chronic pediatric conditions. In P. R. Magrab (Ed.), *Psychological Management of Pediatric Problems,* (pp. 3–14.) Baltimore: University Park Press.

Mattsson, A., & Agle, D. (1972). Group therapy with parents of hemophiliacs. *Journal of the American Academy of Child Psychiatry, 11,* 558–571.

Matus, I. (1981). Assessing the nature and clinical significance of psychological contributions to childhood asthma. *American Journal of Orthopsychiatry, 51,* 327–341.

McCollum, A. (1971). Cystic fibrosis: Economic impact upon the family. *American Journal of Public Health, 61,* 1335–1340.

Meijer, A. (1981). A controlled study on asthmatic children and their families. Synopsis of findings. *Israel Journal of Psychiatry, 18*(3), 197–208.

Melamed, B., & Siegel, L. (1975). Reduction of anxiety in children facing hospitalization and surgery by use of filmed modeling. *Journal of Consulting and Clinical Psychology, 43,* 511–521.

Minuchin, S., Baker, L., Rosman, B., Liebman, R., Milman, L., & Todd, T. (1975). A conceptual model of psychosomatic illness in children. *Archives of General Psychiatry, 32,* 1031–1038.

Minuchin, S., Rosman, B., & Baker, L. (1978). *Psychosomatic families*. Cambridge, MA: Harvard University Press.

Nader, P., & Mahan, J. (1976). Measurement of school behavior and performance of chronically ill children. In G. Grave & B. Pless (Eds.), *Chronic childhood illness: Assessment of outcome* (Vol. 3, pp. 167–174). Washington: DHEW Publications.

Peshkin, M. (1968). Analysis of the role of residential asthma centers for children with intractable asthma. *The Journal of Asthma Research, 6*(2), 59–92.

Peterson, E. (1972). The impact of adolescent illness on parental relationships. *Journal of Health and Social Behavior, 13,* 429–437.

Pless, I., Roghmann, K., & Haggerty, R. (1972). Chronic illness, family functioning, and psychological adjustment: A model for the allocation of prevention mental health services. *International Journal of Epidemiology, 1,* 271–277.

Pless, I., & Satterwhite, B. (1972). Chronic illness in childhood: Selection, activities, and evaluation of nonprofessional family counselors. *Clinical Pediatrics, 11*(7), 403–410.

Purcell, K., Brady, K., Chai, H., Muser, J., Molk, L., Gordon, N., and Meand, J. (1969). The effect on asthma in children of experimental separation from the family. *Psychosomatic Medicine, 31,* 144–164.

Richter, R., & Dahme, B. (1982). Bronchial asthma in adults: There is little evidence for the effectiveness of behavioral therapy and relaxation. *Journal of Psychosomatic Research, 26,* 533–540.

Robinson, G. (1972). The story of parentectomy. *The Journal of Asthma Research, 9,* 199–205.

Rosenbloom, A. L. (1982). Need for residential treatment for children with diabetes mellitus. *Diabetes Care, 5,* 545–546.

Rosenbloom, A. L. (1983). Residential treatment centers for children and youth with diabetes mellitus. *Clinical Pediatrics, 22,* 760–763.

Rubenstein, H., King, S., & London, E. (1979). Adolescent and postadolescent asthmatics' perception of their mothers as overcontrolling in childhood. *Adolescence, XIV*(53), 1–18.

Sadler, J. (1975). The long-term hospitalization of asthmatic children. *Pediatric Clinics of North America, 22,* 173–183.

Satterwhite, B. (1978). The impact of chronic illness on child and family: An overview based on five surveys with implications for management. *International Journal of Rehabilitative Research, 1,* 1–17.

Simonds, J. (1976). Psychiatric status of diabetic youth in good and poor control. *International Journal of Psychiatry, 7,* 133–151.

Simonds, J. (1977). Psychiatric status of diabetic youth matched with a control group. *Journal of The American Diabetes Association, 26,* 921–925.

Spinetta, J., & Maloney, L. (1978). The child with cancer: Patterns of communication and denial. *Journal of Consulting and Clinical Psychology, 46,* 1540–1541.

Staudenmayer, H. (1982). Medical manageability and psychosocial factors in childhood asthma. *Journal of Chronic Diseases, 35,* 183–198.

Stein, R., & Riessman, C. (1980). The development of an Impact-on-Family Scale: Preliminary findings. *Medical Care, XVII,* 465–472.

Steinhausen, H. (1976). Hemophilia: A psychological study in chronic disease in juveniles. *Journal of Psychosomatic Research, 20,* 461–467.

Stone, D. (1961). A study of the incidence and causes of poor control in patients with diabetes mellitus. *The American Journal of the Medical Sciences, 241,* 436–442.

Susman, E., Hersch, S., Nannis, E., Strope, B., Woodruff, P., Pizzo, P., & Levine, A. (1982). Conceptions of cancer: Perspectives of child and adolescent patients and their families. *Journal of Pediatric Psychology, 7,* 253–261.

Tal, A., & Miklich, D. (1976). Emotionally induced decreases in pulmonary flow rates in asthmatic children. *Psychosomatic Medicine, 38,* 190–200.

Tarnow, J., & Silverman, S. (1981–1982). The psychophysiologic aspects of stress in juvenile diabetes mellitus. *Psychiatry in Medicine, 11,* 25–44.

Tavormina, J., Boll, R., Dunn, N., Luscomb, R., & Taylor, J. (1981). Psychosocial effects on parents of raising a physically handicapped child. *Journal of Abnormal Child Psycholog, 9,* 121–131.

Taylor, S. (1980). The effect of chronic childhood illnesses upon well siblings. *Maternal-Child Nursing Journal,* 109–116.

Tew, B., & Laurence, K. (1976). The effects of admission to hospital and surgery on children with spina bifida. *Developmental Medicine and Child Neurology, 18* (Suppl. 37), 119–125.

Tonkin, P. (1979). Parent care for the low risk and terminally ill child. *Dimensions in Health Service, 56,* 42–43.

Turk, J. (1964). Impact of cystic fibrosis on family functioning. *Pediatrics, 34,* 67–71.

Vance, V., & Taylor, W. (1971). The financial cost of chronic childhood asthmma. *Annals of Allergy, 29*(9), 455–460.

Vermilion, B., Ballantine, T., & Grosfeld, J. (1979). The effective use of the parent care unit for infants on the surgical service. *Journal of Pediatric Surgery, 14,* 321–324.

Wikran, R., Faleide, A., & Blakar, R. (1978). Communication in the family of the asthmatic child: An experimental approach. *ACTA Psychiatrica Scandinavica, 57,* 11–26.

Williams, M. L. & Savage, D. C. L. (1979). Glycosylated hemoglobin levels in children with diabetes mellitus. *Archives of Disease in Childhood, 54,* 295–298.

Wright, L., & Fulwiler, R. (1974). Long range emotional sequelae of burns: Effects on children and their mothers. *Pediatric Research, 8,* 931–934.

Yancy, W. (1972). Approaches to emotional management of the child with a chronic illness. *Clinical Pediatrics, 11,* 64–67.

Zlatich, D., Kenny, T., Sila, U., & Huang, S. (1982). Parent-child life events: Relation to treatment in asthma. *Journal of Developmental and Behavioral Pediatrics, 3,* 69–72.

9

Chronic Illness in an Adult Family Member: Pain as a Prototype

Herta Flor

Dennis C. Turk

Chronic pain is typically and somewhat arbitrarily viewed as pain of more than six months' duration that is not due to an acute disease process. Chronic pain conditions involve complaints such as low back pain, headaches, abdominal pain, and arthritis. Millions of people are affected by chronic pain and its often debilitating physical, psychological, and financial consequences. In addition to the degree of suffering experienced by the patient and his or her family, Bonica and Butler (1978) estimate that chronic pain syndromes cost the American taxpayer more than 40–50 billion dollars annually in loss of productivity, income tax, and workman's compensation. Pain syndromes therefore deserve the special attention of

Support for the completion of this chapter was provided by Veterans Administration Merit Review Grants.

255

the health care professionals. The poor results of traditional medical approaches to chronic pain (e.g., Flor & Turk, 1984; Toomey, Ghia, Mao, & Gregg, 1977) have led to the development of biopsychosocial models for the etiology and treatment of chronic pain (e.g., Fordyce, 1976; Sternbach, 1974, 1978; Turk, Meichenbaum, & Genest, 1983). The psychological approaches to chronic pain (for overviews see Kerns, Turk, & Holzman, 1983; Turk & Flor, 1984; Turner & Chapman, 1982a,b) have focused almost exclusively on the individual patient, occasionally taking a dyadic perspective, but generally disregarding the role of the family.

It seems to be intuitively obvious that chronic pain affects the functioning of the entire family when one takes into account that chronic pain often leads to permanent disability, loss of employment, high medical expenses, in addition to psychological consequences for the patient such as depression, preoccupation with health-related issues, irritability, and sexual dysfunction. The following case illustrates the impact of chronic pain on all aspects of the patient's and family's lives.

Mr. L was a 46-year-old self-employed trucker who experienced six years of unremitting pain following an accident when he injured his back loading a heavy crate into his truck. At the time of our intitial interview with Mr. L, he indicated that his pain disrupted all aspects of his life. He reported that he was irritable with his wife and his two sons. Mr. L had not worked since his accident and neglected even the most minor chores around his home. Mr. L reported that he was always fatigued as he was never able to have more than a few hours of sleep without being awakened by his pain.

Mrs. L was frustrated and angry with physicians for not succeeding in curing her husband. She was also distressed with her husband for his "incessant" complaining, generally high state of irritability, and lack of participation in decisions regarding his home and his family. She described life with her husband as one of "walking on egg shells," never knowing what would set her husband off on a tirade. She also indicated that she felt in a bind because she loved her husband and felt sorry for him and thus tried not to express her feelings of anger toward him because she did not want him to suffer any more. She reported feeling guilty whenever she was angry and upset because he was suffering. At the time of the interview, Mrs. L was being treated for a peptic ulcer and admitted that she was depressed.

Mr. L's two teenage sons were confused and angry. They tried to spend as little time at home as possible as it seemed nothing they did ever satisfied their father. The more Mr. L's sons stayed away from home the more Mr. L berated them for being insensitive and uncaring. He reported feeling guilty for "blowing up" at them and his inability to control his temper.

Mrs. L had taken a part-time job to compensate for the loss of Mr. L's income and because his medical care had depleted the family's bank account. Mr. L had difficulty accepting his change in role from breadwinner to dependent and expressed his anger toward his wife when she left for work, complaining about the cleanliness of their home.

Mr. L admitted that his behavior and temper had alienated his friends who no longer came to visit or called him. In general, he had no interest in any previously enjoyed activities—recreational, social, or sexual. He indicated that he was ambivalent. On the one hand he wanted to be left alone and on the other hand he wanted support and attention from his family.

The purpose of this chapter is to apply a family perspective to chronic pain. The theoretical framework of this approach as it applies to pain will be discussed and empirical evidence for the role of family interaction in chronic pain syndromes will be evaluated. The following sections examine the role of the family in the pathogenesis, maintenance, coping with, and treatment of chronic pain. Because of the relatively sparse literature specifically addressing these issues and still less pertinent empirical research results, the review can only be cursory and most assumptions will have to remain tentative. Nevertheless this chapter will attempt to stimulate awareness of the important role of family variables in the management of chronic pain and provide suggestions for further research as well as clinical practice.

ROLE OF THE FAMILY IN THE ETIOLOGY AND PERPETUATION OF CHRONIC PAIN

Little attention has been given to the role of the family in the etiology and maintenance of chronic pain. Weakland (1977) speaks of "family somatics" (i.e., the assumption that family interaction variables influence the physical well-being of individuals in analogy to psychosomatics) as a "neglected edge." Although most pain management programs do involve the spouses to a minimum level, rarely is a theoretical rationale provided for this procedure. The exceptions appear to be Fordyce's (1976) operant approach and the cognitive-behavioral approach of Turk et al. (1983) that will be described in more detail later. Systematic research on the role of the spouse in pain treatment approaches is almost completely lacking, and there is little research on the efficacy of treatment approaches that include the entire family in the treatment of pain syndromes.

The lack of relevant literature directly addressing the role of the family in chronic pain syndromes requires reliance on related areas of research, such as the (a) role of family processes in psychosomatic and physical disorders; (b) impact of chronic illness on the spouse and the family; (c) emerging field of family medicine; and (d) pain literature in general in search of research and treatment approaches that are relevant for the family perspective in chronic pain. Some suggestions exist in the writings on physical and especially psychosomatic illness and family interaction in general. First, a rationale for the search for family interaction variables in the pathogenesis and maintenance of chronic pain will be discussed and then the empirical evidence for these assumptions will be examined.

The basic question concerns whether there is theoretical justification for the hypothesis that family interaction contributes to the development of chronic pain. More specific issues are (a) Why does a specific family member suffer from chronic pain and not another? (b) Why does he or she develop a specific chronic pain syndrome and not another problem? (c) Why does the symptom occur at a specific time? (d) How do family process variables and physical factors interact?

Weakland (1977) proposes three mechanisms of the influence of family interaction on the development of disease: (a) direct causation or causation in interaction with other factors; (b) increase in the susceptibility to disease; (c) influence on the course and rehabilitation of the disease. Various authors have addressed these issues more or less extensively. Basically, the three different viewpoints that can be distinguished are psychoanalytic theory, family systems theory, and behavioral models. All three approaches will be discussed.

Psychoanalytic Approaches

Psychoanalytically oriented authors have traditionally emphasized the role of intrapsychic processes in the development of psychosomatic symptoms. However, increasing consideration is given to the role of the family context and the family history in the development of psychosomatic disorders. Engel (1959) proposed that the presence of pain in a "pain-prone" individual often does not require peripheral stimulation. He suggested that pain may become an important means of regulating the individual's psyche. The pain-prone individual was characterized by him as showing (a) a prominance of guilt; (b) a history of suffering, defeat, and intolerance of success; (c) a strong aggressive drive; (d) development of pain upon loss or a threatened loss; and (e) a family history of aggressive and hostile relationships. Pain is thus viewed as the somatic expression of unresolved conflict.

Recently, Blumer and Heilbronn (1982) have suggested that a subset of chronic pain patients was predisposed to the development of their pain problem at least partially because of family characteristics. They suggest that the families of their groups of pain-prone patients included a history of depression and alcoholism, spouse abuse, and often a close relative with a chronic pain problem.

Apley (1975) and Apley and Hale (1973) report a large body of evidence that chronic abdominal pain in children is related to "pain-proneness" in their families. Chronic abdominal pain is a very frequent childhood disorder with one in nine unselected schoolchildren affected by it (Apley & Hale, 1973). An organic cause of the problem can often be found in only one out of 20 children with abdominal pain (Apley, 1975). The rate of abdominal pain in parents, siblings, and relatives of patients with abdominal pains was almost six times higher than in a group of normal controls.

Furthermore, Apley suggests that a preoccupation with the abdomen may exist in these families because of similar previous pain problem in another family member. Often a dramatic event involving the abdomen had occurred or the family attention became focused on the abdomen during a minor, transient disorder. Similarly, Oster (1972) found a higher incidence of pain-proneness in families of children with abdominal pains, headaches, or "growing pains," but no congruence of the location of the pain complaints. He surveyed 2000 schoolchildren with headaches and abdominal pain out of a population of 18,000 children and mailed questionnaires to about 600 parents. No further details about the study are provided, so that questions about the reliability and validity of his measurements remain unanswerable.

Gentry, Shows, and Thomas (1974) report that 59% of their low back pain patients had close family members with chronic low back pain or another debilitating physical disorder. Similarly, Kreitman and Salisbury (1965) reported that more depressed patients with somatic complaints, many of whom had pain problems, tended to have mothers with similar complaints as compared to depressed patients without somatic complaints. Blumer and Heilbronn (1982) as well as Schaffer, Donlon, and Bittle (1980) also noted a higher incidence of depression in the first-degree relatives of chronic pain patients as compared to a control sample. However, these papers contain a number of conceptual problems mitigating the relationship reported (cf. Turk & Salovey, 1984). Moreover, because the base rate in the population is unknown and controlled studies are lacking, the available data cannot be seen as conclusive evidence to confirm that pain "runs in families" nor to suggest that such a pattern of pain in families is necessarily caused by unresolved psychic conflicts.

Although these psychoanalytically oriented authors emphasize the role of the patient's family history in the development of the pain problem, they still adhere to a model of intrapsychic causality that does not view psychophysiological symptoms as the expression of a familial conflict. In contrast to the intrapsychic "conflict" model of some psychoanalytic theorists, family systems theorists have viewed the entire family as "sick" and the family unit as a target of intervention. However, many of them rely heavily on psychoanalytic concepts in their description of the disturbed family. Development of pain in a familial context has thus been viewed as involving regulation of the "familial psyche."

Family Systems Theory

Family systems approaches view the family as a system of relationships with the functioning of each member depending on the functioning of the other members. This system has a tendency toward homeostasis (Jackson, 1957). Any symptom that develops in the family context is considered as serving a stabilizing role in the familial system. Weakland (1977) points out the large body of evidence for the influence of emotional stress on physical functioning (for chronic pain see Sternbach, 1978; Turk et al., 1983; Weisenberg, 1977). He proposes that this evidence may be viewed as an indication of the importance of interactional variables in disease, because in his view emotional strain stems largely from communicative interaction.

Waring (1977) proposes a model of "significant other specificity" to explain the choice of a pain symptom and of the bearer of the symptom. He suggests that the symptoms of the patient may fulfill the emotional needs of other family members. Symptoms that appear at random—for example, in a child—may be reinforced if the symptom resembles a pain problem in the parents' nuclear family. The acute occurrence of pain may turn into a chronic pain complaint if the symptom fulfills the object-related needs of a family member. The mechanisms at work may be scapegoating, that is, projection to fit unconscious wishes or the embodiment of "splitoff introjects." In this case the symptom is reinforced accordingly. Waring bases his explanations on Framo's (e.g., 1970, 1976; see also Dicks, 1976) concept of projective identification, Bowen's (e.g., 1966) transgenerational hypothesis, and Minuchin's (1974) assumption of conflict avoidance through the symptom bearer (often the child). Both Framo and Bowen (1966) emphasized the importance of the multigenerational transmission of familial dysfunction. Bowen pointed out that the parents tend to project the undifferentiation of their self onto the children in order to stabilize the marital relationship. He believes that the children may repeat this process by marrying someone at their level of differentiation.

Framo (1970) followed the assumption of object relations theory that suggested that the need for a satisfactory relationship is a primary motive for human beings. In early childhood, the "objects" of these relationships—especially their frustrating aspects—are internalized as introjects. He further hypothesizes that in adulthood the spouse or the children may be perceived according to the individual's object-related needs and others are judged in terms of the individual's splitoff traits. Mates are presumably chosen in search of splitoff aspects of primary object relations and this projective identification process enables the reexperience of these primary relations. This process will, however, lead to conflict because unwanted aspects of the self are projected onto the mate or children and thus create stress in them as they are embodying old introjects.

According to Waring (1977), the maintenance of the symptom is due to the stability the symptom may give to the familial system ("sick-role homeostasis"). For example, marital conflict may be avoided by the concern for a sick child. He also describes the family myth of "better sick than dead" as important for regulating interaction in these families because the expression of negative emotions and hatred is not tolerated in these families. Waring further explains that the choice of a *physical symptom* may be preferred in these families as a nonthreatening means to express conflicts. It also allows for better interaction with health care professionals. Instead of saying "you are a pain" it may be communicated as "I am in pain."

In one study, Mohamed, Weisz, and Waring (1978) reported that depressive chronic pain patients and their spouses do have families with substantially higher numbers of pain experiences and more similar locations of the pain problem than do only depressed patients. Mohamed et al. (1978) noted that spouses of chronic pain patients often displayed more pain problems than the identified patient. This raises questions about the labeling processes that may occur in these families and what determines who becomes the identified patient.

The correlations between levels of psychiatric distress in a sample of 36 chronic pain patients and their spouses were examined by Shanfield, Heiman, Cope, and Jones (1979). Besides high distress levels in patients and spouses (as measured with the SCL 90) they noted a high correlation between the patients' and spouses' distress levels. They suggest that individuals with similar levels of complaint find each other in marriage, that is, "gravitate to each other" (Shanfield et al., 1979, p. 349), thus providing some evidence for the notion of projective identification. On the other hand, these elevated distress levels may well be a mere consequence of the pain problem (e.g., Kerns & Turk, 1984). Kerns and Turk noted that, in their sample of predominantly male chronic pain patients, more than 50% of the patients and spouses reported significant levels of depression and marital dissatisfaction. Because neither depression nor marital satisfaction was very highly correlated with the patients' pain levels but were correlated with each other, they suggest that familial variables may be important mediators of a patient's or spouse's reaction to chronic pain. It is not clear to what extent these couples were depressed and dissatified with their marriage prior to the onset of the pain problem and to what extent the pain problem serves as a distractor from marital problems. As long as no prospective studies are available no firm conclusions can be drawn about the direction of the causation.

The concept of family myth and its relation to the maintenance of a symptom in the family has been postulated by Ferreira (1963). A similar construct has been described by Reiss and his colleagues (Oliveri & Reiss, 1982; Reiss, 1982) labeled "family paradigms." Ferreira describes the family myth as a "series of fairly well-integrated beliefs shared by all family members, concerning each other and their mutual positions in family life." (p. 457) The family myth is a homeostatic mechanism that is self-corrective and maintains stability in the family. It is called into action whenever tension and emotional disruptions threaten the equilibrium in the family. It may consist of assigning the sick role to a family member. Generally, the need for homeostasis may be seen as a motivator for maintaining the symptom, whereas the myth can be viewed as a means to accomplish it.

Similarly, Delvey and Hopkins (1982) discussed the role of "collusion" in the maintenance of chronic pain syndromes. They describe collusion as the occurrence of unconscious contracts or agreements between the spouses that determine their respective roles in the relationship. These hidden contracts may mask emotional difficulties in or between the partners and preclude any constructive problem solving or changes in the relationship. Any change endangering the equilibrium the partners may have found through the collusion will be therefore prevented. Thus the giving up of the patient role by one of the partners may be viewed as dangerous to the system and foster resistance to treatment.

Swanson and Maruta (1980) found what they termed "undesirable mutuality" in couples in which one member suffered from chronic pain. They reported a high degree of agreement between patients and spouses on questions concerning their pain and the influence of the pain on their daily lives. The higher the agreement the worse was the treatment outcome. Again, it is not clear to what extent this mutuality is a precondition of the chronic pain problem or a consequence of it (e.g., due to the salience of the problem in the daily lives of the pain patients and their spouses). Delvey and Hopkins (1982) also present anecdotal evidence of the role of "collusion" in the maintenance of chronic pain. They describe how caretakers of pain patients may become instrumental in maintaining the patient's pain behaviors. They assume that the caretaker may alleviate his or her own emotional difficulties or interactional problems by defining the partner as the patient and viewing oneself as the helping spouse. They cite samples from interviews where they found that the partners of pain patients often displayed more emotional problems than the identified patient. They also describe how these problems often seem to have vanished with the onset of the patient's pain problem. However, as with most of the research in this area, only casual examples are presented with a lack of empirical substantiation. "Collusion" might be a way of stabilizing the family system and thus be of pathogenetic significance, but data are not available to draw such a conclusion.

A theoretical rationale for the development of psychosomatic illness from specific patterns of familial interactions and specific emotional dysfunction in the family members is also offered by Meissner (1966). He assumes that a family member becomes sick when he or she is "immature and emotionally overinvolved" in the family. Therefore the member depends entirely on the family for his or her emotional stability and cannot function without the support of the family. The onset of the disease is thought to occur when emotionally significant events disturb the emotional balance of the family (i.e., homeostasis) and thus also of the affected person.

Disruption of the emotional balance of the family is postulated by Meissner (1966) to result in an emotional crisis. This psychological breakdown is subsequently thought to be somatically decompensated, that is expressed in a physical symptom. The choice of the symptom depends on the specific conflict that is externalized. That is, symptom selection is suggested as being directly related to the type of conflict. In a way this is analogous to the traditional psychosomatic approaches applied to individuals (e.g., Alexander, 1951; Grace & Graham, 1952).

Based on his examination of familial factors in psychosomatic symptoms, Grolnick (1972) suggests that a certain pattern of family interaction, specifically rigidity, may be related to the symptom development. This lack of flexibility to adapt to life changes as well as the suppression of affect are, in his opinion, important precursors for the onset of psychosomatic disease. A similar view was expressed by Jackson (1957). The assumption of rigid patterns of family interaction is generally more accessible to empirical testing than is that of unconscious motivations pushing a family member into the sick role.

Minuchin, Baker, Rosman, Liebman, Milman, and Todd (1975) proposed a comprehensive model of psychosomatic illness in children that has also been applied to chronic pain (Liebman, Honig, & Berger, 1976). Following Jackson (1957), Minuchin and his colleagues proposed that certain types of family organization may be related to psychosomatic illness and that psychophysiological symptoms serve an important function in maintaining family homeostasis. Minuchin et al. (1975) identify several preconditions for the development of psychosomatic illness. First, a certain physiological vulnerability is assumed to be necessary. Second, four transactional characteristics of the family must be present: (a) *enmeshment*—a strong interdependence of relationships in the family with excessive "togetherness," weak or confused boundaries with intergenerational coalitions, parental children, and so forth; (b) *overprotectiveness*—a high involvement of family members in each other's lives, thus hindering the development of autonomy; (c) *rigidity*—a view of all change in the family as threatening. The family functions as a closed system with low tolerance for change. All efforts of the system are geared toward avoiding growth and change, with illness often used to detour change; and (d) *lack of conflict resolution*—a low threshold for conflict with the high tendency to avoid confrontation and leave problems unsolved. Third, the child plays an important role in conflict avoidance, thus provoking the reinforcement of the symptomatology. The child may be involved in various coalitions to detour open conflict. Often the child's symptoms are viewed as the only problem leading to the avoidance of confrontation of any other conflicts.

According to Minuchin et al. (1975; see also Minuchin, Rosman, & Baker, 1978), the choice of the symptom is explained by the family history that often reveals similar complaints in other family members or relatives (contagion or vicarious learning being the operative mechanisms) or a preoccupation of the family with the specific bodily functions (e.g., digestion, bowel function in the case of abdominal pain). The precipitating event is described as a threat to the family homeostasis such as (imminent, anticipated) separation. Maintenance of the symptom is suggested to be a function of the new stability the symptom may provide for the family system. Liebman, Honig, and Berger (1976) provide some anecdotal data to support the validity of their model with children suffering from chronic pain problems. However, small sample sizes and the lack of control groups make it difficult to draw firm conclusions from this paper.

The related concepts of adaptability and cohesiveness have been used by Olson, Sprenkle, and Russell (1979) to classify functional and dysfunctional families. Their circumplex model suggests that dysfunctional families show extremely high or low flexibility and cohesiveness, whereas optimal familial functioning is thought to be related to a middle position on these dimensions. These variables may also play an important role in psychophysiological disorders and chronic pain syndromes. However, to date there is no empirical evidence to support the characteristic mode of family function.

There seems to be some agreement among various family systems theorists about important familial variables related to the onset of psychophysiological disorders, including chronic pain. These factors seem to be (a) emotional overinvolvement, enmeshment, collusion of the family members (Delvey & Hopkins, 1982; Ferreira, 1963; Meissner, 1966; Minuchin et al., 1975; Waring, 1977); (b) rigidity, lack of flexibility (Grolnick, 1972; Jackson, 1957; Minuchin et al., 1975; Olson et al., 1979; Reiss, 1982); (c) contagion or vicarious learning (Blumer & Heilbronn, 1982; Engel, 1959; Minuchin, 1974); and (d) reinforcement (Minuchin et al., 1975; Waring, 1977). The various systems theorists differ in the extent to which they rely on psychodynamic concepts in their models. The authors also generally fail to sufficiently address the "translation" of a dysfunctional interaction pattern into a physical symptom and, specifically, the choice of a particular system. Moreover, in many cases their constructs have not been adequately operationalized or been assessed by procedures without demonstrated psychometric properties. Although these models offer interesting suggestions about the familial pathogenesis of chronic pain, no direct empirical evidence to support them is available; rather they rely largely on anecdotal cases.

The empirical research on the influence of the family on the development of chronic pain is scattered, sparse, and often anecdotal or only indirectly related to the issue. Methodological problems, especially the frequent use of retrospective reports or reliance on correlational data, hamper conclusions. Moreover, no prospective, longitudinal studies have been conducted to distinguish between the contribution of constitution and family interaction variables, or between causal and reactive dysfunctional patterns of interaction, nor is it clear what really dysfunctional patterns of interaction entail. That is, there has been a tendency to ignore family interaction patterns of families without a pain problem. It is possible that there are families with dysfunctional interaction patterns who do not have a pain problem and that there are also families with chronic pain and no dysfunctional pattern of communication. A special problem posed by family systems theory is that it adheres to a model of circular causality that assumes reciprocal cause and effect relationships within the family system (cf., Watzlawick, Beavin, & Jackson, 1967). Differentiation of dependent and independent variables as required by the conventional research methodology based on linear causality is thus problematic. Because none of the proponents of a family systems approach to chronic pain provided empirical evidence for this model, most of the research evidence must be extrapolated from other sources.

In summary, there are theoretical justifications for the role of the family in the development and maintenance of chronic pain as well as some limited empirical data. The empirical evidence is in general, however, neither sufficient nor methodologically sound. The reports by Gentry et al. (1974), Mohamed et al. (1979), and Shanfield et al. (1979) point toward the possibility that chronic pain patients select spouses with similar pain complaints because pain-proneness was also found in the families of the spouses. Although not conclusive, these reports are consistent with Waring's assumption of significant other specificity. However, it is also conceivable that exposure to symptoms in significant others may lead to a similar symptomology in other family members through modeling processes (cf. the following section on behavioral models and also Craig, 1978). Nor has the contribution of genetic factors been clarified in these studies. Furthermore, the direction of the causality has not yet been elucidated. That is, it is unclear whether family interactions are a cause or a response to chronic pain or whether both pain and dysfunctional family factors are coeffects caused by some third variable, for example, socioeconomic status. Although the family systems approaches are appealing, they are still relatively vague in their assumptions and often lack testable hypotheses. They especially fail to address the question of the "translation" of maladaptive interactional patterns into physical problems. Moreover, there are limited empirical data available upon which to base any conclusion regarding their validity. An additional problem is that no reliable and valid assessment procedure to evaluate family interaction style has been reported.

Behavioral Approaches

Compared with family systems approaches behavioral models of the pathogenesis of chronic pain offer a more "linear" view because they focus mainly on the contribution of the spouse to the development and maintenance of a chronic pain problem and less on the family system as a whole (with the exception of the cognitive-behavioral model that explicitly addresses the impact of pain on the family) (Turk et al, 1983). The behavioral theories provide more specific and testable conceptualizations of the role of the family in chronic pain, although so far the spouse has been the major focus of discussion. The learning conceptualizations also were formulated specifically for chronic pain and not for psychophysiological disorders in general. This may be a reason why they have found relatively more consideration in research and treatment.

In the operant model of the development and maintenance of chronic pain (Fordyce, 1976, 1978), the transition from an acute to a chronic pain complaint is explained in terms of conditioning of pain behaviors (communications that indicate the patient is suffering, such as, moaning, facial grimacing, rubbing parts of the body). Initially, the expression of acute pain may be an adaptive and appropriate response to noxious stimulation. When the pain exists for a longer period of time, it may come under the control of external contingencies of reinforcement. Pain behaviors may be maintained by (a) direct positive reinforcement of expressions of pain, for example, through attention and sympathetic responses from the spouse and significant others; (b) avoidance of undesirable activities such as work or sex; (c) lack of reinforcement from other sources, so that pain behaviors provide the only means of reinforcement. In these cases pain behaviors may become maladaptive because they lead to increasing inactivity, dependence on medication, increase in pain complaints, and decrease in healthy behaviors. The spouse is characterized by Fordyce as a primary reinforcing agent with power to shape the patient's behavior. The remaining family members are not given specific attention by Fordyce, although they may also become very important reinforcers of pain behaviors.

Craig (1978) reviewed a large body of evidence for the role of social learning factors in chronic pain syndromes. He suggested that vicarious learning from observational processes may play an important part in the acquisition of chronic pain behaviors. Observational learning may inhibit or disinhibit old reactions and instigate new reactions to pain experiences. Factors of potential influence include cultural habits and views, early socialization experiences, as well as any form of social interaction, most of which occurs in the family or is mediated by it. This perspective might account for the papers that report high incidence of family history of chronic pain for the chronic pain patients described earlier.

Several studies provide preliminary evidence to Fordyce's operant model. Fordyce et al. (1973) demonstrated that "well behavior" (e.g., activity) increased and pain behavior (e.g., medication use) decreased when attention was withdrawn from pain behaviors and well behaviors were reinforced. Cairns and Pasino (1977) showed that verbal reinforcement for activity (well behavior) and disattention to pain behavior led to an increase in well behavior. Because pain patients spend the majority of their time in contact with family members, it is assumed that they provide the greatest amount of reinforcement and may contribute to the development and maintenance of a chronic pain problem.

Block, Kremer, and Gaylor (1980) demonstrated that the spouse may not only be an important reinforcer but also an important discriminative stimulus for pain behavior in the patient. They showed that chronic pain patients reported varying pain levels depending on who observed them. If the observers were solicitous spouses, the patients reported higher pain levels as compared to a neutral observer condition (ward clerks). The pain patients with nonsolicitous spouses reported higher pain levels when observed by ward clerks and lower levels when observed by their spouses. Solicitiousness was positively correlated with the duration of the pain problem. This study demonstrates that spouses may serve as cues for pain behavior. The patients altered their pain behavior according to their perception of different observers. Block and his colleagues (1980) conclude that patients might be more likely to develop a chronic pain problem when spouses were reinforcing their pain behavior. Likewise, Flor, Kerns, and Turk (1984) showed that there are high correlations between the amount of pain and interference reported by the pain patients and the amount of reinforcement of pain behaviors as perceived by the patient or reported by the spouse. Thus level of pain as reported by the patient does appear to be associated with the spouse's response.

The finding of high agreement concerning the intensity of pain among patients and their partners (e.g., Kerns & Turk, 1984; Swanson & Maruta, 1980) and its relationship to poor treatment outcome could also be interpreted within an operant framework. The reinforcement by the significant other may be stronger if the patient's report and the spouse's perception are highly similar. That is, patients seem to communicate their distress to the spouse and their communications may induce attention and thereby reinforcement of pain behaviors, thus creating a vicious circle. Also, the more concerned spouses who may also be more convinced of the severity of their partner's pain problem may find it harder to alter their reinforcement patterns.

Turk et al. (1983) describe the very salient quality of pain behaviors—a fact that is often not perceived by the pain patient who assumes that only the verbal expression of pain will reach his or her significant others. The study by Block et al. (1980) demonstrated that the spouses of pain patients may become discriminative stimuli for their partner's pain behavior. Another study by Block (1981), which is described in more detail in the following section, also shows that spouses of pain patients show marked physiological reactions on seeing their partners in pain. This also demonstrates the salience of pain behaviors and their high likelihood of being shaped by the environment, and especially the family. The communicative role of pain behaviors and the interdependence of the reactions of the patient's environment and his or her pain expression has also been discussed by Sternbach (1974).

In summary, there is some research evidence for the relationship between the reinforcement of pain behaviors and the development and maintenance of chronic pain. There remain, however, a number of problems in these studies that preclude any firm conclusions about a causal relationship—especially the fact that they were usually conducted following the identification of a chronic pain problem. One strength of the behavioral approach is the operationalization of the relevant constructs such as reinforcement of pain behaviors (cf. Cairns & Pasino, 1977; Turk, Wack, & Kerns, in press). The evidence so far is, however, suggestive and further research seems warranted.

IMPACT OF CHRONIC PAIN ON THE FAMILY

It is obvious that chronic pain with its often debilitating character for the patient may have important consequences for the patient and his or

her family. The following excerpt from a letter sent by the wife of the pain
patient (Mr. L), described previously, after an initial family interview illustrates this very well:

> This letter is in regard to my recent visit to your clinic with my husband who
> has back pain. Whether or not I will be able to visit you again because of my
> working nights, I don't know but that perhaps if I could explain my hus-
> band's attitudes it might help you understand his problems, which I could
> not discuss in his presence without causing him embarrassment.
>
> The questionnaire you gave him to complete and send back became a tre-
> mendous ordeal for him. Why, I'll never know, because the questions were
> simple, but in the state of mind he is in, everything gets to be a chore. Would
> you believe one day I left for work at one o'clock and returned 11:30 and he
> still hadn't completed the questionnaire. . . . Since his back operation five
> years ago he has become increasingly impatient and progressively slower
> with no ambition at all to even try to help himself. He had made himself an
> invalid and it has become very difficult for me or my family to tolerate his
> constant complaining. He blames me, blames our two sons, who he says
> don't help him around the house when in fact he does little or nothing to
> help himself. He does exactly the same things day after day with projects he
> starts and never completes and always because of his health.
>
> Even with pain, having had operations, I have been forced to do the many
> things required as a mother and a wife, but my husband cannot seem to
> forget his problems and put some effort into accomplishments instead of
> complaints. . . . To dwell on his illness is what he wants and only that he will
> do, believe me. He needs psychiatry of some kind and . . . I hope that per-
> haps you can convince him even to get some work outside the home which
> I'm sure will help him understand the pressure the family has been under
> for many years now. If you can convince him to get out of the lounge chair
> that he sits in half a day and sleeps the other half, we would be extremely
> grateful.

Despite what may appear obvious, little attention has been focused
upon the impact of chronic pain on the family. In the following the theoretical rationale as well as the empirical evidence for the impact of chronic
pain on the family will be discussed and the nature of the family's reaction
to chronic pain described.

The first formulations of the family's adaptation to stress were presented in the 1930s and 1940s and dealt with the adaptation to unemploy-
ment or war-induced separation. Hill's (1949) ABC-X model of the family's
reaction to crisis was widely used. In this model, A represents the crisis-
inducing event that interacts with B, the family's resources to deal with it,
and C, the family's definition of the event. These three factors together
will determine X, the crisis. Hill (1949) described the adjustment of the
family to a crisis in three stages—disorganization, recovery, and new level
of organization. He emphasized especially the role changes that may be
required in a crisis situation. These role changes, Hill (1958) suggests, in-

variably lead to temporary disorganization requiring readjustment. Parsons (1951) likewise described how the adoption of the "sick role" by a patient impacts on his or her relationship with other family members and their interaction.

Burr (1973), in a reformulation of Hill's model, added the concepts of vulnerability and regenerative power of the family a important intervening variables between the stress stimulus and the stress reaction. Bruhn (1977) and Turk et al. (1983) specifically addressed the changes in roles and task allocation a family has to undergo when a family member becomes chronically ill. These role changes are thought to lead to tension, conflict, and distress. It is also pointed out that the changes in roles may lead to forming new symptoms in the partner or old symptoms may be revived. The family's adaptability to change seems to be of utmost importance in the reaction to crisis.

As noted, family systems theory assumes that due to the interrelationship of all the members of the family, the illness of one member will affect the entire constellation in the system and thus illness can not be viewed separate from the system. Chronic illness will upset the homeostatic balance in the family system, will cause tension, and will require reorganization of the family relationships Bauman & Grace, 1977; Jackson, 1957). Somewhat paradoxically, family theorists will also argue that a symptom may serve as a stabilizing factor in the family system (see previous sections). The role of the symptom will depend on the state of the family interrelations at the point of the development of the symptom and its consequences. A functional analysis and/or a longitudinal examination of the development of the chronic pain problem in a family system might differentiate between the two conflicting views.

As noted above, the operant approach generally disregards the question of the impact of chronic pain on the family system but focuses rather on the development and maintenance of pain behavior in the patient. In contrast, the cognitive-behavioral perspective (e.g., Kerns & Turk, 1984; Turk et al., 1983) places equal emphasis on the impact of illness on the patient and the family and the way families cope with the associated life changes. Turk and his colleagues suggest that following the development of a chronic pain problem, all aspects of the family change—social, recreational, marital, vocational, and financial. Moreover, the family roles are often greatly altered so that a formerly nonemployed spouse may have to become the source of finances or a working spouse may have to assume new roles related to household chores and caretaking of the partner. They suggest that it would not be surprising to find that spouses become upset, frustrated, angry, and perhaps depressed. Interestingly, however, the spouse may feel unable to express his or her feelings directly because their spouse is suffering already and expressing negative feelings might often serve to exacerbate the patient's distress (recall the description of Mrs. L presented earlier).

There are several research findings to support these assumptions.

Klein, Dean, and Bogdonoff (1967) found new or increased preexisting symptoms as well as increased role tension scores when they examined chronically ill patients and their spouses. The spouses often even displayed more symptoms than the identified patient. Thus they raised the question of how a family member may become the identified patient. They assume that some spouses may be symptomatic before the partner develops a physical problem and they may be "waiting in the wings" to become a patient.

The few studies that have examined the impact of chronic pain on the family have focused on the impact of chronic pain on the spouse rather than on the entire family system. Mohamed et al. (1978) found considerable marital maladjustment in their sample of depressed pain patients, but fail to report any prepain levels. They also noted a significant amount of pain problems in the spouses of pain patients. Kerns and Turk (1984), Merskey and Spear (1967), Schaffer, Donlon, and Bittle (1980), Shanfield and Killingsworth (1977), and Waring (1977) all report marital dissatisfaction in their studies.

Maruta and Osborne (1978) report that over 60% of their chronic pain patient sample reported deterioration in sexual adjustment (reduced frequency and satisfaction from sexual activity) and more than 30% also reported deterioration in their marital relationship following the beginning of the chronic pain problem. In a subsequent study, Maruta, Osborne, Swanson, and Hallnig (1981) interviewed 50 married pain patients and their spouses who participated in a pain treatment program. More than 50% of the patients reported significant dissatisfaction with the present frequency and quality of their sexual activity. Seventy-eight percent of the patients reported an elimination or reduction in sexual activity as compared to 84% of the spouses. The change in marital adjustment subsequent to the pain problems was viewed as more of a problem by the spouses than by the patients. Although 75% of the patients reported no change in marital satisfaction after the onset of the pain problem, 65% of the spouses reported a deterioration of their marital relationship. It is conceivable that the considerable reinforcement pain that patients tend to obtain from their spouses will maintain their marital satisfaction, whereas the spouses, in contrast, will experience a significant loss of reinforcement due to the extreme limitations that chronic pain problems will often impose on the marital relationship. This assumption is consistent with the findings of Kerns and Turk (in press) who report a significant association between the patient's marital satisfaction and depression but no sign of this association in the spouses.

Shanfield et al. (1979) report high levels of psychological distress in the spouses of chronic pain patients as measured with the SCL 90, especially when the patients also displayed high levels of distress. Kerns and Turk (1984) found moderate levels of depression in both pain patients and their spouses. They also emphasized the importance of spouse support in decreasing the likelihood of depression in chronic pain patients. They found marital satisfaction to be a mediating variable in the pain–depression relationship and strongly encourage the inclusion of spouses in both the assessment and the treatment of chronic pain.

In a recent study, Block, Kremer, and Gaylor (1981) report that spouses of chronic pain patients showed considerable phasic skin-conductance changes and a tendency toward heart rate increases when viewing videotapes that displayed painful facial expressions versus the neutral expressions of their pain–patient spouses, other pain patients, or actors. Moreover, spouses who reported high levels of marital satisfaction showed greater skin conductance responses when exposed to videotapes of their partners in pain than the dissatisfied spouses, although the patients gave identical ratings of the perceived pain. Thus the display of pain behaviors may elicit physiological arousal in the spouse of the chronic pain patient that is directly related to the quality of the marital relationship. Autonomic reactions appear to lead to heightened distress and may be precursors of later physical symptoms in the spouse. These results may explain the high frequency of pain among family members noted by Gentry et al. (1974) and Mohamed et al. (1978).

The available evidence suggests that the inclusion of the spouses of pain patients in treatment may be important for the spouse as well as for the pain patient. Summarizing, there are theoretical concepts as well as empirical findings that underscore the impact of the chronic pain on the spouse of the patient. The nature of the impact includes deterioration of marital adjustment, loss of or deterioration of sexual functioning, distress and depression, as well as physiological arousal and physical symptoms in the spouse. The extent to which children are affected by their parents pain problems has received minimal attention. The research and theoretical conceptualization regarding contagion and modeling (e.g., Apley, 1975; Blumer & Heilbronn, 1982; Craig, 1978) suggest that this is an area that is greatly in need of empirical investigation. Clearly, more research is needed on the impact of chronic pain on the entire family system.

ROLE OF THE FAMILY IN THE TREATMENT OF CHRONIC PAIN

The theoretical models of family systems theory as well as the behavioral models provide theoretical rationales for the inclusion of the family in the treatment of a chronic pain problem. They argue that the consideration of other family members in the treatment may not only be useful but even necessary for a successful treatment outcome (cf. Fordyce & Steger, 1979; Liebman, Honig, & Berger, 1976; Turk et al., 1983). If the pain problem serves a function in the family or is the expression of a familial problem, treatment of the identified patient alone will not be successful, because the constellation of the existing system may perpetuate the symptom. This is consistent with the notion of sick-role homeostasis (Waring, 1977). Resistance to treatment might, according to this model, occur when changes in the identified patient take place without concomitant change in the family system, resulting in destruction of the familial equilibrium and provoking the sabotage of change.

The operant model explicitly implicates the reinforcing agents in the patient's environment in the development of the chronic pain problem. The person who provides the greatest amount of reinforcement is the spouse; however, all family members may contribute. If the family plays an important role in reinforcement, then the inclusion of the family into the treatment process is vital for the success of the treatment. Otherwise the reinforcement of well behaviors and the extinction of pain behaviors, usually the focus of operant inpatient treatments, will be reversed as soon as the patient returns to his or her home environment. From a family systems perspective, it may, however, be problematic merely to teach the spouse how to extinguish pain behaviors and reinforce well behaviors. This poses a problem if the symptom serves a purpose in the family system and contributes to maintaining a homeostatic balance. In this case, teaching the spouse extinction of pain and reinforcement of well behaviors may not in itself be sufficient to provoke long lasting change. Any change in this situation may be undermined by the needs of the family system. The family systems view may explain some treatment failures. However, much speculation is still involved in these arguments because empirical research is lacking.

Turk et al. (1983) also emphasize the importance of including the family in treatment. The considerable impact of chronic pain on all aspects of familial functioning and the necessity for the patient as well as his or her family to adapt to new demands and to develop new ways of coping will often require therapeutic intervention. It also seems important to assess all family members' views of the pain problem in order to assure cooperation in the treatment process. The spouses of chronic pain patients are often confused about the nature of their partners' pain problem due to the conflicting diagnoses and messages they may have received from health care providers who were unable to provide help. Long-standing disability in the patient, irritability, and role conflicts often create the potential for considerable marital problems that need to be taken into consideration to avoid treatment resistance by the spouse (recall the case of Mr. and Mrs. L described earlier).

The operant treatment focuses on the existing contingencies of reinforcement of pain behaviors by the spouse and teaches patient and spouse how to acquire and reinforce well behavior. The spouse participation is combined with a number of additional therapeutic steps such as medication reduction and reinforcement by the hospital staff. Because often additional treatments, such as biofeedback, relaxation, and vocational counseling are added, the value of including the spouse into treatment cannot be ascertained. Examples for this treatment approach are presented by Fordyce (1976), Gottlieb et al. (1977), and Roberts and Reinhardt (1980).

Another comprehensive treatment program based on the cognitive-behavioral perspective (Khatami & Rush, 1978, 1982) included structural family therapy (Minuchin, 1974; Minuchin & Fishman, 1981). Here too the contribution of the inclusion of the family in treatment cannot be assessed. Studies have not been conducted that compare treatment outcome with and without family participation.

A treatment model for the therapy of chronic abdominal pain in children, using a combination of behavior therapy and structural family therapy, has been proposed by Liebman et al. (1976). The treatment is conducted in cooperation with the pediatrician and emphasis is put on deemphasizing the patient's role as the symptom bearer. Further treatment goals include the establishment of competence in the symptom bearer to control the system, disengaging her or him from parental conflict, thus changing the family system. The successful treatment of ten cases was described. However, there was no control for spontaneous remission of the symptom or any other important variables (e.g., attention) nor were any statistical analyses presented. It remains unclear therefore what may have caused the impressive results reported by the authors.

Waring's (1977, 1980) suggestions for the treatment of adult chronic pain patients follow guidelines similar to Liebman et al. (1976). He suggests that a change in the system must occur through the diffusion of the presenting symptom. He points out that the primary physician, who is often involved in the conflicts of the family system, should become a participant in the family therapy. He also suggests that the encouragement of open expression of anger, sadness, and similar emotions may be very helpful in the course of the therapy. In his more recent article, Waring (1980) describes cognitive family therapy as a treatment approach that focuses on the facilitation of self-disclosure. He characterizes patients with psychophysiological symptoms as unable to discuss personal matters and private beliefs in their interpersonal relationships. Enhanced self-disclosure is believed to improve the couple's level of intimacy and to increase the patient's sense of psychological control over symptoms. Unfortunately, Waring does not provide any empirical evidence for the clinical efficacy of his treatment suggestions (see also Jaffe, 1978).

Hudgens (1979) describes the treatment of 24 patients with a combination of operant treatment and counseling that involved at least one significant other in the treatment process. She reports that 75% of the patients and their families were able to live "normally active and satisfactory lives" after treatment and maintained the success at six months to two years follow-up. However, this study lacks a control group as well as statistical analysis. Furthermore, only 33% of the patients evaluated for the program were admitted because of the very narrow selection criteria that included the prerequisite that at least one significant other was willing to participate in the program, that identifiable and modifiable pain behaviors were present, and that reinforcers for healthy behaviors could be identified.

Also following an operant orientation, Lieberman (1970) suggests that treatment of migraine headaches should focus on redirecting the spouse's attention from pain behaviors to well behaviors. In a case study of chronic back pain, Scheiderer and Bernstein (1976) report that the unilateral treatment of marital problems through the patient resulted in improvement of the patient's functioning. They instructed the pain patient to change the contingencies of reinforcement for the partner and they could thus improve the marital relationship as well as the functioning of the pain patient.

In summary, research evidence on the usefulness of family therapy or the integration of family members in the therapeutic process is practically nonexistent, although this approach is used in clinical practice. No controlled treatment outcome study featuring family systems approach or manipulating the inclusion of the spouse in the treatment has yet been published.

IMPLICATIONS FOR RESEARCH AND CLINICAL PRACTICE

Although there is some theoretical foundation as well as empirical evidence for the role of the family in chronic pain, the evidence is scattered and far from conclusive. What is necessary is more basic research on interaction patterns in chronic pain patients, their perception of and reaction to the pain problem, and the ways families cope with crises. This research must at the present stage necessarily be exploratory and flexible—as Weakland (1977) points out—due to the very rudimentary basis that exists so far. Direct observation of the interaction between family members, and observing and recording the subjective, behavioral, and physiological responses to pain behaviors in the family members are necessary as well as the interview and questionnaire studies on the impact of the pain problem on the family. Better formulated theoretical models with testable hypotheses could guide empirical studies and conversely better designed and controlled research could facilitate the formulation of theoretical models.

Much more reseach is needed to develop and test psychometrically sound instruments to measure such important constructs as family interaction patterns, pain behaviors, and collusion. None of the theories presented has provided sufficient detail to support the operationalization of these theoretical constructs. Without such instruments and procedures it will be impossible to evaluate the validity of competing theories.

The family systems approach must necessarily address the problem of circular causality that is hard to approach with current research methodology. Longitudinal studies are needed to assess the contribution of family variables to chronic pain syndromes. Prospective studies are needed to answer questions of etiology that cannot be answered from working only with identified patients whose problem has existed, by definition, for at least six months and often as long as 20 years.

In the field of therapy research, family approaches and individual approaches should be contrasted. The contribution of family therapy could also be assessed by the use of treatment packages with or without spouse or family involvement. It would be especially interesting to assess differential effects of the treatments and find criteria for the assignment of family versus individual therapy.

The treatment of chronic pain should focus more on the contribution of family variables to the pain problem as well as its impact on the family. It seems crucial to include at least the family in the assessment in order to obtain a picture of factors that may contribute to the maintenance of a chronic pain problem and to assess its impact on the family members (Turk & Kerns, 1983). The family must at least be informed of the treatment rationale and goals or they may wittingly or unwittingly sabotage the patient's treatment. To reiterate a major theme of this chapter and to state the obvious, more research is needed to come to valid conclusions about chronic pain and the family.

REFERENCES

Alexander, F. (1951). *Psychosomatische medizin.* Berlin: de Gruyter.

Apley, J, (1975). *The child with abdominal pains.* Oxford: Blackwell.

Apley, J., & Hale, B. (1973). Children with recurrent abdominal pain: How do they grow up? *British Medical Journal, 3,* 7–9.

Bauman, M., & Grace, N. (1977). Family process and family practice. *Journal of Family Practice, 4,* 1135–1140.

Block, A. (1981). An investigation of the response of the spouse to chronic pain behavior. *Psychosomatic Medicine, 43,* 415–422.

Block, A., Kremer, E., & Gaylor, M. (1980). Behavioral treatment of chronic pain: The spouse as a discriminative cue for pain behavior. *Pain, 9,* 243–252.

Blumer, D., & Heilbronn, M. (1982). Chronic pain as a variant of depressive disease. *The Journal of Nervous and Mental Disease, 170,* 381–406.

Bonica, J., & Butler, S. (1978). The management and functions of pain centers. In M. Swerdlow (Ed.), *Relief of intractable pain.* Amsterdam: Elsevier-North Holland Medical Press.

Bowen, M. (1966). The use of family theory in clinical practice. *Comprehensive Psychiatry, 7,* 345–359.

Bruhn, J. G. (1977). Effects of chronic illness on the family. *Journal of Family Practice, 4,* 1057–1060.

Burr, W. (1973). *Theory construction and the sociology of the family.* New York: Wiley.

Cairns, D. & Pasino, J. A. (1977). Comparison of verbal reinforcement and feedback in the operant treatment of disability due to chronic low back pain. *Behavior Therapy, 8,* 621–630.

Craig, K. (1978). Social modeling influences on pain. In R. A. Sternbach (Ed.), *The psychology of pain* (pp. 73–110). New York: Raven Press.

Delvey, J., & Hopkins, L. (1982). Pain patients and their partners: The role of collusion in chronic pain. *Journal of Marital and Family Therapy*, (January), 135–142.

Dicks, H. V. (1976). *Marital therapy*. New York: Basic Books.

Engel, G. L. (1959). "Psychogenic" pain and the pain prone patient. *American Journal of Medicine, 26*, 899–918.

Ferreira, A. J. (1963). Family myth and homeostasis. *Archives of General Psychiatry, 9*, 457–463.

Flor, H., Kerns, R. D., & Turk, D. C. (1984). *The spouse and chronic pain: A behavioral analysis.* Unpublished manuscript, Yale University.

Flor, H., & Turk, D. C. (1984). Etiological theories and treatments for chronic back pain: I. Somatic factors and interventions. *Pain, 19*, 105–122.

Fordyce, W. E. (1976). *Behavioral methods in chronic pain and illness.* St. Louis, MO: Mosby.

Fordyce, W. E. (1978). Learning processes in chronic pain. In R. A. Sternbach (Ed.), *The psychology of pain* (pp. 49–72). New York: Raven Press.

Fordyce, W. E., Fowler, R. S., Lehmann, J., DeLateur, B., Sand, P., & Treischmann, R. (1973). Operant conditioning in the treatment of chronic pain. *Archives of Physical Rehabilitation, 54*, 486–488.

Fordyce, W. E., & Steger, J. C. (1979). Chronic pain. In O. F. Pomerleau & J. P. Brady (Eds.), *Behavioral medicine: Theory and practice.* Baltimore: Williams & Wilkins.

Framo, J. L. (1970). Symptoms from a family transactional viewpoint. In N. W. Ackerman, J. Lieb, & J. K. Pearce (Eds.), *Family therapy in transition.* Boston: Little, Brown.

Framo, J. L. (1976). Families of origin as a therapeutic resource for adults in marital and family therapy: You can and should go home again. *Family Process, 15*, 193–210.

Gentry, W. D., Shows, W. D., & Thomas, M. (1974). Chronic low back pain: A psychological profile. *Psychosomatics, 15*, 174–177.

Gottlieb, H., Strite, L. C., Koller, R., Madorsky, A., Hockersmith, V., Kleeman, M., & Wagner, J. (1977). Comprehensive rehabilitation of patients having chronic low back pain. *Archives of Physical Medicine and Rehabilitation, 58*, 101–108.

Grace, W. J., & Graham, D. T. (1952). Relationship of specific attitudes and emotions to certain bodily diseases. *Psychosomatic Medicine, 14*, 243–251.

Grolnick, L. A. (1972). Family perspective of psychosomatic factors in illness: A review of the literature. *Family Process, 11*, 457–486.

Hill, R. (1949). *Families under stress.* New York: Harper & Row.

Hill, R. (1958). Generic features of families under stress. *Social Casework, 39*, 139–150.

Hudgens, A. (1979). Family-oriented treatment of chronic pain. *Journal of Marital and Family Therapy*, 67–78.

Jackson, D. D. (1957). The question of family homeostasis. *Psychiatric Quarterly, 31*, 79–90.

Jaffe, D. (1978). The role of family therapy in treating physical illness. *Hospital and Community Psychiatry, 29*, 169–174.

Kerns, R. D. & Turk, D. C. (1984). Depression and chronic pain: The mediating role of the spouse. *Journal of Marriage and the Family, 46*, 845–852.

Kerns, R. D., Turk, D. C., & Holzman, A. D. (1983). Psychological treatment for chronic pain: A selective review. *Clinical Psychology Review, 3*, 15–26.

Khatami, M., & Rush, A. J. (1978). A pilot study of the treatment of outpatients with chronic pain: Symptom control, stimulus control, and social system intervention. *Pain, 5*, 163–172.

Khatami, M., & Rush, A. J. (1982). A one-year follow-up of the multimodel treatment for chronic pain. *Pain, 14*, 45–52.

Klein, R. F., Dean, A., & Bogdonoff, M. (1967). The impact of illness upon the spouse. *Journal of Chronic Diseases, 20*, 241–248.

Kreitman, N., & Salisbury, P. (1965). Hypochondriasis and depression in outpatients at a general hospital. *British Journal of Psychiatry, 3,* 607–615.

Lieberman, R. (1970). Behavioral approaches to family and couple therapy. *American Journal of Orthopsychiatry, 40,* 106–118.

Liebman, R., Honig, P., & Berger, H. (1976). An integrated treatment program for psychogenic pain. *Family Process, 15,* 397–406.

Maruta, T., & Osborne, D. (1978). Sexual activity in chronic pain patients. *Psychosomatics, 19,* 531–537.

Maruta, T., Osborne, D., Swanson, D. W., & Hallnig, J. M. (1981). Chronic pain patients and spouses. Marital and sexual adjustment. *Mayo Clinic Proceedings, 56,* 307–310.

Meissner, W. W. (1966). Family dynamics and psychosomatic processes. *Family Process, 5,* 142–161.

Merskey, H., & Spear, F. G. (1967). *Pain: Psychological and psychiatric aspects.* London: Balliere, Tindall and Cassell.

Minuchin, S. (1974). *Families and family therapy.* Cambridge, MA: Harvard University Press.

Minuchin, S., Baker, L., Rosman, B., Liebman, L., Milman, L., & Todd, T. C. (1975). A conceptual model of psychosomatic illness in children. Family organization and family therapy. *Archives of General Psychiatry, 32,* 1031–1038.

Minuchin, S., & Fishman, H. (1981). *Family therapy techniques.* Cambridge, MA: Harvard University Press.

Minuchin, S., Rosman, B., & Baker, L. (1978). *Psychosomatic families. Anorexia nervosa in context.* Cambridge, MA: Harvard University Press.

Mohamed, S. N., Weisz, G. N., & Waring, E. M. (1978). The relationship of chronic pain to depression, marital adjustment and family dynamics. *Pain, 5,* 285–292.

Oliveri, M. E., & Reiss, D. (1982). Families' schemata of social relationships. *Family Process, 21,* 245–311.

Olson, D. H., Sprenkle, D., & Russell, C. (1979). Circumplex model of marital and family systems: Cohesion and adaptability dimensions, family types and clinical application. *Family Process, 8,* 3–27.

Oster, J. (1972). Recurrent abdominal pain, headache and limb pains in children and adolescents. *Pediatrics, 50,* 429–436.

Parsons, T. (1951). *The social system.* New York: Free Press.

Reiss, D. (1982). The working family: A researcher's view of health in the household. *American Journal of Psychiatry, 139,* 1412–1420.

Roberts, A. H., & Reinhardt, L. (1980). The behaviorial management of chronic pain: Long-term follow-up with comparison groups. *Pain, 8,* 151–162.

Schaffer, C. B., Donlon, P. T., & Bittle, R. M. (1980). Chronic pain and depression: A clinical and family history survey. *American Journal of Psychiatry, 137,* 118–120.

Scheiderer, E. G., & Bernstein, O. A. (1976). A case of chronic pain and the "unilateral" treatment of marital problems. *Journal of Behavior Therapy and Experimental Psychiatry, 7,* 47–50.

Shanfield, S., Heiman, E., Cope, D., & Jones, J. (1979). Pain and the marital relationship: Psychiatric distress. *Pain, 7,* 343–351.

Shanfield, S., & Killingsworth, R. N. (1977). Psychiatric aspects of chronic pain. *Psychiatric Annals, 7,* 24 35.

Sternbach, R. A. (Ed). (1978). *The psychology of pain.* New York: Raven Press.

Swanson, D. W., & Maruta, T. (1980). The family viewpoint of chronic pain. *Pain, 8,* 163–166.

Toomey, T. Ghia, J. N., Mao, W., & Gregg, J. (1977). Acupuncture and chronic pain mechanisms: The moderating effect of affect, personality, and stress on response to treatment. *Pain, 3,* 137–145.

Turk, D. C., & Flor, H. (1984). Etiological theories and treatments for chronic back pain: II. Psychological models and interventions. *Pain, 19,* 209–234.

Turk, D. C., & Kerns, R. D. (1983). Conceptual issues in the assessment of clincial pain. *International Journal of Psychiatry in Medicine, 113,* 57–68.

Turk, D. C., Meichenbaum, D. H., & Genest, M. (1983). *Pain and behavioral medicine: A cognitive-behavioral perspective.* New York: Guilford Press.

Turk, D. C., & Salovey, P. (1984). Chronic pain as a variant of depressive disease: A critical reappraisal. *The Journal of Nervous and Mental Disease, 172,* 398–405.

Turk, D. C., Wack, J. T., & Kerns, R. D. (in press). An empirical examination of the "pain behavior" construct. *Journal of Behavioral Medicine.*

Turner, J. A., & Chapman, C. R. (1982a). Psychological interventions for chronic pain: A critical review. I. Relaxation training and biofeedback. *Pain, 12,* 1–21.

Turner, J. A., & Chapman, C. R. (1982b). Psychological interventions for chronic pain: A critical review: II. Operant conditioning, hypnosis, and cognitive-behavioral therapy. *Pain, 12,* 23–46.

Waring, E. M. (1977). The role of the family in symptom selection and perpetuation in psychosomatic illness. *Psychotherapy and Psychosomatics, 28,* 253–259.

Waring, E. M. (1980). Marital intimacy, psychosomatic symptoms, and cognitive therapy. *Psychosomatics, 21,* 595–601.

Watzlawick, P., Beavin, J. H., & Jackson, D. D. (1967). *Pragmatics of human communication: A study of interactional patterns, pathologies and paradoxes.* New York: Norton.

Weakland, J. H. (1977). "Family somatics": A neglected edge. *Family Process, 16,* 263–272.

Weisenberg, M. (1977). Pain and pain control. *Psychological Bulletin, 84,* 1008–1014.

10

Aging and the Family

Lori C. Bohm

Judith Rodin

Throughout the life cycle, the way in which the family contributes to the well-being of an individual develops and changes. Much has been written about the impact of family interaction upon the psychological development and health of children and adolescents (e.g., Ainsworth, 1979; Bachman, 1970; Croog, 1970; Nye, 1957). Less attention has been paid to familial effects on the health and well-being of people during the early and middle stages of adulthood, perhaps because these periods have only recently been conceptualized as having special significance (Waring, 1978; Panel on Youth, 1974). The role of the family during the final stages of the life cycle has been the concern of many investigators interested in the well-being of elderly individuals (Shanas, 1979; Shanas, Townsend, Wedderbun, Friis, Milhoj, & Stehouwer, 1968; Rosow, 1967). Although recognizing that "aging" is a process that begins at birth and continues throughout life, in this chapter on aging and the family we have chosen to focus on the effects of family on the well-being of its most senior members, because people at this period of the life cycle appear so vulnerable to health de-

279

cline. In so doing we will also consider the ramifications for middle-aged adults and their children of dealing with the problems of an aging parent or grandparent.

In order to appreciate the important health-promoting functions the family may serve in the lives of older adults, it is instructive to consider the family to be one crucial form of social support. Recent research has documented the effects of social support as a buffer against disease development in people under stress (Pilisuk & Froland, 1978; Kaplan, Cassel, & Gore, 1977; Cobb, 1976). The mechanism by which this buffering effect occurs has not been determined, but several theorists have considered certain functions of social relationships that may promote health.

FUNCTIONS AND ATTRIBUTES OF SOCIAL SUPPORT NETWORKS

According to Cobb (1976), a social relationship can provide several types of *information*, which then becomes helpful to the participants in the relationship in a nondependency-producing way. His definition of social support excludes the actual provision of goods and services, which may foster dependency. Cobb defines social support as information belonging to one or more of the following three classes:

1. Information leading a participant to believe he is cared for and loved;

2. Information leading a participant to believe he is esteemed and valued;

3. Information leading a participant to believe he belongs to a network of communication and mutual obligation. (p. 300)

Other theorists have similarly delineated the functions of social support, but have not excluded potentially dependency-producing functions, such as the provision of "tangible support" (Kaplan et al., 1977) and "nurturance" (Berger & Wuenscher, 1975).

Although the value of the first two types of information—that one is loved and that one is valued—to the well-being of people throughout life is self-evident, the mechanism by which the third type of information becomes supportive requires further explanation. Belonging to "a network of communication and mutual obligation" may be helpful for several reasons. It is through communicating with others that people obtain information about what is expected of them in ambiguous or otherwise stressful situations (Caplan, 1974). For example, an early study by Schacter (1959) on "the affiliative tendency" demonstrated that subjects experiencing experimentally induced states of anxiety often preferred to be with others in the same situation as a means of socially evaluating and determining the appropriate reaction. What often makes a situation stressful is the inability of the person experiencing it to obtain information that his or her actions are leading to desired outcomes (Kaplan et al., 1977). Some types of social relationships can provide needed information, thus lessening stress. In addition, communicating with others allows for transmission of other facts that may have an impact upon well-being, such as information about beneficial health practices (Pennebaker & Funkhauser, 1981).

Kaplan and his colleagues (1977) also emphasize the importance of having a social network that is dependable, that is, relationships that can be counted on to provide social evaluation information, crisis intervention, a sense of "community," or whatever else an individual may need at the moment. Knowing that one's social network is reliable may or may not be implicit to "belonging" to a network of communication, but that knowledge clearly has an impact upon the supportiveness of a social network.

Finally, the feeling of *mutual* obligation, which includes the possibility of helping others as well as of obtaining help, appears to be far more beneficial than being engaged in a one-sided relationship. In fact, there is some evidence that when individuals find themselves in inequitable relationships (i.e., ones where there is little reciprocity), they actually become psychologically distressed (Walster, Berscheid, & Walster, 1976). This happens when a person gets less out of the relationship than he or she puts in, resulting in anger, or gets more from the relationship than he or she contributes, resulting in guilt.

Also, especially for older adults, feelings of responsibility and efficacy have an impact upon morale and health (Kurtz & Kyle, 1977; Rodin & Langer, 1977). A network of mutual obligation offers more opportunities to exercise control and responsibility. Conversely, Engel (1968) describes the "giving-up-given-up" complex of feelings, a precursor to disease development, which is characterized by psychological impotence—the absence of feelings of efficacy. People experiencing the giving-up-given-up complex do not perceive themselves to be embedded in a network where they can be helpful and obtain help.

To summarize, social relationships, including those with family members, theoretically become social supports when they:

(1) Fulfill emotional needs (e.g., for intimacy and love)
(2) Reassure participants of their worth and value
(3) Provide the opportunity for feedback and clarification of expectations
(4) Transmit other valuable information
(5) Are dependable
(6) Provide opportunities for exerting responsibility and feeling efficacious while allowing for reciprocity in the relationship. Provision of instrumental needs may not necessarily be supportive if it fosters dependency and limits opportunities for reciprocity.

Growing older presents certain life situations that potentially increase the need for social support (Pilisuk & Minkler, 1980) while simultaneously making these functions of social relationships more difficult to obtain. We will highlight the environmental and personal concomitants of aging that affect the homeostasis of the family system and the ability to obtain social support. These changes in turn may increase the possibility for illness development. We will describe the effects of four types of life experiences commonly associated with old age:(a) retirement,(b) bereavement, (c) deterioration of certain physical capacities, and (d) the lessening of authority and feelings of control. These are often pivotal experiences of the aging process, each of which profoundly affects and is affected by interaction with family. Following a description of these aging-connected life events and their interrelationship with family process is a discussion of the historical perspective and current knowledge on aging and the family, as well as sections covering methodological issues and future directions for research.

Retirement

One major task of later life is to adapt to retirement (Sheldon, McEwan, & Ryser, 1975). Retirement, an event that is often mandated by the rules and regulations of various employing organizations, may introduce profound changes in the balance of familial relationships. Described by Oppenheimer (1981) as a "life-cycle squeeze," retirement brings a decline in income and the loss of possibilities for interpersonal interaction that give meaning and purpose to an individual's life. Upon retirement, a person loses a major reference group as well as opportunities for social contact and for feeling useful and competent (Sheldon et al., 1975). The retired person may become more dependent upon the family, especially the spouse, to provide for certain needs left unfulfilled by the cessation of full-time employment. In a traditional family in which the wife is the "homemaker" and the husband the "breadwinner," the newly retired husband is, to some extent, a stranger in the household. He risks, for example, feeling like an intruder in the roles that belong to his wife if he attempts to help her with household chores and decision making. If both spouses retire together, they are likely to become increasingly interdependent. However, these changes in family interaction patterns brought about by retirement may not necessarily have negative effects upon the health of family members. The effects of increased interdependence of the aging couple, for example, will depend upon the degree of preretirement interdependence (Kelley, 1981). As with all the issues to be discussed here, individual differences in the prior structure of family interaction, in the personal resources of the individual family members, and in the availability of community and other resources outside the family will shape the form of the impact of age-related transitions on family functioning.

In addition to the work-related losses of relationships and roles for the retiree, the loss of income that accompanies retirement may also influence family process. Life on a meager fixed income may limit choices of leisure activities. Retirement income may in fact not be sufficient to provide for basic requirements of food, clothing, and shelter. If so, middle-aged children may have to be relied upon for financial support at a time when they must pay for college for their children and save money for their own retirement (Buck, Furukawa, & Shomaker, 1982; Oppenheimer, 1981). This may contribute to resentment on the part of adult children and, at worst, to abuses perpetrated by children against their aging parents (Buck et al., 1982). Insufficient income, a possible by-product of retirement, may thus affect the quality of family interaction, such that the family may cease to be a source of support for its members.

The above suggests that there are many routes whereby family relationships can be affected by retirement. Depending upon many factors, the family may be a vital source of strength during this transitional period or may be a detriment to the well-being of the retiree.

For example, family members may provide new roles and tasks for the retirees or may make them feel as if they are "in the way." The family may also be a source of inexpensive recreational activities and may cheerfully and nonintrusively lessen the economic liability of a fixed income for retired members. Geographic proximity of relatives, the quality of preretirement family relationships, and the economic status of all family members are some of the factors that may determine the helpfulness of the family when its older members retire (Buck et al., 1982; Sheldon et al., 1975). Other factors await specification in future empirical research.

In addition, the retirement of an older family member may have negative ramifications for the well-being of young family members. Middle-aged children may be torn between their desire to provide emotional and financial sustenance to their own families and to be available in these ways to their retired parents (Oppenheimer, 1981). How the interaction between older people and their families has been and should be studied will be described in later sections.

Bereavement

"Successful" aging includes in its crucial tasks the ability to come to terms with loss and separation (Zung, 1980), for bereavement becomes more and more likely as people grow older. Loss of significant others has been associated with heightened illness and mortality risk, especially for men (Rowland, 1977). (See also Chapter 11 by Jacobs, Kasl, & Kosten, this volume). This risk is highest during the first year of bereavement, and is greatest among those with fewer social contacts (Rowland, 1977). For example, Parkes, Benjamin, and Fitzgerald (1969) studied a sample of more than 4400 widows, 55 years of age and older, and found that 213 of the respondents died during the first six months of bereavement. This number represents a 40% increase over the rate expected for married men of the same age. Incidence of disease in the bereaved group was a full 67% higher than in the general population.

Rees and Lutkins (1967) studied a group of 903 people who had experienced the death of a close relative (spouse, parent, child, or sibling) and compared their death rates with those of a control group who had living relatives in the area. The bereaved group experienced a mortality rate seven times greater than that of the control group (4.76% as compared with .68%). Widowed persons in the bereaved group experienced the greatest mortality impact, a 12.2% death rate. Death rates for the widowed were highest during the first six months following loss of spouse, and mortality rate for widowers was significantly higher than for widows.

However, "social support" can moderate the ill effects of bereavement (Garrity & Marx, 1979; Raphael, 1977). Family members may have the potential to be especially effective sources of support at a time of loss. A recent study by Bankoff (1983) found that widowed elderly mothers were the most crucial source of support for newly widowed middle-aged daughters. This was largely because the bereaved daughters felt that their mothers could empathize with them, having experienced widowhood themselves. Those widows who did not receive strong support from living parents had the lowest sense of well-being. For these people, support provided by other network associates did not improve their psychological states. These findings emphasize the important role that older family members can play as *sources* of support for their relatives in addition to being recipients of support.

The homeostasis of the family system will also be disrupted when the loss is of an important family member. For example, for an older adult, the loss of a spouse may represent the loss of the key relationship in which independence and dependency needs were taken care of in a balanced way (Cantor, 1980). Relationships with children may then become the arena in which these issues are played out, with the newly widowed parent relying upon her children to "take care of" her. This in turn may compromise the middle-aged children's ability to care for their own families or continue their own work as desired. Again, prior family patterns, personal and social/community resources will help shape the outcome for all family members when they experience a loss.

Heightened Possibility for Physical Decline

Late adulthood is characterized by the increased likelihood of chronic and acute disease as well as declines in perceptual acuity (Butler & Lewis, 1982). These difficulties can sap the strength of the older person and, in the case of eyesight and hearing loss, can contribute to social isolation. However, as Butler and Lewis (1982) point out, 95% of older persons are able to live in the community despite the fact that 86% have one or more chronic health problems. Eighty-one percent need no outside assistance in order to maintain daily life patterns. How older people adapt to the aging changes in their bodies is a critical determinant of the extent and rapidity of further emotional and physical decline. Reactions and support of family members can mediate the adaptational process in a variety of ways. For example, family members can tailor their interactions to deal with the older person's perceptual difficulties and can reassure older members of their worth and value by providing them with opportunities to contribute to family life in ways that are not physically challenging. There is also evidence suggesting that family and social support may help promote adherence to medication regimes (Cobb, 1976; Pennebaker & Funkhauser, 1981) and encourage participation in a rehabilitation program (Gray, Kesler, & Newman, 1964). The precise mechanisms whereby familial support effectively bolsters adaptation are many and varied, and have only begun to be investigated empirically.

Families may also have negative effects on adaptation to illness in elderly family members. Kelley (1981) proposes that one potentially negative sequence of interpersonal interaction following acute illness is unequal dependency in the relationships. Research on familial interaction following a heart attack (Bilodeau & Hackett, 1971; Croog & Levine, 1977; Skelton & Dominian, 1973) or cancer (Wortman & Dunkel-Schetter, 1979) provides a model in considering the development of unequal dependency:

> After treatment, the victim (usually the husband) returns home feeling worried, depressed and helpless. He becomes irritable, impatient and demanding with his wife . . .[or middle-aged child]. . . . Being concerned to promote his recovery, the wife . . .[or child] . . . becomes overly protective, seeking to limit his activities and enforce his adherance to medical regimens. Protectiveness heightens the husband's irritability, and this creates a severe internal conflict for her. . . . (Kelley, 1981, p. 292)

This is only one possible scenario depicting how family members may inadvertently retard adaptation to recovery from illness. In the extreme, the older parents' poor physical health has been linked with "parent abuse," a practice believed to be as prevalent as child abuse (Buck et al., 1982). Family members, when available, may enhance or hamper the ability of older people to cope with physical decline. Health may also be affected when these supports are not accessible. The loss or absence of networks of familial support has been associated with a variety of chronic and acute physical problems including heart disease, ulcers, and lack of recovery from some types of cancer (Pilisuk & Froland, 1978).

Lessening of Authority/Loss of Perceived Control

One frequent by-product of aging in modern American society is the transition from a position of control and authority to one of a relative lack of power and influence. This transition comes about as a result of several environmental and personal concomitants of aging, including retirement, bereavement, and decline in physical abilities. As a result the individual, who has been accustomed to making choices and exerting authority in the worlds of work, family, and community, is gradually relegated to a position of uselessness relative to his or her past position. The results of the loss of a sense of control and importance in day-to-day life can be physically and emotionally devastating (Engel, 1968). Conversely, research with elderly people in nursing homes and in the community has shown that when older adults either report having or are made to feel that they can have greater personal control in their lives, they are more likely to be happier and healthier (Kurtz & Kyle, 1977; Kuypers, 1972; Langer & Rodin, 1976; Palmore & Luikart, 1972; Reid, Haas, & Hawkings, 1977; Reid & Ziegler, 1980; Rodin & Langer, 1977; Schulz, 1976). Again, the family may be a context in which feelings of control and responsibility may be fostered, thus contributing to better health.

Cicirelli (1980) has demonstrated that the types of family relationships older people have are related to their sense of control. Specifically, older people with fewer living brothers and with more "cohesive" relationships with siblings and children tended to feel a greater sense of internal control. "Cohesiveness" of relationship was indicated by a composite factor score of three interview items dealing with frequency of contact, perceived closeness, and perceived agreement in values with the given family member. However, these data are correlational, yielded from a single interview protocol. Thus the possibility that stronger feelings of control cause different perceptions about family relationships, rather than the reverse, cannot be ruled out.

The finding (Rosen, 1973) that older adults who live with their children tend to have lower morale than those living by themselves has also been explained in a way that highlights the potential impact of family upon feelings of control. Rosen suggests that children may reinforce feelings of helplessness and loss of identity, whereas independent living may help foster successful aging. His data, too, were correlational, and the explanation offered for his findings was not empirically tested.

Certainly, living with a family member may not necessarily lead to helplessness. Similarly, some families may reinforce dependency in older family members who do not live with them. When older adults are physically disabled, Sussman (1976) has found that their adjustment and that of their families are enhanced if the older members are able to continue to contribute to family activities. It is in the context of this type of family life that older people may maintain the sense that they can be productive and useful. In general, the older person who is allowed to remain an active, differentiated participant in the family system will experience fewer negative emotional symptoms and will cope more effectively with other life crises (Hall, 1976).

The preceding discussion of four major life-stage-related issues—retirement, bereavement, decline in physical health, and the lessening of authority—point up the important role the family can play in enhancing or damaging the health and general well-being of its older members. In addition, the difficulties of dealing with the changes of older family members may increase the stress on their relatives, possibly affecting the health of younger family members. Middle-aged children may be especially vulnerable in that they must "take care of" their own families as well as of their aging parents.

In order to understand how the complicated relationship between family interaction and well-being in older adults has been empirically investigated, we will consider first the approaches that have been used historically in the field of social gerontology. We will then highlight current approaches to research in this area.

HISTORICAL PERSPECTIVE

Empirical investigations that were the forerunners of studies that are now yielding a rich and complex picture of the importance of the family for well-being in later adulthood did not begin with this research goal in mind. Instead, early research was concerned with testing the importance of social interaction and integration for the well-being of older adults (e.g., Tobin & Neugarten, 1961). Implicit in this research was the idea that the previously described events of later adulthood—retirement, bereavement, and loss of physical capacities—were detrimental to well-being because they meant "role loss" for the older adult (Lemon, Bengston, & Peterson, 1972; Rosow, 1967). The resulting "role ambiguity" could presumably be alleviated by having increased contact with others, whether peers or family members (Rosow, 1967). This sociological perspective on the remedies for the pitfalls of aging was formalized as "activity theory." The theory proposed that activity can contribute to the well-being of older people by increasing "role support," which in turn would lead to a more positive "self-concept" (Lemon et al., 1972). Although the original activity theory suggests that the way activity is effective is through its contribution to the maintenance of social roles, studies often investigated a derivative hypothesis that the more activity an older person engages in, the happier he or she will be, regardless of whether the activity is social or solitary in nature (e.g., Lemon et al., 1972; Markides & Martin, 1979).

Activity theory is in direct opposition to another historically prominent theory in social gerontology, the "disengagement perspective," which suggests that life satisfaction in old age is bolstered by a gradual withdrawal by the aging individual from social roles. This process is considered to be mutually advantageous for the older person and the society (Cumming & Henry, 1961). Given the fact that both of these diametrically opposed per-

spectives on what is "good for" the aging individual vis à vis social interaction and integration were developed empirically from longitudinally collected interview data, it is not surprising that research on the two
perspectives ultimately concluded that disengagement and activity represent two of many possible responses to aging (George, 1978; Sheldon et
al., 1975). Whether or not these responses or others will be most adaptive
for a particular individual and that individual's family will depend upon a
variety of factors.

In the context of exploring the activity and disengagement theories of
adaptation to old age, several questions in regard to the role of the family
were indirectly considered. Cross-cultural research on aging in three societies conducted by Shanas and her colleagues provided information about
structural and demographic features of the relationship between older
adults and their families (Shanas et al., 1968). From the findings of these
lines of inquiry, we will describe how early research addressed three important questions in regard to aging, the family, and psychological and
physical health:

1. What affects family/social interaction?
2. What is derived from family/social interaction?
3. What features of family/social interaction affect well-being?

What Affects Family/Social Interaction?

The original research pertaining to this question was carried out by sociologists who were interested in social status variables and indices that
are defining characteristics of the social structure. These variables are considered important in shaping the social forces that pattern interpersonal
interaction and influence the social integration of older adults (George,
1978). Social status variables include socioeconomic status (SES), marital
status, health status, sex, and whether or not an older person has children.
Characteristics of the social structure are aspects of the older person's
housing situation (e.g., proportion of age peers) and community size.

For example, studies were conducted that considered the impact upon
social interaction of living in housing developments with only older persons (age-segregated settings). In summarizing this work, Teaff, Lawton,
Nahemow, and Carlson (1978) determined that living in age-segregated
housing affects participation in organized activities but is not associated
with differences in contact with family or friends. Variation in community
size also does not affect social interaction patterns (Conner & Powers,
1975).

Family interaction patterns in particular have been the focus of extensive research efforts by Shanas and her colleagues (e.g., Shanas et al., 1968;
Shanas, 1979). Shanas was concerned with whether and under what social

circumstances families abandon their elderly members or, conversely, care for them. She determined that, contrary to popular myth, families rarely forsake their older members. Certain characteristics of the relationship between families (e.g., whether or not the old person lives with a child or other family member and the frequency of interaction with them) are related to social status factors, including marital status, sex, and age of both the old person and the child. As long as families of older adults have adequate financial resources, they are usually willing to care for their older members (Shanas & Sussman, 1981).

There are sex differences in interaction patterns among older people. Men apparently have more frequent social contacts than women but are less likely to have an intimate friend (Powers & Bultena, 1976). When disabled, older women are more likely than men to expect to be invited to live with their children (Seelbach, 1977). These conclusions were drawn from self-report data, gleaned from community surveys. Although the sample in Powers and Bultena's (1976) study appears to have been representative of noninstitutionalized older adults, Seelbach's sample consisted solely of lower-income urban minority elderly, thus limiting the generalizability of his results.

In general, differences in both social status and social structure are connected with variability in patterns of social interaction among older adults. Moreover, there appears to be an assortment of interactions among social structure and social status characteristics, resulting in differing patterns of social interaction. A major study concerned with these issues was conducted by Rosow (1967). He found that socially disadvantaged older adults (e.g., widowed people, poor people, women) tend to rely more heavily upon local associates for interaction when in age-peer-dense housing situations than do their advantaged counterparts. For example, women are more responsive than men to differences in the concentration of age peers in their residences. The social interaction patterns of single and widowed women are particularly sensitive to residential density. Also, people from working class backgrounds tend to rely heavily on locally available associates, whereas middle-class people are more likely to have significant relationships with friends and relatives who live in other areas (Rosow, 1967).

This theoretical framework is very useful for documenting the fact that "role loss," in interaction with availability by the propinquity of age peers, affects frequency of social involvement and the identity of those with whom older adults involve themselves. However, it is unsuccessful in accounting for differences in the quality of those interactions. Emotional dependence of the elderly upon their children is not a function of role loss, but is "a stable psychological relationship" (Rosow, 1967, p. 213). Similarly, mutual assistance between families and their older members and between older people and their neighbors is not a function of residential or social status parameters. Instead, help-seeking and giving behavior appears to be a function of personality differences. The elderly who rely upon their children for help and also provide help to them tend to be the ones who rely upon and help neighbors (Sherman, 1975). Thus the historically important approach of trying to understand what affects social interaction by considering social status and social structure variables has its obvious limitations. Current approaches to what affects interaction between older adults and their family members and peers have begun to remedy these limitations by taking a more in-depth descriptive approach to conceptualizing differences in family structure.

What Is Derived from Family/Social Interaction?

In correspondence with earlier conceptualizations of older people's problems as deriving from role loss and lack of social integration, the "roles" of older adults vis à vis their family members and friends were the focus of inquiry. Typical questions addressed were (a) Who provides what services/help for whom? (b) What are the comparative functions of older people's family members versus those of their friends?

In regard to the first question, a cross-sectional study by Hill (1965) compared the help given and received in five domains (economic, emotional gratification, household management, childcare, and illness) across three adult generations in the same family. Data were collected through semistructured interviews with the wives of each of three generations of couples from the given family—married adult children, married parents, and married grandparents. Thus the findings in regard to help exchanged among the generations may be generalized only to married people who already have a significant source of support in their own spouses. Grandparents were found to be "both meager givers and high receivers," in contrast to the middle generation who gave more than they received in all areas except illness. Only the youngest family members, the married children, engaged in balanced, reciprocal relationships with other family members, giving more in some domains and receiving more in others.

Even as recently as the early 1980s most studies of social support and older adults continue to view the process as a one-way street, with the elderly as recipients of help and others as potential sources of support (e.g., Palmore, 1980; Pilisuk & Minkler, 1980; Shanas et al., 1968). These studies uniformly cite the family as the most important and frequent source of aid for older adults, followed by friends and neighbors, and last by social service agencies (e.g., Palmore, 1980; Freed, 1975). Although Hill's work provides some empirical justification for this bias, it is likely that a broader definition of support would permit a fuller view of the true process of exchange among the generations. Taking a more detailed approach to the process of interaction is characteristic of the way the relationship between older adults and their families is currently being studied. Later in this chapter these newer approaches will be described in greater detail.

The other major question in this domain has been concerned with the comparative functions of family and peers for the elderly. Blau (1973) suggested that friendships would be more important to older adults than relationships with family members because friendship results from mutual choice and mutual need and is voluntary. In addition, Blau and others have noted that the generations have little in common, and thus older parents may feel like "outsiders" to their childrens' families (Arling, 1976; Blau, 1973). Finally, it has been proposed that relationships with family may foster dependency, whereas those with friends may promote feelings of usefulness (Arling, 1976; Rosen, 1973).

A study by Arling (1976) provided some meager empirical support for feelings of usefulness in association between elderly peers rather than between older people and their children. In a survey of elderly widows, Arling determined that frequency of contact with children and having children living within an hour's drive were not related to less loneliness or greater feelings of usefulness. However, being able to visit neighbors and having friends in the neighborhood were correlated with these measures. Because this study's design was correlational, it is impossible to conclude from the findings that family members necessarily *foster* dependency and feelings of uselessness. Furthermore, measures of contact frequency and family proximity may not accurately reflect what is important to old people about their family relationships. It is significant that in contrast to the above suggestions, other work cited previously pointed up the important role the family plays as a source of support for older people. Indeed, Rosow (1967) found that "the aged have a much stronger orientation to their adult children than to friends and neighbors" (p. 25), thus making relationships with children and those with friends noncomparable. As is clear from this discussion, early work on the differential function of relationships between the elderly and types of significant others barely began to explore this issue with respect for its true complexity. This may have stemmed in part from the emphasis on "roles," and the tendency to assign specific roles to certain relationships and not to others. As we will discover, current work on what is derived from family/social interaction is attempting to elucidate the process through which these relationships can be important to health.

What Features of Family/Social Interaction Affect Well-Being?

Information pertinent to this question is also drawn mainly from work on the activity theory/disengagement controversy. Much investigative effort was spent in quantifying "activity" levels and correlating these measures with indices of psychological well-being (e.g., life satisfaction and morale). Interaction with family was only one type of activity that received attention, and it was often combined with other activity measures, both social and nonsocial. One outcome of mixing social and nonsocial activity together and attempting to show that the sheer quantity of activity was significant to morale was the finding that "morale and activity are not consistently, predictably correlated" (George, 1978, p. 840).

Some investigators used measures of frequency of interaction to consider separately the correlations of "informal" social activity (e.g., "visiting" with neighbors and family), "formal" social activity (e.g., club and church participation), and/or solitary activity with life satisfaction. The majority of these studies found some statistically significant relationships between the frequency of various kinds of social, rather than nonsocial, activity and psychological well-being. However, many of these studies also featured caveats and cautions as to the limiting conditions under which the relationship between social activity and psychological well-being holds. For example, both Graney (1975) and Knapp (1976) found frequency of social interaction to be more significant to "happiness" or to "life satisfaction" than were measures of frequency of solitary pursuits. Although Knapp's (1976) findings held after controlling for SES and degree of mobility (an interviewer-rated indicator of health), an earlier study by Cutler (1973) had found that when health and SES were controlled, the correlation between organization participation ("formal activity") and life satisfaction disappeared. To compound the confusion, Smith and Lipman (1972) found that frequency of peer interaction did not affect life satisfaction for those with an adequate income and relatively good health, but was helpful to those who were in poorer health and/or were strained financially. Finally, Bultena and Oyler (1971) concluded that both frequency of social contact and good health were related to life satisfaction, but that the type of interaction changed depending on the health status of the respondent. Specifically, those in poor health tended to interact more with family, whereas those in good health saw more of friends.

It is apparent from the number of qualifications as to when and with whom frequency of contact remains correlated with well-being that the process whereby social interaction becomes an effective mediator of emotional health is more complex than mere measures of frequency of contact have the power to convey. This point is particularly salient in work by Sherman (1973) who, in comparing the social support networks of older people living in various types of retirement housing, noted that it was "ironic that at the site where residents interact most with each other they would expect the least support in time of crisis." (p. 8) Clearly, frequency of contact is a relatively inelegant measure of the value of the relationship to the older person.

Operating from different theoretical frameworks, other investigators attempted to consider the impact upon well-being of several qualitative features of interpersonal relationships. The classic study of this type is that of Lowenthal and Haven (1968), who documented the ameliorative effects of having a confidant. Having a confidant was operationalized as an affirmative response to the question "Is there anyone in particular you confide in or talk to about yourself or your problems?" In attempting to understand

earlier findings that neither the forced decline in social interaction associated with widowhood and retirement nor voluntary reduction of social
activity consistently led to poor morale or mental illness (Lowenthal, 1965;
Lowenthal & Boler, 1965), Lowenthal and Haven (1968) discovered that
having a confidant served to mediate the development of emotional malaise in people experiencing changes in social interaction. Men usually relied on wives as confidants, whereas women were more likely to confide
in a child, another relative, or a friend.

Other early studies were concerned with another index of relationship
quality—expectations of support. These investigators exclusively considered the relationships between older parents and their children. Kerckhoff
(1966) studied patterns of family relationships following retirement and
found that morale was highest for older people who expected and received
little support from their children. Similarly, Seelbach and Sauer (1977) investigated the relationship between parental expectation of children's obligations for support and found that for black, low-income urban elderly
high filial expectations were associated with low morale. An early review
of the literature on the sociology of family interaction of the aged proposed
the hypothesis that psychological well-being is a function of a match between performance and expectations in the interaction between older parents and their adult children (Smith, 1965). This hypothesis found empirical support in work by Muhs (1977). Data for Muhs's study were collected
through a 123-item self-administered questionnaire that subjects received
in the mail. Response rate was 56%. Questions about quality and quantity
of interaction with family and friends were included, in addition to the
questions assessing degree of consistency between the expectations for
support of the parents and perceived performance of support by children.
The data were analyzed by stepwise multiple regression, with life satisfaction as the measure of well-being. Quality of family interaction emerged
as the most important predictor of life satisfaction, followed by the variable
measuring congruence between expectations and perceived support.

The attempt to consider what actually goes on in relationships between
older adults and their families as a predictor of well-being foreshadows the
direction taken by current research on aging and the family. However, the
impact of family relationships upon the *physical* health of older adults is
conspicuously absent from this earlier research. Considerably more research effort has been directed at this important issue recently and will be
discussed in the section to follow.

One way in which historically relevant research did address the influence of family upon the health of older adults was in regard to how older
adults, with various family situations, used health services. For example,
Shanas et al. (1968) demonstrated a link between the utilization of institutional and community services by the elderly with family structure and
relationships. Family factors play an important role in determining
whether or not an older person will enter a long-term care institution

(Brody, 1971). When ill, older people with few or limited family relationships are the ones most likely to enter a nursing home (Shanas, 1979). Childless or low fertility women have a 15% higher chance of institutionalization before age 75 than do women who bore three or more children (Soldo & Myers, 1976).

Family relationships also have implications for the use of social service agencies by aged adults. Freed (1975) found that "where the family support system is not available or is too weak, indecisive, or conflicted, the family agency virtually becomes the surrogate family" (p. 581). Elderly people who are without reliable family supports apparently use the social service system much more frequently than those who can get help from family members.

But simply having family members available does not necessarily prevent people from displaying illness behavior, including seeking help from health and social service professionals. Kasl and Cobb (1966) reviewed studies of health and illness behavior and found that in some families there was an "obligation" for the ill person to remain sick. In these families, the members neither expected the patient to get well nor genuinely desired improvement. Having an ill member served some homeostatic function in these families. In certain families, voicing trivial illness complaints and going to the doctor may be the only socially acceptable means to seek reassurance and support (Mechanic, 1968). Current research is now being directed at determining the ways in which families support health-relevant rather than illness behavior on the part of older family members.

Summary

Historically, research yielding information about the impact of family upon the health of older members came primarily from studies on the activity and disengagement theories of adaptation to old age. Interaction with family members and others was viewed as salutary because it provided involvement in the social process and thus relief from the role ambiguity. However, these studies were poor at explaining why social involvement did not necessarily lead to happiness and in explaining qualitative differences in family relationships that included comparable amounts of contact. The impact of family relationships upon the physical health of older adults was not investigated in this early research.

CURRENT KNOWLEDGE

The current approach to understanding the importance of the family for the health and well-being of older adults differs in several ways from the historically prominent methods and theories discussed above. No longer is "role loss" considered to be a sufficient explanation of why pivotal events of aging—retirement, bereavement, physical decline, and the potential lessening of authority—are problematic. There is increased awareness that these events have varying influences on family life and upon the health of older people including, in some instances, positive effects. Factors such as prior family structure and values, the personal strengths of individual family members, and the availability of community resources will help shape familial and individual responses to these life-stage-related events.

In correspondence with a greater appreciation for the complexity of the forces affecting the family and its response to aging members, there is a greater focus on description of family process and on delineation of mediating mechanisms consistent with the development of new data analytic techniques (e.g., path analysis). There is also an increased awareness of "cohort effects," that is, differences in the issues faced by a given group of aging adults that are related to the historical time period in which they are living (Cherlin, 1983). Finally, there is more information available on how the family may affect the physical as well as the emotional health of its older members.

What follows is a description of the knowledge we currently have about the three questions posed previously. From this description, the differences between the historical and the contemporary approaches to these issues will become clear.

What Affects Family/Social Interaction?

Our present understanding of this question shows the increasing importance of taking a "systems approach" to family interaction. One theme that emerges from diverse sets of data is that social/family supportiveness is a function of the needs of various family members. When the family system is strained by having an excessively needy older member in conjunction with having its own unfulfilled needs or insufficient resources, it ceases to be a willing source of support. This situation may be even more taxing when younger family members are called upon to provide aid with "marital household services" (such as providing meals and cleaning) to their formerly independent parents or relatives (Litwak & Kail, in press). The potential for family conflict is heightened as the balance of independence and dependence needs in older members shifts (Cantor, 1980). Retirement, bereavement, decline in physical capacities, and societally imposed lessening of authority may each serve to shift this balance, thereby disrupting the homeostasis of the family system. Families who are flexible, prepared to take on new tasks vis à vis older members, while still providing them with a meaningful role, will contribute positively to the elderly person's health and well-being (Hall, 1976).

Familial (or individual) attitudes about particular age-related events will also affect responses to those events. For example, attitudes about the causes and dangers of certain illnesses (e.g., cancer) will affect family members' responses to the elderly patient with that disease. Family members may believe that they should be cheerful and encouraging when the patient may really want to discuss the disease's more unpleasant ramifications. Serious illnesses, such as cancer, have been shown to provoke ambivalence in people who are potential sources of support for the victim (Wortman & Dunkel-Schetter, 1979). This ambivalence, coupled with conflicts between the patient's needs and the family members' beliefs about the role they should take in response to the patient, may then affect the frequency and quality of family interactions with the patient, leaving him or her without needed support (Rodin, in press).

Although the current approach to the causes of family support variation still recognizes the impact of social status variables (e.g., age and income), there is increased attention to why and how these variables are important. Social structure characteristics, for example, whether a person lives in age-segregated housing, have often been shown to be themselves a function of family situation and health rather than being direct causes of differences in social interaction. It appears that older adults choose to have the institutionalized protection provided by age-segregated housing when their health is poor and they have little locally available support (Bohm, 1983).

There is also an awareness of the limitations of social and community structure features to explain differences in interaction quantity and quality. For example, Shanas (1979) notes that "joint living is not the most important factor governing the relationship between old people and their grown children. Rather it is the *emotional bond* between parents and children that is of primary importance" (p. 169). Shanas (1979) does not operationalize "emotional bond," however, a step that must be taken in order to further research in this area. Discovering how that bond can be strengthened when parents become elderly should be a focus of future work.

Finally, it has become clear that certain family patterns including the high divorce rate and the increased participation of women in the labor force that have become more prevalent in American society of the 1970s and 1980s are affecting the type and extent of support families can provide their older members. The older members are also being called upon to provide new kinds of support for their children and grandchildren as a result of these changes. For example, adult children are increasingly turning to their parents for emotional and often financial support in the aftermath of divorce. Grandparents are finding it more difficult to continue viable relationships with their grandchildren when the divorced daughter-in-law or son-in-law is granted custody of the children (Cherlin, 1983).

The employment of women also affects family interaction in several ways. Daughters, who previously would have been the major caretakers of ailing parents, are no longer as available because of their work schedules. On the other hand, elderly women are increasingly likely to have been employed, giving them greater retirement income and improved skills for dealing with events outside the home sphere. This may make them less dependent, in old age, upon their children, thus improving their family relationships (Cherlin, 1983).

Although the family support offered to this cohort of older adults is greatly influenced by the contemporary trends in family structure, policy makers often use traditional conceptions of the family in making decisions that affect elderly peoples' lives (Shanas & Sussman, 1981). Policy making frequently is guided by the acceptance of three popular myths about old people and their families: (1) older people and their children are alienated; (2) older people are isolated; and (3) families do not care for ailing elderly members (Shanas & Sussman, 1981). The increased employment of women and the higher divorce rate may change the patterns of family availability for taking care of ill aged parents, but policy should not be based on the false idea that older people are alienated and isolated from their families. This could lead, for example, to monies being targeted for long-term care facilities and other specialized elderly housing facilities rather than into forms of assistance that would allow younger family members to participate more fully in the care of their parents and grandparents. Such misguided policies would in turn create problems for old people and for their support networks of family members.

What Is Derived from Family/Social Interaction?

Research that is uncovering new information about the process of interaction between older adults and their family members and peers has continued to address the two questions highlighted above, but with a new twist. Current work on (a) who provides what help for whom and on (b) the comparative functions of family members versus peers now acknowledges the importance of situational variables in shaping the answers for a given individual. The theoretical speculations about the relative roles of family members versus friends or neighbors in the lives of older adults (e.g., Blau, 1973; Rosen, 1973) have also been put to empirical test, yielding a more complex picture than was originally hypothesized.

There is now empirical evidence that many of the supportive tasks generally believed to be solely within the purview of the family are taken on by friends and neighbors in the absence of family members (Bohm, 1983). Regardless of whether friends/neighbors are age peers, they are likely to be the ones to offer assistance with needs that surface sporadically (e.g., help in emergencies, accompaniment to the bank or doctor). In situations where family members do not live nearby or when the older person is childless, friends and neighbors may also take on supportive functions of a longer-term nature (e.g., care of the older person during an extended illness) (Cantor, 1980).

Relationships between older people and their children and grandchildren may also be more reciprocal than formerly believed. In a recent study, Cantor (1980) again considered the question of reciprocity among the generations. However, unlike Hill (1965), she included more tasks that older people might be best able to assist with (e.g., giving advice about child rearing and major family decisions) as "help." She found that older adults do exchange favors with younger neighbors, family members, and peers, offering assistance with child care, decision making, and nursing others through illness. Thus there appears to be more reciprocity as well as more occasions in which neighbors/friends compensate for the absence of family than was originally believed.

The older person's choice of a supportive person may also depend upon the type of crisis or problem that has occurred. For example, recently widowed people find other widows to be the greatest source of support (Walker, MacBride, & Vachon, 1977). This points up the inadequacy of asking "Do older adults rely on children, other relatives, or friends most often for emotional support?" The answer to this question will often be dictated by why they need emotional support at that particular time.

There are a few tasks that are more relationship-specific, however. Older people tend to rely upon family members only for financial assistance, and on family members or hired persons for help with personal affairs such as tax or insurance forms (Bohm, 1983). Friends are especially important for socialization, tension reduction, and "reaffirmation of personal worth." (Cantor, 1980, p. 138). In general, however, current work supports one historically drawn conclusion: That family members, especially children or spouses, are seen as the most appropriate first source of help, regardless of task (Cantor, 1980). What is different in the current view is the recognition that people without family do get a wide variety of supportive functions satisfactorily fulfilled by friends and neighbors.

What Features of Family/Social Interaction Affect Well-Being?

Again, what distinguishes current approaches to this question from those of the past is recognizing the multifaceted way in which the family and other social supports can have an impact upon the health of older adults. There are beginning attempts to specify, both theoretically and empirically, some of the complex mechanisms underlying this process.

Because there is little evidence that the relationship between family/social support and well-being is different for older adults than for people of other age groups (Kasl & Berkman, 1979), some of the theories about this process that have been developed without regard to the age of support recipients will be discussed. Part of the work to be reported has yet to be empirically tested, but will be described here because of its prominent place in our current conceptualization of these issues.

There are at least four ways that the family and other sources of support can have an impact upon the health of older adults: (a) promotion of health maintenance behavior; (b) elevation of mood; (c) reduction of anxiety and its physiological concomitants; and (d) provision of direct, instrumental support in areas of need. Conversely, the family can exacerbate illness by (a) reinforcing maladaptive behavior; (b) aggravating sources of depression; (c) creating and reinforcing worry and anxiety; and (d) being unavailable to provide instrumental support when needed. The research evidence and the hypotheses regarding each of these issues will be discussed separately.

There are numerous ways that individuals can contribute to the maintenance of their own health. This is especially important for the elderly who are at an increased risk of developing disease. Adherence to prescribed medical regimens, including proper diet and exercise, appropriate taking of medication, and routine "checkups" can promote better health (Hamburg, Elliott, & Parron, 1982). Family and other social support may encourage adherance (Cobb, 1976; Pennebaker & Funkhauser, 1981) and, at the very least, can often provide transportation to health care professionals when needed. In addition, the family can be a ready source of information about helpful health practices and warning signs of illness. By modeling healthy behaviors and coping responses, they may further bolster health.

Elevation of mood by family members is a contribution to well-being in its own right. There is also evidence that depression may be connected with illness development (Ostfeld, in press; Engel, 1968), and thus mood elevation may improve physical health as well. It has been hypothesized that depressed moods may interfere with immune functioning and thus make the depressed person more vulnerable to the development of disease (Ostfeld, in press; Rodin, 1983; Solomon, 1981; Visintainer, Volpicelli, & Seligman, 1982). At this point, however, specific mechanisms underlying the ability of the family to influence the mood of older people have not been determined.

Anxiety also has physiological ramifications (e.g., overactivation of the autonomic nervous system) that over time produce disease (Krantz, Glass, Contrada, & Miller, 1981). Family and social interaction may reduce anxiety by providing feedback and clarification of expectations and of the appropriateness of feelings in ambigious situations (Kaplan et al., 1977).

Finally, by providing assistance when needed, the family can contribute in a variety of ways to the health and well-being of its older members. Not only does knowing that someone will be available to help relieve anxiety, but it may also prevent an older person from taking on a task that would be physically harmful. There are certainly myriad ways that having help with instrumental needs can protect an older person from stress and possibly promote better health.

Unfortunately, most of the above mechanisms by which family support contributes to well-being have not been fully specified either empirically or theoretically. It is clear that engaging in helpful health practices, avoiding depression and anxiety, and having help with important tasks can each contribute to better health; however, the way the family actually plays a role in these functions is as yet unclear. We know from work discussed above that families can also support a variety of maladaptive behavior patterns (Kasl & Cobb, 1966; Mechanic, 1968; Minuchin, 1974), including helplessness and dependency. Just as family members can model beneficial health practices and provide helpful information about illness warning signs, they can be poor models and inadequate information sources. Family members are often significant causes of distress for their older parents or grandparents instead of providing them with relief. In terms of empirical evidence, as yet, efforts of applied psychologists to improve health by increasing social (including family) support have not produced uniformly positive results (Harrison, Caplan, French, & Wellons, 1982). This is one area for future research, which will be discussed more fully later in the chapter.

In addition to these ideas about ways that the support of family members may contribute positively and negatively to the well-being of older adults, some empirical research has been conducted that does specify a few of the possible mechanisms underlying this relationship. One group of investigators has continued to work on the theory that morale is strongly influenced by social integration, which is in turn a function of social status and other variables. These researchers have employed path analysis to specify the relationships among the variables of interest. Although path analysis cannot definitively establish the "final cause" of a phenomenon because it is always impossible to eliminate all other possible causal factors (or "third variables") (Asher, 1976), it is the best technique available for suggesting cause-and-effect relationships in correlational data. The main contribution of the Liang group path model for the present concern is that it demonstrates the role of psychological or cognitive mediators in determining how social interaction relates to well-being. "Objective social integration," which was operationalized as a composite of amount of interpersonal interaction and organizational participation, was shown to influence morale indirectly only, through its impact upon "subjective social integration" or the subjective belief that one is not isolated (Liang, Dvorkin, Kahana, & Mazian, 1980). This model provides further proof for the inadequacy of the historically important idea that family members and others influence the well-being of older people simply via their frequent presence.

There is one other factor that has emerged as particularly important in influencing whether family relationships will support or damage the physical and emotional health of older adults. In a recent study, Bohm (1983) hypothesized that a critical mediator of the relationship between family and social interaction and well-being was the degree to which older adults felt in control of and able to mobilize support from their relationships when desired. The findings confirmed the hypothesis by demonstrating that the significant association between various relationship features (e.g., frequency of contact, expectations for support) and psychological and physical well-being shown in earlier studies was dramatically attenuated when differences in feelings of interpersonal control on the part of the elderly person were taken into account. This study suggests that if family relationships become an important source of feelings of efficacy for older adults, the deleterious effects of the experience of the lessening of authority in other domains may be countered. Bohm (1983) also showed that old people who feel more efficacious in their relationships are healthier and happier than their peers who do not feel the same degree of control.

Summary

Our current understanding of the role the family plays in the well-being of its older members reflects an increased awareness of the many factors impinging on the family that shape its ability to be supportive. Included are situational factors (e.g., geographic proximity), cohort-related issues (e.g., the women's movement and the high divorce rate), and psychological variables (e.g., feelings of interpersonal control and a subjective belief that one is socially integrated). By viewing the family as a system, researchers may be better able to focus on these and other influential factors. Although attempts are being made to specify the mechanisms that make family relationships supportive ones for older people, this work is only in the initial stage of development.

CONCEPTUAL AND METHODOLOGICAL ISSUES

Several major methodological issues limit, to some extent, the conclusions we may draw from the research previously cited. Many of the findings derive from correlational studies, thus limiting knowledge of cause and effect relationships. Most of the studies employ self-report measures exclusively. Finally, all the inferences drawn from these studies on family and social interaction and well-being in older adults are time limited: They cannot be generalized beyond the cohort sampled because the historical conditions of future cohorts of elderly people may be significantly different. Variability in the social and historical events shaping the world in which a person ages will also have a profound impact on family relationships.

Correlational Nature of the Research

The data collected in almost all the studies reported in this chapter derive from questionnaires and interviews, analyzed via multiple regression, factor analysis, and other correlational procedures. With the exception of studies using path analysis, few permit causal inferences to be drawn. The use of correlational survey research in this area was largely a product of the fact that until recently only nonmanipulable variables (i.e., social status and social structure measures) were of concern. Current research has, however, continued to use the same methodology. This may be due in part to an interest in being able to compare findings more easily across studies and in part to the fact that at this point investigators have only a beginning understanding of what are the relevant family system, situational, and psychological variables. Because it is not yet obvious what variables to manipulate, investigations have remained correlational in nature.

There are clear disadvantages to having only correlational data when one is asking questions about psychological and physical well-being and their relationships to family and social support. First, it is impossible to determine from these data whether or not patterns of helping behavior by families occur in response to or are productive of certain health problems in aging relatives. For example, Mrs. X is interviewed to determine her health, the quality and quantity of contact she has with family members, and her morale. Her family members are also interviewed to determine the quality and quantity of contact they feel they have with Mrs. X. It is discovered that Mrs. X has a heart condition, and she stays home most of the time. She believes her health is very poor, and she is often quite unhappy. Her children do everything for her, including cleaning her house, buying her groceries, and making her meals. Mrs. Y, another subject in the study, also has a heart condition, but she remains actively involved in the community. She believes her health is good, and she is rarely lonely or depressed. She seems to have a relationship with her children that includes reciprocity in helping: She babysits for them several times a week, and they drive her to the grocery store and other places. Assuming that these data are representative of all the subjects, is the appropriate conclusion that Mrs. X's children have fostered dependency and contributed to her poor morale and poor evaluation of her health unlike Mrs. Y's children? Or are Mrs. X's children simply acting responsibly, given a depressed, ailing mother?

This dilemma can be partly addressed by longitudinal data collection, which is the approach used by some of the studies discussed in this chapter. However, unless there are significant changes in the health status or family support patterns during the period of the study, it will remain impossible to make causal inferences.

Another unresolvable confound, given correlational data, is offered in the following example. It has been found that depressed older parents see their children less and go to the doctor more than nondepressed parents (Gurland, Dean, & Cross, in press). It is impossible to determine whether seeing children less *causes* depression or if the depression causes less contact between generations.

It is essential that studies in this area eventually attempt to manipulate certain crucial variables in order to test cause and effect relationships; however, it is difficult to delineate and manipulate important family systems variables. Suggestions for future research of this type will be described in the last section of the chapter.

Limitations of Self-Report Measures

Most of the studies described in this chapter rely on self-report data. This is problematic for several reasons. Self-report data, especially when it involves health problems and family relationships, is subject to distortions. Respondents may, for example, wish to appear "normal," not to be "complainers," or for any other reason may give a socially desirable rather than an accurate response. This limits the validity of the data on which the conclusions of the studies are based.

Self-reported health, in particular, is clearly influenced by mood and by feelings of loneliness (Rubenstein & Shaver, 1980). By using self-report measures of health, it is impossible to determine whether a lonely person is really less healthy or simply reports being less healthy than happier peers. In fact, self-reported health may be an excellent index of psychological status in older adults (Bohm, 1983). In a study in which demographic indices, family and peer relationship quality, quantity of social contact, and feelings of control and efficacy were used in regression models to account for the variance in multiple self-reported indices of emotional and physical health, Bohm (1983) found that after controlling for psychological well-being virtually no other variables were significant in accounting for differences in self-reported physical health. Physical health measures included a physician-rated index of the overall severity of all illnesses reported by subjects, frequency of somatic complaints, degree of interference in daily activities due to physical illness, and responses to two questions, "How has your general health been during the last year and a half?" and "In comparison with people you know who are the same age as you, how would you rate your general health?" This finding suggests that psychological well-being plays a very significant role in older adults' ratings of their physical health. If, however, it is objective health status that is of interest, other indices should be used. Health data may be collected from physician's records and hospital charts. In addition, other data collection methods can be used to bolster inferences drawn from self-report data. For example, daily behavioral checklists could be used to cross validate self-report from interview data. To record family contacts, a "social diary" could be kept by subjects. In general, however, investigators in this area should be prepared to design innovative ways of gathering information appropriate to the given study in addition to self-report measures.

Cohort Effects

Our modern society is characterized by rapid technological and social changes. People who are now in their eighties experienced, in their lifetimes, the invention of the "horseless carriage," of the airplane, of radio and television—in short, they experienced a technological revolution that brought vast, sweeping changes to the way people live their daily lives. Earlier in the chapter, we touched upon two contemporary shifts—the high divorce rate and the increase in the employment of women—that will have a profound impact upon the lives of people who are nearing retirement age today. Certainly, what contributes to the emotional and possibly physical health of the group of elderly people who are now the "old-old" (85 years of age and older) will be different from that for people who are now the young-old (65 to 75 years of age) when they become 85. Variations in educational and job opportunities, the increased prominence of the nuclear rather than the extended family, and other changes make the worlds of these two cohorts quite distinct. Being able to specify and separate cohort effects from more stable age/family relationship variables remains an important research challenge.

FUTURE RESEARCH

Ultimately, research on aging and the family should yield information to help social service agencies and health care professionals design interventions that will maximize the ability of the family to promote the health and well-being of its older members. Suggestions for social policy changes involving, for example, home health care, Medicare, and nursing home legislation may also emerge from work in this area. However, before interventions are designed and legislation written, we must achieve a more thorough understanding of the process whereby family interaction affects health. In order to achieve this intermediate step, future studies should address the concerns raised earlier in this chapter in several ways.

Using the conceptual framework that views the family as a system, research should be designed to analyze family process as it occurs in regard to (a) encouragement of helpful health practices; (b) elevation of mood; (c) relief of anxiety; and (d) provision of instrumental support. These are the four previously described ways that the family may have an impact upon health. Observational techniques could be employed to bolster inferences drawn from interview data. As has been done in research on mother-child interaction, relevant family members could be given a standard set of tasks around which to interact. Their behavior could be videotaped and scored according to relevant interaction parameters. It is likely that such a research program would also uncover other ways that the family influences the health of its members, which could then be investigated further.

A second research approach could involve evaluating the effectiveness of preexisting programs that provide outreach family counseling for families with older members and of programs that were designed especially for older adults and their families. Our recent review of this literature (Rodin,

Desiderato, & Cashman, in press) found no studies where actual outcome measures such as those specified below have been taken. Indeed, there has been little systematic evaluation research in this area at all. In conducting such evaluations, it would be important to focus not only upon health and well-being outcomes but also upon the way in which family members interact and upon the way their interaction changes during the course of the programs. This would facilitate further specification of process-of-interaction variables that could then be applied in research designs of the first type.

The information provided from the second research approach would provide convergent validity for the inferences drawn from the first approach. With the results from these studies, new interventions to bolster the supportiveness of the family could be designed and evaluated. Increased specification of the critical family process variables would also permit the designing of experimental studies in which these variables could be manipulated.

Future research should also be directed at the effects of cohort-specific patterns that affect family life. In order to consider the impact of the increased employment of women upon the care of older adults, we should compare, for example, groups of elderly with both employed and unemployed daughters in regard to how each group gets health and other needs met. Career women who are now retiring could also be compared with women who have always been homemakers as to the qualitative features of their respective patterns of family interaction. In this way, the hypothesis that the enhanced skills of the previously employed group would decrease dependency upon family and generally improve relationships could be tested.

Similarly, studies should be conducted of older adults with divorced children to determine (a) the effects on family interaction patterns and (b) how families cope with the issues presented by divorce. By determining which coping efforts are successful and which are not, preventative interventions could be designed to teach effective ways of handling divorce-related problems to older adults whose children are getting divorced.

Finally, policy makers could be the target of research efforts, as well as the recipients of newly gleaned research conclusions. It would be important to determine how policy makers conceptualize the relationship between the family and older adults. Information could then be provided to update their conceptualizations, if necessary.

The family is clearly an important resource for the health and well-being of all of its members. Older adults, because of their special vulnerabilities, may especially stand to benefit from our increased understanding of how the family contributes positively to health. Although progress has been made in this area, much work remains to be done before health practitioners and social scientists will be able to readily mobilize the supportive potentials of the family to improve the health of the aging population.

REFERENCES

Ainsworth, M. D. S. (1979). Infant-mother attachment. *American Psychologist*, 34(10), 932–937.

Arling, G. (1976). The elderly widow and her family, neighbors and friends. *Journal of Marriage and the Family* (November), 757–768.

Asher, H. B. (1976). *Causal modeling*. Beverly Hills, CA: Sage Publications.

Bachman, J. G. (1970). The impact of family background and intelligence on tenth-grade boys. *Youth in transition* (Vol. 2). Ann Arbor: University of Michigan, Institute for Social Research.

Bankoff, E. A. (1983). Aged parents and their widowed daughters: A support relationship. *Journal of Gerontology*, 38(2), 226–230.

Berger, M., & Wuenscher, L. (1975). The family in the substantive environment: An approach to the development of transactional methodology. *Journal of Community Psychology*, 3(3), 246.

Bilodeau, E., & Hackett, T. P. (1971). Issues raised in a group setting by patients recovering from myocardial infarction. *American Journal of Psychiatry*, 128, 73–78.

Blau, Z. S. (1973). *Old Age in a changing society*. New York: New Viewpoints.

Bohm, L. C. (1983). *Social support and well-being in older adults: The impact of perceived control*. Unpublished doctoral dissertation.

Brody, E. M. (1971). Long-term care for the elderly: Optimums, options, and opportunities. *Journal of the American Geriatrics Society*, 9, 482–494.

Buck, J., Furukawa, C., & Shomaker, D. (1982). Relationship with aged parents. In C. Furukawa & D. Shomaker (Eds.), *Community health services for the aged*. Rockville, MD: Aspen Systems Corp.

Bultena, G. L., & Oyler, R. (1971). Effects of health on disengagement and morale. *Aging and Human Development*, 2, 142–148.

Butler, R. N., & Lewis, M. I. (1982). *Aging and mental health* (3rd ed.). St. Louis, MO: Mosby.

Cantor, M. H. (1980). The informal support system: Its relevance in the lives of the elderly. In E. F. Borgatta & N. G. McCluskey (Eds.), *Aging and society* (pp. 131–144). Beverly Hills, CA: Sage Publications.

Caplan, G. (1974). *Support systems and community mental health: Lectures on concept development*. New York: Behavioral Publications.

Cherlin, A. (1983). A sense of history: Recent research on aging and the family. In M. W. Riley, B. B. Hess, & K. Bond (Eds.), *Aging in society: Selected reviews of recent research* (pp. 5–23). Hillsdale, NJ: Erlbaum.

Cicirelli, V. G. (1980). Relationship of family background variables to locus of control in the elderly. *Journal of Gerontology*, 35(1), 108–114.

Cobb, S. (1976). Social support as a moderator of life stress. *Psychosomatic Medicine*, 38, 300–314.

Conner, K. A., & Powers, E. A. (1975). Structural effects and life satisfaction among the aged. *International Journal of Aging and Human Development*, 6, 321–327.

Croog, S. H. (1970). The family as a source of stress. In S. Levine & N. A. Scotch (Eds.), *Social stress*. Chicago: Aldine.

Croog, S. H., & Levine, S. (1977). *The heart patient recovers*. New York: Human Sciences Press.

Cumming, E., & Henry, W. E. (1961). *Growing old*. New York: Basic Books.

Cutler, S. J. (1973). Voluntary association participation and life satisfaction: A cautionary research note. *Journal of Gerontology*, 28, 96–100.

Engel, G. L. (1968). A life setting conducive to illness: The giving-up-given-up complex. *Bulletin of the Menninger Clinic*, 32, 355–365.

Freed, A. O. (1975). The family agency and the kinship system of the elderly. *Social Casework* (December), 579–586.

Garrity, T. F., & Marx, M. B. (1979). The relationship of recent life events to health in the elderly. In J. Hendricks & C. D. Hendricks (Eds.), *Dimensions of aging* (pp. 98–112). Cambridge, MA: Winthrop Publishers.

George, L. K. (1978). The impact of personality and social status factors upon levels of activity and psychological well-being. *Journal of Gerontology, 33,* 840–847.

Graney, M. (1975). Happiness and social participation in aging. *Journal of Gerontology, 30,* 701–706.

Gray, R. M., Kesler, J. P., & Newman, W. R. E. (1964). Social factors influencing the decision of severely disabled older persons to participate in a rehabilitation program. *Rehabilitation Literature, 25,* 162–167.

Gurland, B. J., Dean, L. L., & Cross, P. S. (in press). The effects of depression on individual social functioning in the elderly. In L. D. Breslau & M. R. Haug (Eds.), *Depression and aging: Causes, care, and consequences.* New York: Springer.

Hall, C. M. (1976). Aging and family processes. *Journal of Family Counseling, 4,* 28–42.

Hamburg, D. A., Elliott, G. R., & Parron, D. L. (1982). *Health and behavior: Frontiers of research in the biobehavioral sciences.* Washington, D.C.: National Academy Press.

Harrison, R. V., Caplan, R. D., French, J. R. P., & Wellons, R. V. (1982). Combining field experiments with longitudinal surveys: Social research on patient adherence. In L. Bickman (Ed.), *Applied social psychology annual* (Vol. 3, pp. 119–150). Beverly Hills, CA: Sage Publications.

Hill, R. (1965). Decision-making and the family life cycle. In E. Shanas & G. F. Streib (Eds.), *Social structure and the family: Generational relations* (pp. 114–126). Englewood Cliffs, NJ: Prentice-Hall.

Kaplan, B. H., Cassel, J. C., & Gore, S. (1977). Social support and health. *Medical Care, 15* (Suppl. 5), 47–58.

Kasl, S. V., & Berkman, L. F. (1979). *Some psychosocial influences on the health status of the elderly: The perspective of social epidemiology.* Paper presented at the National Academy of Sciences Conference on Aging.

Kasl, S. V., & Cobb, S. (1966). Health behavior, illness behavior, and sick-role behavior. *Archives of Environmental Health, 12* (April), 531–540.

Kelley, H. H. (1981). Marriage relationships and aging. In R. W. Fogel, E. Hatfield, S. B. Kiesler, & E. Shanas (Eds.), *Aging: Stability and change in the family* (pp. 275–300). New York: Academic Press.

Kerckhoff, A. C. (1966). Family patterns and morale in retirement. In I. H. Simpson & J. C. McKinney (Eds.), *Social aspects of aging.* Durham, NC: Duke University Press.

Knapp, M. R. J. (1976). Predicting the dimensions of life stability. *Journal of Gerontology, 31*(5), 595–604.

Krantz, D. S., Glass, D. C., Contrada, R., & Miller, N. E. (1981). Behavior and health. In *The five-year outlook on science and technology* (Vol. 2, NSF). Washington, D.C.: U.S. Government Printing Office.

Kurtz, J. J., & Kyle, D. G. (1977). Life satisfaction and the exercise of responsibility. *Social Work, 22*(4), 323–324.

Kuypers, J. A. (1977). Internal-external locus on control, ego functioning, and personality characteristics in old age. *The Gerontologist* (Summer, Pt. 1), 168–173.

Langer, E. J., & Rodin, J. (1976). The effects of choice and enhanced personal responsibility for the aged: A field experiment in an institutional setting. *Journal of Personality and Social Psychology, 34,* 191–198.

Lemon, B. W., Bengston, V. L., & Peterson, J. A. (1972). An exploration of the activity theory of aging: Activity types and life satisfaction among in-movers to a retirement community. *Journal of Gerontology, 27,* 511–523.

Liang, J., Dvorkin, L., Kahana, E., & Mazian, F. (1980). Social integration and morale: A re-examination. *Journal of Gerontology, 35*(5), 746–757.

Litwak, E., & Kail, B. (in press). Some social costs to primary group helpers of aged depressives. In L. D. Breslau & M. R. Haug (Eds.), *Depression and aging: Causes, care, and consequences.* New York: Springer.

Lowenthal, M. F. (1965). Antecedents of isolation and mental illness in old age. *Archives of General Psychiatry, 12,* 245–254.

Lowenthal, M. F., & Boler, D. (1965). Voluntary vs. involuntary social withdrawal. *Journal of Gerontology, 20,* 363–371.

Lowenthal, M. F., & Haven, C. (1968). Interaction and adaptation: Intimacy as a critical variable. *American Sociological Review, 33,* 20–30.

Markides, K. S., & Martin, H. W. (1979). A causal model of life satisfaction among the elderly. *Journal of Gerontology, 34,* 86–93.

Mechanic, D. (1968). *Medical sociology.* New York: Free Press.

Minuchin, S. (1974). *Families and family therapy.* Cambridge, MA: Harvard University Press.

Muhs, P. J. (1977). *The psychological well-being of the aged individual in interaction with the family and the larger social and environmental system.* Unpublished doctoral dissertation.

Nye, F. I. (1957). Child adjustment in broken and in unhappy unbroken homes. *Marriage and Family Living, 19,* 356–361.

Oppenheimer, V. K. (1981). The changing nature of life-cycle squeezes: Implications for the socioeconomic position of the elderly. In R. W. Fogel, E. Hatfield, S. B. Kiesler, & E. Shanas (Eds.), *Stability and change in the family* (pp. 47–81). New York: Academic Press.

Ostfeld, A. M. (in press). Depression, disability and demise in older people. In L. D. Breslau & M. R. Haug (Eds.), *Depression and aging: Causes, care, and consequences.* New York: Springer.

Palmore, E. (1980). The social factors in aging. In E. W. Busse & D. G. Blazer (Eds.), *The handbook of geriatric psychiatry* (pp. 222–248). New York: Van Nostrand Reinhold.

Palmore, E., & Luikart, C. (1972). Health and social factors related to life satisfaction. *Journal of Health and Social Behavior, 13* (March), 68–80.

Panel on Youth. (1974). *Youth: Transition to adulthood.* Chicago: University of Chicago Press.

Parkes, C. M., Benjamin, B., & Fitzgerald, R. G. (1969). Broken heart: A statistical study of increased mortality among widowers. *British Medical Journal, 1,* 740.

Pennebaker, J. W., & Funkhauser, J. E. (1981). *Influences of social support, activity, and life change on medication use and health deterioration among the elderly.* Unpublished manuscript.

Pilisuk, M., & Froland, C. (1978). Kinship, social networks, social support, and health. *Social Science and Medicine, 12B,* 213–228.

Pilisuk, M., & Minkler, M. (1980). Supportive networks: Life ties for the elderly. *Journal of Social Issues, 36*(2), 95–116.

Powers, E. A., & Bultena, G. L. (1976). Sex differences in intimate friendships of old age. *Journal of Marriage and the Family* (November), 739–747.

Raphael, B. (1977). Preventive intervention with the recently bereaved. *Archives of General Psychiatry, 34,* 1450–1457.

Rees, W., & Lutkins, S. (1967). Mortality of bereavement. *British Medical Journal, 4,* 13–16.

Reid, D. W., Haas, G., & Hawkings, D. (1977). Locus of desired control and positive self-concept of the elderly. *Journal of Gerontology, 32*(4), 441–450.

Reid, D. W., & Ziegler, M. (1980). Validity and stability of a new desired control measure pertaining to psychological adjustment of the elderly. *Journal of Gerontology, 35*(3), 395–402.

Rodin, J. (in press). Applications of social psychology to pressing human concerns. In G. Lindzey & E. Aronson (Eds.), *Handbook of social psychology* (3rd ed.). Reading, MA: Addison-Wesley.

Rodin, J. (1983). Behavioral medicine: Beneficial effects of self-control training in aging. *International Review of Applied Psychology, 32*, 153–181.

Rodin, J., Cashman, C., & Desiderato, L. (in press). Enrichment interventions in aging. In A. Baum, J. Matarazzo, & M. Riley (Eds.), *Perspectives on behavioral medicine* (Vol. 4). New York: Academic Press.

Rodin, J., & Langer, E. J. (1977). Long-term effects of a control-relevant intervention with the institutionalized aged. *Journal of Personality and Social Psychology, 35*, 897–902.

Rosen, D. H. (1973). *Social relationships and successful aging among the widowed aged.* Unpublished doctoral dissertation.

Rosow, I. (1967). *Social integration of the aged.* New York: Free Press.

Rowland, K. F. (1977). Environmental events predicting death for the elderly. *Psychological Bulletin, 84*(2), 349–372.

Rubenstein, C. M., & Shaver, P. (1980). Loneliness in two northeastern cities. In J. Hartog, J. R. Audy, & Y. A. Cohen (Eds.), *The anatomy of loneliness* (pp. 319–337). New York: International Universities Press.

Schacter, S. (1959). *The psychology of affiliation.* Palo Alto, CA: Stanford University Press.

Schulz, R. (1976). Effects of control and predictability on the physical and psychological well-being of the institutionalized aged. *Journal of Personality and Social Psychology, 33*, 563–573.

Seelbach, W. C. (1977). Gender differences in expectations for filial responsibility. *The Gerontologist, 17*(5), 421–425.

Seelbach, W. C., & Sauer, W. J. (1977). Filial responsibility expectations and morale among aged parents. *The Gerontologist, 17*(6) 492–499.

Shanas, E. (1979). The family as a social support system in old age. *The Gerontologist, 19*(2), 169–173.

Shanas, E., & Sussman, M. B. (1981). The family in later life: Social structure and social policy. In R. W. Fogel, E. Hatfield, S. B. Kiesler, & E. Shanas (Eds.), *Stability and change in the family* (pp. 211–231). New York: Academic Press.

Shanas, Townsend, Wedderburn, Friis, Milhoj, & Stehouwer. (1968). *Old people in three industrialized societies.* New York: Atherton Press.

Sheldon, A., McEwan, P. J. B., & Ryser, C. P. (1975). *Retirement: Patterns and predictions.* Rockville, MD: National Institute of Mental Health.

Sherman, S. (1973). Housing environment for the well-elderly: Scope and impact. Paper presented at *Man-environment interaction among the elderly: An assessment of the impact of housing.* Symposium conducted at the meeting of the American Psychological Association, Montreal.

Sherman, S. R. (1975). Mutual assistance and support in retirement housing. *Journal of Gerontology, 30*(4), 479–483.

Skelton, M., & Dominian, J. (1973). Psychological stress in wives of patients with myocardial infarction. *British Medical Journal, 2*, 101.

Smith, H. E. (1965). Family interaction patterns of the aged: A review. In A. Rose & W. Peterson (Eds.), *Older people and their social world* (pp. 143–161). Philadelphia, PA: Davis.

Smith, K. J., & Lipman, A. (1972). Constraint and life satisfaction. *Journal of Gerontology, 27*(1), 77–82.

Soldo, B. J., & Myers, G. C. (1976). *The effects of total fertility on living arrangements among elderly women: 1970.* Paper presented at the annual meeting of The Gerontological Society, New York.

Solomon (1981). Immunologic abnormalities in mental illness. In R. Ader (Ed.), *Psychoneuroimmunology.* New York: Academic Press.

Sussman, M. B. (1976). The family life of old people. In R. H. Binstock & E. Shanas (Eds.), *Handbook of aging and the social sciences*. New York: Van Nostrand Reinhold.

Teaff, J. D., Lawton, M. P., Nahemow, L., & Carlson, D. (1978). Impact of age integration on the well-being of elderly tenants in public housing. *Journal of Gerontology,, 33*, 126–133.

Tobin, S. S., & Neugarten, B. L. (1961). Life satisfaction and social interaction in the aging. *Journal of Gerontology, 16*(4), 344–346.

Visintainer, M. A., Volpicelli, J. R., & Seligman, M. E. P. (1982). Tumor rejection in rats after inescapable or escapable shock. *Science.*

Walker, K. N., MacBride, A., & Vachon, M. L. S. (1977). Social support networks and the crisis of bereavement. *Social Science and Medicine, 11*, 35–41.

Walster, E., Berscheid, E., & Walster, G. W. (1976). New directions in equity research. In L. Berkowitz & E. Walster (Eds.), *Advances in experimental social psychology* (Vol. 9). New York: Academic Press.

Waring, J. (1978). *The middle years.* New York: Academy for Educational Development.

Wortman, C. B. & Dunkel-Schetter, C. (1979). Interpersonal relationships and cancer: A theoretical analysis. *Journal of Social Issues, 35*, 120–155.

Zung, W. W. K. (1980). Affective disorders. In E. W. Busse & D. G. Blazer (Eds.), *Handbook of geriatric psychiatry* (pp. 338–367). New York: Van Nostrand Reinhold.

11

Terminal Illness, Bereavement, and the Family

Thomas R. Kosten

Selby C. Jacobs

Stanislav V. Kasl

The simplest family system in which to study bereavement has been the spousal dyad, and most studies have indeed focused on spousal bereavement. Losses of other family members have received less attention in controlled studies, but loss of a young child has generated several important clinical observations. These observations help to illustrate certain patterns of bereavement for different types of family losses and at different points in the life of families. In particular, spousal loss has usually been studied in older family members while child loss has focused on young families. Child loss has also provided a setting for some unique studies of intervening biological variables during grief and anticipatory mourning. It is these studies of intervening variables, including not only biological but also behavioral and social variables, that need expansion and replication in future research.

The response to a loss may also be conceptualized in terms of interactional process, and outcomes such as separation, divorce, change in status or change in functioning may be specified for the family as a whole. The individual always exists in interaction with the social environment and, in fact, a rich interplay of personal and social needs and abilities takes place. Given a paucity of methods for assessing the family as a social system, a tendency exists to define hypotheses about the family as a system with reference to the individual, but future studies should consider the family as a system during bereavement.

HISTORICAL PERSPECTIVE AND CURRENT STATE OF KNOWLEDGE

A variety of epidemiological studies have been done since the nineteenth century on the mortality patterns of widows and widowers. In 1858 Farr (1858) observed, "Young widowers under the age of 30, and even under the age of 40, experience a very high rate of mortality; and after 60, the widowers die more rapidly, not only than husbands, but more rapidly than older bachelors." Another approach utilized by Pearson in 1903 and Ciocco (1940) was to show that there was a correlation between the ages at death of the first spouse and the surviving spouse. This correlation could be artifactual, however, as Myers (1963) has pointed out, because in considering only paired deaths in a limited area and time period ignores those spouses who have *not* died during this period and who are most likely not to die soon after the death of their spouse. More recent epidemiological studies have addressed this limitation in mortality studies and have also assessed the morbidity associated with bereavement.

Four study designs have been used in the more recent investigations of the mortality and morbidity of bereavement. The first study design uses *vital statistics* data to compare mortality rates for each marital status group. For example, widowed male death rates are compared with rates for married and never married males within different age strata. From these comparisons conclusions about the steady state of the population are possible, but any excess deaths among the widowed are not necessarily due only to the *acute* stress of bereavement, but can also be due to the widowed state per se. A second design is the *historical cohort*, a longitudinal design allowing an investigator to reconstruct without bias a cohort of subjects from the past and collect some follow-up data on them. Because the investigator did not assess these people before their bereavement, this design is limited by the quality and quantity of data originally collected. Medical charts or other sources might be used in such a study. The third design is a longitudinal *follow-up* that includes de novo, tailor-made data collection on subjects who are first seen sometime *after* the loss has occurred. The fourth is the longitudinal, fully *prospective* study in which persons are identified and assessed *before* the event, such as death of the spouse, and then followed for a specific length of time. The end point of mortality provides the strongest outcome for fully prospective studies, because this can be determined without a "detection bias" of missing some ill people in either the bereaved or nonbereaved comparison group. Morbidity as an outcome runs this risk of missing some ill persons in either of these two groups when the monitoring for morbidity is not complete. Hereafter we shall refer to these four designs as vital statistics, historical cohort, follow-up, and prospective studies, respectively; the last three can be collectively called cohort studies.

The Effect of Death of a Spouse on the Health Status of the Conjugal Partner

The Mortality of Surviving Spouses.   A basic pattern of excess mortality in the widowed, especially in males, is discernible in the studies summarized in Table 11.1. This table summarizes first the vital statistics studies and then the historical and follow-up cohort studies. The studies are listed in the left column of the table with the authors, year completed, and the location of the study. In the center column is a description of the bereaved subjects used in each study. The year or years during which the spousal loss occurred is followed by the number of subjects in each study, the age range (or mean) of the subjects, and the percentage of widowers (versus widows). The refusal rate of people approached for the follow-up cohort studies is also given. For example, 42% of the people that Clayton et al. asked to participate in their study refused to complete any questions. This is a high rate of refusal and suggests that a highly self-selected sample was obtained. The third column compares the mortality rates of the bereaved with a nonbereaved group. In several studies, these comparisons have been stratified by sex and by duration since the loss. For example, in the Rees and Lutkins study the female mortality rates are 8.5 deaths per year over the first year and 6.7 per year over the second year as compared to the nonbereaved mortality rates of 1.2 per year for the first year and 3.0 deaths per year for the second year. Comparison of these rates indicates that bereaved women have much higher mortality rates, particularly during the first year after the loss. The other studies may be surveyed similarly using this table.

The duration of the elevated risk varies by sex and it may be greater than two years for men (Helsing, Szklo, & Comstock, 1981), although the peak risk for men is generally in the first six months of widowhood. For women the peak risk may be in the second year, although there are studies that have failed to confirm any such elevated risk for women. The period

TABLE 11.1 Mortality of Conjugal Bereavement: Selected Vital Statistics and Cohort Studies

Study	Publication Year	Place	Bereaved Subjects Year	No.	Age, yr.[a]	Sex, % men	Mortality (%) Bereaved <12 mo.	Bereaved <24 mo.	Controls <12 mo.	Controls <24 mo.
Kraus Lilienfield	1959	USA	1949–1950	All Deaths	Not Specified	Not Specified	Annual rates, mortality ratios, from 1.14 to 4.32 compared with married		No control for duration of bereavement	
Young et al.	1963	Great Britain	1957	4,486	>55	100	8.7	15.5	6.2 Based on total British population	1.5
Cox & Ford	1964	Great Britain	1927	60,000	<70	0	1.4	2.9	1.41	2.68
McNeill	1973	Conn., USA	1965–1968	9,247	20–74	32	F[b]1.2 M[c]3.7	2.5[c] 6.9[c]	1.2 3.5	2.6 7.2
Helsing et al.	1982	Md., USA	1963–1974	2,016	18–75	30	F[b]— M[b]—	24.1[c] 65.3[c]	— —	23.2 51.8

TABLE 11.1 (Continued)

Publication Study	Year	Place	Bereaved Subjects No.	Bereaved Subjects Year	Age, yr.[a]	Sex, % men	Refusals, %	Mortality (%) Bereaved <6 mo.	6–12 mo.	13–24 mo.	Controls <12 mo.	<24 mo.
Rees & Lutkins	1967	Llanidloes Wales	156	1960–1966	69.7	32.7	None	F[b] ← 8.5 → M[b]13.7	5.9	6.7 4.9	1.2 —	3.0 —
Clayton et al.	1974	St. Louis, Mo.	109	1968	62	30	42%	F[b] ← 2.6 → M[b]3	3	5.2 3	5	—
Gerber et al.	1975	New York, NY	169	Early 1970s	67	28	6–26%, no difference from participants.	"No increase," 2.4% in the first 15-month period.			Rates for controls not reported.	
Ward	1976	Sheffield, England	366	1971–1972	64	23.8	None	F[c]0.4 M[b]8	1.8 0	1.8 2.2	← 4 → ← 6.9 →	

[a] Average age of those in the cohort who died.
[b] F = Female. M = Male.
[c] Although these figures do not demonstrate an elevated risk in the widowed, when age and specific cause of death were controlled, the characteristic pattern of elevated risk among the bereaved emerged.
[d] Study reported *no* change in mortality rates in relationship to length of time bereaved.

of excess risk for suicide in the widowed of both sexes may be several years. For all causes of death other than suicide, there may be a slight dip in observed mortality by comparison with expected mortality in the fourth and fifth years. Cohort studies of the young widowed are notably absent from the literature, and therefore this part of the picture is incomplete. However, in studies using vital statistics, the elevated risk for the young of both sexes, but particularly for men, is consistent.

Although the follow-up cohort studies generally do not have large enough sample sizes to permit cause-specific analyses of mortality rates, vital statistics studies have shown a broad effect that includes, in the main, conditions that are manifest in middle and late life. Cause specificity varies by sex. For men there is excess mortality from tuberculosis, influenza and pneumonia, cirrhosis and alcoholism, suicides and accidents, and heart disease. For women, there is elevated mortality from tuberculosis, cirrhosis and alcoholism, heart disease, and cancer. For women over 60 years of age, there is a suggestion of elevated risk of mortality from suicide and accidents, and diabetes (MacMahon & Pugh, 1965; Maddison & Viola, 1968). The infectious causes of death observed in the first half of this century before antibiotics are apparently no longer important.

A recent historical cohort study (Helsing & Szklo, 1981) contradicts these cause-specific rates in previous studies. This study fails to confirm an elevated risk of mortality from cardiovascular diseases, alcoholism, and cirrhosis in men and documents higher rates of infectious diseases, accidents, and suicide. For widowed women, only cirrhosis of the liver proved to be a specific cause of death that differentiated them from married women. However, the study's use of proportional mortality with no significant excess mortality overall for women weakens these cause-specific excess rates, because this would imply a protective effect of bereavement for some other causes of death. Overall the studies are not completely consistent in the specific causes of excess mortality among the bereaved and may be influenced by temporal changes in mortality rates and differences in the length of follow-up of the widowed and the comparison populations.

Table 11.1 also presents four major follow-up cohort studies of mortality following conjugal bereavement. The essential finding is that both widows and widowers have higher mortality rates than their nonbereaved comparison groups. Other findings have related to risk factors for death following bereavement.

The largest follow-up cohort study is the six-year survey of Rees and Lutkins (1969) who followed 903 survivors of 371 deceased residents in a semirural area of Wales with a population of 5184. The 903 survivors were matched with 878 area residents on age, sex, and martial status. The survey found a sevenfold increase in risk within one year between the bereaved and control group, which was highly significant. The risk was greatest for widowed spouses who had mortality rates that were ten times higher than the rates for parents, siblings, and children of deceased residents. Bereaved male relatives had the highest rates of mortality. Widowers were subject to the greatest risk of all, especially in the first six months. A histogram of the age distribution of relatives who died in the first year of bereavement demonstrated a biphasic curve. One peak at age 80 was expected based on the age distribution of all the people who died in the area. The second peak between 60 and 70 was unexpected and suggested that deaths in this age group contribute substantially to the excess number of deaths observed.

The site of death was an important determinant of risk for bereaved relatives in the Rees and Lutkins study (1967). If death occurred in a public place such as in a shop, or a road, or in a field as opposed to at home or in the hospital, there was a higher risk. This last observation raises questions about an additional factor, the expectedness of death, which is probably an important element that underlies the influence of site.

Factors that are thought to influence the risk of death are the duration of illness in the deceased spouse and preexisting illness in the survivor. A common assumption is that a prolonged terminal illness in the deceased may permit the survivor to prepare himself or herself through anticipatory grief. However, in the one study that compares the widowed on this factor, there was no salutory effect from a long terminal illness (Ward, 1976). Two other studies of the physical and psychological morbidity of bereavement support this absence of effect (Gerber, Rusalem, & Hannon, 1975; Clayton et al., 1971, 1972, 1973). This absence of effect may reflect a canceling out of opposing effects. The burden that a prolonged illness of the deceased may have had on the surviving spouse may cancel out any salutory effect of being able to prepare for the loss. Young widowed are not well represented in the samples involved here and this conclusion should not be generalized to them, because prolonged terminal illnesses may detrimentally affect the health of young surviving spouses (Glick, Weiss, & Parkes, 1974). Preexisting illness in the survivor may contribute to the elevated risk of mortality in the survivor independent of widowed status (Ward, 1976). This may be particularly true of survivors with major psychiatric disorders who ultimately die themselves by suicide (Shepherd & Barraclough, 1974). Hospital versus home as the site of death of the deceased spouse is a risk factor for subsequent death of the survivor (Rees & Lutkins, 1967), but it is also a function of preexisting illness in the survivor (Ward, 1976). The ill surviving spouses cannot care for their terminally ill spouse at home and will put them in the hospital. Thus these survivors with hospitalized spouses are often ill before becoming widowed and at greater risk of dying.

In summary, bereaved persons are at higher risk for multiple specific diseases, various in etiology and organ site, including for the most part chronic conditions of middle and late life. The excess risk of mortality due to bereavement is higher among widowed men than widowed women at all ages. However, the period of excess risk is unclear. Earlier studies indicate that for men risk peaks in the first six months after a loss and for women in the second year. A more recent study indicates that the period of risk may be considerably extended in time, at least for men, and women may not have an excess mortality.

Stress Response to Death: Bereavement

A general picture of grief in adult life resulting from conjugal loss emerges from several cohort studies that are most convincing for women of age 65 and under. Men, the elderly, and social minorities are poorly represented in the groups that have been studied. Although these under-represented persons may vary in specific elements of their grief, there is no suggestion in the available literature that their pattern of grief might be fundamentally different.

Some studies focus on grief that results from unexpected death and thus cannot adequately take into consideration the phenomenon of anticipatory grief and its effect on grief. In general, grief is recognized as a basic human response that is, practically speaking, universal and inevitable.

Several authors (Clayton, 1972; Parkes, 1972b) agree that the most important, distinctive feature of grieving is the widowed person's preoccupation with the deceased and the pining associated with it. A central component of grief is searching for the lost person that is associated with separation anxiety. Conjugal loss provokes a response that is characterized by a progression of changes if not distinct phases. As such, it is identified as an active, evolving process and not a steady state that simply diminishes in intensity over time. The duration of grief on the average is several months although for some it is over for the most part after four months (Bornstein, Clayton, & Halikas, 1973; Parkes, 1972). No clear end point is established although some point after one year and not exceeding two years is the most likely. The peak intensity is usually passed by the fifth to sixth month, although two thirds of widows may still be actively grieving one year after a loss.

Grief has various manifestations including anxiety, dejection, anger, hallucinations or illusions, and nonspecific somatic symptoms. Current understanding of biological and physiological processes underlying the psychological picture is highly inferential. Grief evolves in a social context that has an important influence on some overt behavior during grief. The mourning ritual of society shapes the response (Krupp & Kligfeld, 1962; Mathison, 1970). For example, in Japan the hallucinatory experiences of feeling the dead spouse's presence is facilitated by the religious tradition of a shrine at which the spirit of the lost spouse dwells (Yamamoto, et al., 1969). In addition, the grieving person must adjust to new roles and changed status. The changed social environment may result in loneliness and cause a sense of insecurity.

Variation in the manifestations of grief among individuals is considerable in normal grieving. Extremes of variation are defined as patterns of atypical grief characterized by delay, prolongation, intense separation anxiety, intense avoidance, and other features. Atypical grief is believed to carry a higher risk of prolonged suffering that is secondary to unresolved grief and other nonspecific psychological complications. The variation in grieving is determined by multiple factors that have been summarized by Parkes.

Phases of Bereavement.   Parkes (1972) who owes a debt to Bowlby (1973) for his conceptualization of normal grieving, has played a central role in the modern study of adult grief. His conclusions are based on extensive clinical work with bereaved patients and the follow-up study of two small London cohorts. One cohort of 22 widows with an average age of 49 was referred through general practitioners (Parkes, 1970a); the other cohort of 21 bereaved patients at the Bethlem Royal and Maudsley Hospitals had a mean age of 49 and included four men (Parkes, 1964, 1965). Direct observations on this small sample were supplemented by chart reviews on an additional 94 patients. Although the first cohort was followed using a standardized interview, it was self-selected by having consulted with a general practitioner and by the women's willingness to participate in Parkes' study. The second cohort of psychiatric patients was selected after being hospitalized for mental disorder. Hence neither sample was representative of the general population of bereaved, and both were very small and not fully prospective cohorts.

Based on his work, Parkes proposed that bereavement be viewed as a process characterized by a progression of changes or phases. Table 11.2 summarizes these phases and compares Parkes' phases with similar conceptualizations of grief by Freud, Lindeman, Clayton, Glick, and Schmale. The first phase is a period of numbness that lasts from a few hours up to a few days. Widows sometimes report the state of feeling stunned, dazed, and shocked, leading to a sense of feeling blunted or numb that is sometimes experienced as a relief from the painful feelings evoked by the loss.

The second phase begins after a relatively clear-cut transition from the initial brief period of numbness. This phase is characterized by separation anxiety, the hallmark of which was preoccupation with thoughts of the deceased. It is this preoccupation along with its affective component of pining that Parkes considers the essential component of the grief reaction. Active, mostly unconscious, searching for the deceased is linked to separation anxiety that is presumably generated from a basic motivating need to recover the lost person. Feelings of anger (protest) and guilt are possible additional parts of this phase. In recognition of the prominence of angry feelings, Bowlby (1973) has characterized this stage of grieving as one of yearning and protest. The angry feelings diminish in intensity, alternating with and finally giving way to feelings of sadness and apathy. The searching phase peaks in two to four weeks following the death.

Further progression of the grieving process into feelings of apathy and

TABLE 11.2 Phases of Bereavement

Parkes	Freud	Lindeman	Clayton et al.	Glick	Schmale
Process with progressive changes if not three stages: 1. Numbness punctuated by pain (peaks in several hours).	"Grief work: gradual dissolution of ties, with the withdrawal of libido from the deceased	A process involving:		A process including: disbelief and shock: cold, numb, dazed, empty, confused	
2. Searching a. Preoccupation with the deceased and pining.	Loss of capacity to adopt new love objects	Preoccupation with the deceased and pangs of somatic distress		Recurring thoughts of the deceased	
b. Attention to place and objects of the deceased	Inhibition of activity or turning away from activity not connected with thoughts of deceased				
c. Crying	Painful dejection		Crying	Sorrow	
d. Anger, protest, and guilt (peaks in 2–4 weeks; no clear end point).		Guilt, hostile reactions			
e. Perceptual set for the deceased.					

3. Despair and sadness	Painful dejection	Depressed mood; normal depressive reaction; Loss of interests; poor concentration		Conservation-withdrawal response with affects including depression, helplessness, hopelessness, and giving up. Presumed to be a sympathetic response / Pervasive sadness "Depressive complex of symptoms"
a. Apathy and aimlessness	Loss of interest in the outside world if not associated with the deceased			Loneliness (social isolation) and deprivation (change in status to single parent and unmarried)
b. Disorganization. Leads to reorganization (Bowlby) gaining a new identity and finding a new life.	Loss of patterns of conduct			
Duration: not more than 2 years, still active at 1 year.	Duration not specified	Duration about 4 months	Duration: reduced intensity after 4 to 5 months, continues for a year	Duration: reduced emotional intensity after 2 months. The social consequences last several months

despair associated with aimlessness and disorganization of behavior patterns is the next change. Here the change is subtle, and it is difficult to recognize the end of one phase or the beginning of another. Intense, yet less frequent and briefer episodes of yearning for the deceased person occur for several months. At the same time that the separation anxiety slowly subsides, the expression of anger becomes variable and finally diminishes. This seems to occur concomitantly with growing feelings of depression. The period of depression that has been denoted as a period of disorganization by Bowlby (1973) because of apathy, and aimlessness does not establish itself as a well-demarcated phase of grief. Rather it occurs repetitively in one context or another. When the depression becomes minimal or when circumstances force it (and partially through the process of identification with the deceased), the bereaved person relinquishes the old bond and ventures out into new roles and a new life. A year after the death of a spouse the majority of subjects in the cohort from the general practice group were still grieving and for eight (of 22) the severity of the emotional disturbance remained moderate or severe.

This review has emphasized the chronological unfolding of the human response to loss in order to suggest that atypical emotional responses to loss may be different at various time periods after the loss. For example, an anxious person searching for the lost spouse ten months after the loss would be quite atypical, but at one month after the loss would be usual and expected.

It warrants additional emphasis that the phasic development presented in this review is not in actuality as clear as a summary might suggest. Moreover, the various features of grief and progression of changes that Parkes described were not universal; most occurred in the range of 50–75% of subjects in varying intensities. Yet Parkes' conceptualization is convincing because of its clarity, its consistency with observations made by Bowlby and his associates, and its basic consistency with other observations of grieving reported in the clinical and the sociological literature.

Other clinical observations.   Freud's *Mourning and Melancholia* (1917) is the origin for several current concepts that are central to our understanding of grief. He identified these four distinguishing features of the condition as part of an idealized account of "normal" mourning: (a) a profoundly painful dejection; (b) a loss of capacity to adopt new love objects; (c) an inhibition of activity or turning away from activity not connected with thoughts of the loved person; and (d) a loss of interest in the outside world insofar as it does not recall the deceased (Siggins, 1966).

Subsequently, Cobb and Lindeman (1943) and Lindeman (1944) reported observations on 101 survivors of the Coconut Grove fire. These survivors had the dual trauma of family loss and having gone through the same fire that killed their family members. They defined five characteristics of normal grief that were considered essential. Included were somatic

distress, preoccupation with the image of the deceased, guilt, hostile reactions, and loss of established patterns of conduct. It seems they preferred to characterize the anxiety in terms of somatic distress. In addition,
they suggested that normal grieving was a process of four months average
duration. No description of the sample was provided other than the information that the loss resulted from a sudden, violent death. Lindeman's
characterization of the main features of grief, although lacking a quantified
basis in his clinical writing, corresponded to parts of Freud's description
and was borne out in the studies of grief by Parkes.

Clayton and associates have reported on a random sample of 109 adult
survivors of spouses who died either at Barnes Hospital or in the St. Louis
area (Clayton et al., 1971; Clayton et al., 1972; Bornstein et al., 1973). This
follow-up cohort study is limited in its contribution to understanding the
natural history of grief by virtue of its focus on psychopathological symptoms.

The occurrence of depressive symptoms is given thorough attention.
The high frequency of depressive symptoms, not to mention primary depressive syndromes in Clayton's cohort, is convincing support for Parkes'
concept of a phase of bereavement characterized by depressed emotion
and despair. There is less convincing affirmation of a phase of anxious
searching partly because Clayton did not directly address the question.
Only 10% of subjects in her study report anxiety as a symptom. Of course,
anxiety may be experienced in many ways and in fact Lindeman preferred
to characterize it as somatic distress. Furthermore, separation anxiety as
defined by Parkes (1972) is not the same as clinical anxiety as assessed by
Clayton (1971). Thus future studies need to assess separation anxiety in
order to test Parkes' hypothesis because clinical anxiety is relatively un-
common during grief.

The grief of the elderly has features that are thought to distinguish it
from that in younger persons (Stern & Williams, 1951; Gramlich, 1968;
Tunstall, 1966; Gerber, Weiner, & Battin, 1975b; Heyman and Gianturec,
1973). Specifically, a loss in the elderly is faced with more acceptance, is
associated with more psychosomatic symptoms, and is characterized by
less numbness, denial, and guilt. However, hallucinations and illusions
occur with greater frequency in the elderly (Rees, 1971). It is plausible to
assume that some of these features—the acceptance, the reduced numbness, denial, and guilt—are related to the anticipation of death in older
people before the actual death. Anticipation of the death may be due to
the chronicity of the illnesses from which older people are more likely to
die and to the timeliness of death when people get older. Anticipatory
grief may play an important role as a determinant of the content and pattern of actual grieving independent of the age of the bereaved person, but
this issue has not been systematically addressed.

A comparison of the types of the lost family members can clarify the
importance of particular family relationships. Four main types of family

relationships can be affected: child loses parent, parent loses child, sibling loses sibling, and spousal loss. The acute effects of parental, child, and sibling losses are relatively understudied compared with spousal loss; however, these other types of losses have been clinically studied. A recent study has found that in comparison with spousal loss or parental loss in adults, child loss produced significantly higher intensities of grief following the loss (Sanders, 1979–1980), and a review of the grief response to stillbirths has concluded that these parents can experience an intensity of grief equal to that of other child losses (Kirkley-Best & Kellner, 1982). Comparative studies of this type suggest that our understanding of grief responses, which is rooted in spousal bereavement, may be limited by the type of loss that has been studied. However, critical studies of these other types of losses are available.

Parental loss in young children has been of particular interest for psychoanalytic theory. The psychoanalytic consensus seems that children do not pass through mourning, when defined as the painful, emotional detachment from the inner representation of the lost person, whether a parent or sibling (Wolfenstein, 1966). However, Bowlby (1961) is a notable exception to this consensus because he considers adult mourning an extension of a childhood process of anger and protest at any separation. Most other observers consider denial of the loss as the central psychological process in children, but children can clearly respond acutely to parental loss, as Bowlby's studies demonstrate.

The loss of a child has usually been studied from the standpoint of the preparation of parents for the loss, but some attention has been given to the siblings of the dying child. Childhood leukemia and the pediatric intensive care unit have been the focus of most studies. A series of stages or phases in the parental response to the potential loss has been described. These stages are very similar to the more systematically studied phases that Parkes (1972) has described following spousal loss (Futterman & Hoffman, 1973; Friedman et al., 1963; Walker, MacBridge, & Vachon, 1979; Binger et al., 1969) and that we have reviewed in detail. The interaction of siblings with their parents has been addressed in two studies of family functioning after child loss. These studies follow the earlier case descriptions of Cain et al. (1964) and others who reported a wide range of disturbed reactions to the death of a sibling. Psychosomatic and behavioral problems have been reported in siblings following sibling loss from cancer (Tietz, McSherry, & Britt, 1977) or from drowning (Nixon & Pern, 1977). The drowning study was particularly useful, because it included a control group and studied some simple aspects of parental functioning as a family system. The grieving families did worse on a variety of indices including a 24 % parental separation rate over five years (compared with 0 % for the controls). Parental substance abuse also increased. This controlled study of 77 families clearly needs replication and other causes of death need study, but nevertheless a focus on the family as a system is useful.

The family as a system has also been studied clinically in terms of family interaction before and after loss of a family member. In several case histories Shanfield (1981) indicated that some marital interaction variables may predict poor response to spousal loss. In those family systems that discouraged the affective expression or that had a "skewed decision-making apparatus" in which one spouse dominated the other, conjugal loss was followed by poor physical and emotional health in the surviving spouse. Other family workers have suggested that scapegoating of a surviving family member may occur as a displacement of the guilt and anger following a loss (Goldberg, 1973). Maladaptive family interactions and pathological family roles that follow "incomplete mourning" of a family member have been implicated in a variety of psychopathological states (Paul, 1967), but no systematic study has related family interaction before the loss to any health outcomes.

Sociological Studies.   Sociological studies of widowhood have introduced into consideration the widow's social status, social roles, and social adjustment. In one follow-up study, the deprivation as a result of change in status and the loneliness as a result of social isolation were important elements of bereavement that caused suffering and problems in their own right (Glick, Weiss, & Parkes, 1974). Whereas these investigators noted a reduction in the intense emotional response associated with a loss in most widows after two months, impairment in social functioning was prolonged and lasted several months. Other sociological studies reporting on single assessments after the loss support the conclusions above about changes in status and disruption of social roles resulting from conjugal loss (Tunstall, 1966; Lopata, 1973; Berardo, 1968, 1970). In general, the social environment of the bereaved is changed and appears insecure and threatening.

Faced with the loss and a changed social environment, the bereaved person turns for support to his or her established social network (Walker et al., 1977). No empirical literature of social supports of the bereaved exists currently, with the exception of how the social network is perceived by the bereaved (Maddison & Walker, 1967; Raphael & Maddison, 1976). Perceived nonsupportiveness of the social network has proven to be a powerful variable in predicting poor outcome of the grieving process. Clinical observations from the follow-up studies affirm the accuracy of these perceptions. Nevertheless, the actual social network is not described and, based on this work alone, it is possible that perceived nonsupportiveness may reflect a quality of personal social functioning (including being part of a depressive reaction) rather than an actual deficiency in the social network of the individual.

Taken together, the studies described above provide a basis for the importance of studying social expectations, roles, and relationships in the process and consequences of grief. However, the research in this area has been primarily focused on women. Sex differences in the effect of bereavement on social ties have been addressed in one study (Bock & Webber, 1972). This study suggested that men may suffer greater social disruption than women. Furthermore, the epidemiologic studies reviewed earlier have shown that the risk of mortality, including suicide, following the loss of a spouse is much higher for males than for females (Jacobs & Ostfeld, 1977; Klerman & Izen, 1977). Sex differences have also been found in the risk of specific types of disorders, particularly in mental disorders. Women have been found to have a higher risk of depressive disorders, whereas men have been found to have a higher risk of alcoholism (Stein & Susser, 1969; Clayton, Halikas, & Maurice, 1972; Parkes & Brown, 1972). Whether this pattern following a loss is specific to bereavement is questionable because it roughly corresponds to the pattern by sex of psychiatric disorders that has been observed in general prevalence surveys (Dohrenwend & Dohrenwend, 1974, 1976, 1977).

In considering role-related explanatory factors for sex differences in outcome, the higher risk of a more severe outcome for males after the loss of a spouse is consistent with the findings of sociological studies of marital satisfaction and social psychiatric studies of marital status and mental illness. In research on marital satisfaction, men have consistently been found to have higher levels of satisfaction with marriage than women (Gerstel, 1978). And in studies comparing married and single men and women on mental health, married men have been found to be much healthier than single men, whereas single women are healthier than their married counterparts (Gove, 1972; Radloff, 1975). On this basis, it has been concluded that marriage is better for men than for women in general and that, more specifically, marriage has a protective effect on the mental health of men (Durkheim, 1951; Gerstel, 1978).

Differences in sex roles are also associated with different coping patterns between men and women. The sex role expectations for men of appearing strong and independent imply a greater need for control among men and a greater tendency toward the avoidance of feelings that might be interpreted as weak or dependent. In relation to these tendencies, one might expect men to be more likely, in reaction to the loss of a spouse, to use denial or suppression defenses. In fact, although the sample of men was quite small, Glick, Weiss, and Parkes (1974) found men to go through less obsessional review of their spouses' death than their female subjects, for they saw it as pointless. Men also had a slower emotional recovery from the death than women, which is consistent with avoidance of feelings. Because of this need of the average man for emotional control, it is suggested that the type of social support perceived as helpful would be expected to be quite different for men than for women. Again, Glick, Weiss, and Parkes (1974) did find such differences, specifically, that men less often wanted to talk about the death of their wives to family or friends and that, in contrast to support found to be positive for women, they wanted help in controlling rather than expressing their emotions.

Other sex role-related differences can affect social and health outcomes after the loss. In terms of both division of labor and power relations, the loss of a spouse has different implications for males and females. For women, the loss of a husband can represent a financial loss and possibly a loss in social status. For men, the loss of a wife is often a loss also of emotional support and of social relations outside the home. The possibility of retirement coinciding with the loss of a spouse in older men involves a potentially crucial focus for concern, as retirement represents an additional loss of a central role function and definition of identity among men. Loss of an occupational role aggravates the risk of social isolation among widowers (Berardo, 1970). These role losses imply different foci of worry and concern for widowers in contrast to widows. Glick, Weiss, and Parkes (1974) captured some of these differences when they found that men defined the loss of their wives in terms of feelings of dismemberment, whereas women defined the loss of their husbands in terms of feelings of abandonment.

In summary, certain dimensions of sex roles are discussed as factors that would distinguish the process of grief for men from that for women. Sex roles are also potential explanatory factors for sex differences found in outcomes of bereavement. Sex roles distinguish how the threat of a conjugal loss may be perceived differently by sex, and how one's coping style or adjustment may differ by sex. Also, they underscore the possibility of differential risks by sex of social isolation after a loss. These differences may explain the higher risk of negative consequences of bereavement for men.

Biological Studies. In general, there has been very little systematic work reported on biological aspects of grieving in adults. One exception is the prospective follow-up study by Hofer, Wolff, Friedman, and Mason (1972a, 1972b) in which urinary corticosteroid levels in parents were examined before the death of a child from leukemia and during the bereavement period at intervals of six months and two years following the child's death. This study indicated that an individual's characteristic adrenal cortical excretion level during a period of impending object loss can be significantly different from that during the bereavement period and that the direction of the difference is an important characteristic of the individual subject, particularly with regard to the style and effectiveness of psychological defenses and the intensity of grief experienced. This study was, however, not primarily concerned with the postloss period and was limited with regard to sampling intervals and in the scope of the endocrine, psychological, and social variables that could be assessed.

A recent study of the dexamethasone suppression test (DST), a biological marker for major depressive disorders, gave normal results in bereaved people who met criteria for a major depressive disorder six months after spousal loss (Kosten, 1984). However, the post-DST serum cortisol levels were positively correlated with depression scores. Thus the more depressed widows and widowers had less serum cortisol suppression by dexamethasone. This is consistent with some relationship between adrenal cortical hyperactivity and depressive symptoms during bereavement. A follow-up study of growth hormone (HGH) following spousal loss demonstrated a large rise in HGH when the loss was reviewed with the surviving spouse (Kosten et al., 1984). The effect on health is unclear, but HGH is normally not secreted during the daytime in adults. A companion analysis of prolactin showed a direct correlation between a rise in serum prolactin and the separation anxiety of grief (Brown et al., 1983).

Another study dealing with biological aspects of grieving is the recently finding of depressed T-cell function in a prospective follow-up study of 26 bereaved spouses six weeks after the loss, indicating an abnormality in immune function which might be secondarily related to psychoendocrine reactions (Bartrop et al., 1977). This finding has been confirmed by Stein and collaborators (1983) in 15 bereaved males.

A follow-up study of young widows provides a measure of automatic symptoms, but it has no convincing validation with concurrent biological measures (Parkes & Brown, 1972). In this study, Parkes and Brown demonstrate a high frequency of automatic symptoms during the first year, especially in women, that diminish to normal levels by the third year. A study of six depressed female patients with a clear apparent psychological loss is also relevant to bereavement (Sachar et al., 1967). In these patients confrontation with the loss precipitated a major corticosteroid elevation. No study has yet addressed the usefulness of these biological measures as predictors of distal health outcomes following loss. This is a major limitation in this area.

METHODOLOGICAL ISSUES

In studies of health outcomes following loss, family heterogeneity is a major methodological issue. Heterogeneity occurs both within and between families. Between families the type of loss and "age" of the family are important sources of heterogeneity. Loss of a child to leukemia in a young family is not only a different type of loss from spousal loss, but it occurs in a family with different tasks and relationships than an isolated, bereaved spouse. The family tasks around bereavement and terminal illness may also differ as the family members pass through the various stages of grief or anticipatory mourning (Parkes, 1975). This concept of stages is a source of heterogeneity within families, because each member may pass through these stages at a different rate. This time perspective must be used to standardize assessments of family functioning and communication so that an assessment of family interaction can be placed in a meaningful context for relating it to health outcomes. For example, a family that seems to be anxiously searching for a member to take the place of a lost child at four weeks after the loss may be normal, but this same response at one year after the loss may be associated with a variety of poor health outcomes. This same response at one year after the loss in a woman of 65 who lost her husband and is searching for a replacement husband may be associated with a good health outcome, and apathy toward such a search might be associated with a poor outcome in this older "family."

Family assessment scales have used both self-report measures and direct observation rating scales by trained raters to focus on the family therapy more than on the natural history of families or on families' response to crises (Gurman & Kniskern, 1981). Although these instruments have not been used to relate family interaction to a pathological outcome during bereavement, evaluation instruments such as the Beavers Timberlawn Guide to Family Assessment (Lewis, Beavers, & Gossett, 1976) or the more comprehensive Yale Family Evaluation Guide (Fleck, personal communication) measure relevant factors such as family communication, problem solving, and generational and power structures. Futhermore, the explicit time perspective of the Yale Guide emphasizes the broad family life cycle of marriage—child rearing–retirement and might accommodate the shorter time span over which grief occurs. Thus family assessment instruments might be made sensitive enough for predicting distal health outcomes in bereaved families. Impairment in family problem solving or communication might reduce the usage of important health services by the family and lead to illness. In particular, in young families the children might miss some preventative health care when one parent or even a sibling dies, whereas in older families a bereaved spouse might not continue his or her own health care. Family assessments could detect these relative impairments in problem solving through longitudinal studies of families during the crisis of loss and bereavement.

The assessment of family interaction holds more promise for future studies of bereavement than its current limited use would suggest, but individual assessments are also necessary in any study of grief. These individual assessments have been much more fully developed and have been specifically targeted for grief in several studies. The Texas Inventory of Grief is a seven-item scale used to assess unresolved grief (Faschingbauer et al., 1977) and has been recently followed by a more extensive grief scale of 58 items (Zisook, De Vaul, & Glick, 1982). This new scale purports to measure normal grief responses, not just the pathological grief assessed by the Texas Inventory. Neither of these scales has been related to distal health outcomes except that nonspecific psychiatric disorders are associated with higher scores on the Texas Inventory. Another recent scale developed by Horowitz, Wilner, and Alvarez (1982) measures emotional numbness and intrusion as responses to acute traumatic events such as loss of a family member. Although this scale does not specifically assess grief, it provides an important instrument for future studies of bereavement. The most recent addition to this area is a new grief scale that we have developed and tested in a large epidemiological study of the health consequences of bereavement. This scale specifically measures emotional numbness and separation anxiety as different components of the grief response and has used a subset of the 20 items from the Center for Epidemiological Studies Depression Scale (CES-D) (Radloff, 1977) to assess the despair associated with grief (Jacobs et al., submitted for publication). This new instrument will be used to predict health outcomes in this study and may be an important addition to the assessments available for health studies of bereavement.

With all these instruments research designs that provide adequate control groups are important for the interpretation of any family scores. Normative data for bereavement responses either in individuals or families are not available in a form that allows researchers to use cross-sectional research designs to compare individuals with some standard response after a loss. Selection of families at high risk for poor health outcomes after a loss is also not possible, because the instruments used in the studies reviewed here have not given any clear high risk markers. Thus longitudinal study designs need to gather normative data and to determine the variation in emotional response over time. Parkes (1972) has provided a conceptual model, but only larger longitudinal studies will be able to test the available bereavement scales and provide the needed normative data for cross-sectional and "case-control" studies of high risk families for poor health outcomes after a loss.

FUTURE DIRECTIONS

Pathogenesis of Complications: Considerations

Based on an understanding of the process of grief and a knowledge of the pattern of mortality associated with conjugal bereavement, three conceptual levels of pathogenetic mechanisms appear relevant: physiological, behavioral, and social. Assuming that Ciocco's (1940) observation that death is rare before the elapse of four months after a conjugal loss is true and not a methodological artifact, it appears most promising to look for pathogenetic forces in the phase of despair.

On a physiological level, the postulated parasympathetic activation of the conservation-withdrawal reaction, a state thought to be associated with increased vulnerability to illness, may have cardiovascular and other consequences (Engel, 1968). Depression and the accompanying physiological changes both in endocrine functioning and in monoamine neurotransmitters may prove to be a mediating mechanism leading to illness and death through suicide, cardiovascular disease, infectious disease, or general susceptibility to disease (Lebovits, Shekelle, Ostfeld, and Paul, 1967; Kasl, Ostfeld, & Brody, 1980; Markus et al., 1977; Imboden, Canter & Cluff,

1961). Alterations in immune mechanisms may lower vulnerability to infectious diseases that increases the risk of morbidity and mortality from these diseases (Bartrop et al., 1977; Ciocco, 1940; Amkraut & Solomon, 1975). Finally, the neuroendocrine system, as an effector system with far-reaching biochemical regulatory actions on virtually every tissue in the body including the brain, provides a particularly promising view of a major mediating linkage through which psychological processes can exert pathogenetic influences upon bodily processes (Mason et al., 1967).

On a behavorial level of conceptualization, changes in health practices of the surviving spouse may lead to illness and death. This idea is consistent with the observation that most of the causes of mortality among the bereaved are conditions of middle and late life. Such changes in health practices such as the neglect of early signs of disease, the neglect of the proper management of disease, or the excessive use of alcohol may be related to several aspects of grief. These aspects include the disorganization and the aimlessness of the despair phase of grief, the exhaustion of searching unsuccessfully in a sustained state of high arousal, the challenge to adapt the new roles in a threatening social environment, or a change in socioeconomic status in a society in which the highest quality of health care is usually purchased privately at high cost. The potential importance of health practices is compatible with the idea that bereavement increases the risk of premature illness or death in bereaved persons who were already vulnerable by virtue of a diathesis or preexisting disease. This is consistent with the observation that mortality rates among the bereaved drop below comparison group rates in the third, fourth, and fifth years after their conjugal loss.

On a social level of conceptualization, the loss of care suffered by a child or by a bereaved spouse in circumstances in which the conjugal partner who has died was the medically responsible member of the family may be another pathogenetic mechanism. The social isolation of widowhood and the widowed person's loss of power to purchase care may be related to this mechanism. The clinical literature on the morbidity of bereavement gives some attention to these risk factors (Parkes, 1972; Clayton, 1973; Shepherd & Barraclough, 1974). In younger families the children's health care is also at risk, and social isolation, depression, and poor finances, if a parent is lost, may all be important mechanisms.

Research Designs and Assessment Instruments. *Prospective* or at least *follow-up* research designs with repeated biological assessments in conjunction with psychological and medical illness outcomes for families need to be implemented over one to two year follow-up periods. The leads available from Hofer et al.'s (1972) study of cortisol in child loss suggest a model for neuroendocrine assessments both before and after the loss of a family member. Although anticipatory mourning may affect these hormonal measures, these authors have provided a model for understanding psychoendocrine relationships during bereavement. Future work needs to extend the assessment to include family interaction, particularly in child loss. Studies will also need to be larger or targeted toward family members at high risk of becoming ill (e.g., having preexisting disorders) in order to elucidate the relationship of these intervening variables to health outcomes. Large epidemiological studies, particularly the vital statistics designs, seem to be of limited usefulness in future work, but small intensive studies of the presumptive biological, behavioral, and social mediating factors have a role in the future understanding of illness and its relationship to loss. As suggested in the section on methodology, several new instruments are available to assess grief and should be used in any future studies to standardize what have usually been more clinical evaluations. Biological mediators also need consideration and appropriate assessment. Neuroendocrine and immunological assessments seem the most promising at present.

Recommendations for Additional Research

Several major areas of research are suggested by the content and the deficiencies of the literature. They include:

1. Studies of the process of grief in its psychological, social, and biological dimensions and interactions, such as Parkes (1972) has begun.
2. The studies of the biology of grief may appropriately be concerned with the neuroendocrinology and immunology of grief, the understanding of biological correlates and determinants of the psychological and social dimensions of the process, and the causes of the increased susceptibility to illness that accompanies grief.
3. Cohort and particularly prospective studies of the social, psychological, and biological features of grief are essential to an understanding of the causes of the morbid and mortal consequences of the process because grief is too global a concept and needs specification as Parkes (1972) has suggested in his model. Such studies should delineate the characteristics of those at high and low risk for these consequences.
4. Studies of both young and elderly grieving men to elucidate the particularly high risk of morbidity and mortality in them.
5. Studies of parents whose children die before full maturity to elucidate for the survivor the risk of illness and death.
6. Studies that elucidate the relationship of loss to the depressive symptoms of bereavement and of both of these to clinical depression.
7. Clinical trials of various treatments such as brief psychotherapy and

antidepressant drugs for grieving persons at high risk of morbidity and mortality or already impaired in functioning as a consequence of severe grief.

8. Studies that compare the human response to loss with the general response to stress and to the anticipation of a loss with the aim of understanding the human response to various environmental stressors.

REFERENCES

Amkraut, A., & Solomon, G. F. (1975). From the symbolic stimulus to the pathophysiologic response: Immune mechanisms. *International Journal of Psychiatric Medicine 5*, 541–563.

Anonymous. (1903). Assortive mating in man: A cooperative study. *Biometrica 2*, 481–498.

Bartrop, R. W., Luckhurst, E., Lazarus, L. et al. (1977). Depressed lymphoctye function after bereavement. *Lancet 1*, 834–836.

Berardo, F. M. (1968). Widowhood status in the United States: Perspective on a neglected aspect of the family life cycle. *Family Coordinator 17*, 191–203.

Berardo, F. M. (1970). Survivorship and social isolation: The case of the aged widower. *Family Coordinator 19*, 11–25.

Binger, C. M., Ablin, A. R., Feverstein R. C. et al. (1969). Childhood leukemia—Emotional impact on patient and family. *New England Journal of Medicine 280*, 414–418.

Bock, E. W., & Webber, I. L. (1972). Suicide among the elderly: Isolating widowhood and mitigating alternatives. *Journal of Marriage and Family*. (February), 24–31.

Bornstein, P. E., Clayton, R., Halikas, J. A. et al. (1973). The depression of widowhood after thirteen months. *British Journal of Psychiatry 122*, 561–566.

Bourne, P. G., Rose, R. M., & Mason, J. W. (1968). 17–OHCS levels in combat—special forces "A" team under threat of attack. *Archives of General Psychiatry 19*, 135–140.

Bowlby, J. (1961). Childhood mourning and its implications for psychiatry. *American Journal of Psychiatry, 118*, 481–498.

Bowlby, J. (1973). *Attachment and loss. Vol. II: Separation, anxiety, and anger*. New York: Basic Books.

Brown, S., Jacobs, S. C., & Mason, J. W. (1983, March). *Prolactin as a stress responsive hormone*. Presented at the American Psychosomatic Society.

Cain, A. C., Fast, I., & Erickson, M. (1964). Children's disturbed reactions to the death of a sibling. *American Journal of Orthopsychiatry 34*, 741–752.

Ciocco, A. (1940). On the mortality in husbands and wives. *Human Biology, 12*, 508–531.

Clayton, P. J. (1973). The clinical morbidity of the first year of bereavement: A review. *Comprehensive Psychiatry 14*, 151–157.

Clayton, P. J. (1975). The effect of living alone on bereavement symptoms. *American Journal of Psychiatry 132*, 133–137.

Clayton, P. J., Halikas, J. A., & Maurice W. L. (1971). The bereavement of the widowed. *Diseases of the Nervous System 32*, 597–604.

Clayton, P. J., Halikas, J. A. & Maurice, W. L. (1972). The depression of widowhood. *British Journal of Psychiatry 120*, 71–78.

Cobb, S., & Lindeman, E. (1943). Neuropsychiatric observations about the Coconut Grove fire. *Annals of Surgery 117*, 814–824.

Cox, R. P., & Ford, J. R. (1964). The mortality of widows shortly after widowhood. *Lancet, 1*, 163.

Dohrenwend, B. P., & Dohrenwend, B. S. (1974). Social and cultural influences on psychotherapy. *Annual Review of Psychology 25*, 417–457.

Dohrenwend, B. P., & Dohrenwend, B. S. (1976). Sex differences in psychiatric disorders. *American Journal of Sociology 81*, 1447–1459.

Dohrenwend, B. P., & Dohrenwend, B. S. (1977). Reply to Gove and Tudor's comment on sex differences in psychiatric disorders. *American Journal of Sociology 82*, 1336–1345.

Durkheim, E. (1951). *Suicide: A study in sociology*. New York: Free Press.

Engel, G. L. (1968). A life setting conducive to illness: The giving-up-given-up complex. *Bull Menninger Clinic, 32*, 355–365.

Farr, W. (1858). Influence on marriage on the mortality of the French people. *Transactions of the National Association for the Promotion of Social Science*, 504–512.

Faschingbauer, T. R., Devaul, R. A., & Zisook S. (1977). Development of the Texas inventory of grief. *American Journal of Psychiatry, 134.* 696, 698.

Fleck, S. Yale. Family Evaluation Guide. Personal communication.

Freud, S. (1957). *Mourning and Melancholia (1917)* (standard Ed.). *Complete Works, 14*, 237.

Friedman, S. B., Chokoff, P., Mason, J. W. et al. (1963). Behavioral observations on parents anticipating the death of a child. *Pediatrics 32*, 610–625.

Futterman, E. H., & Hoffman, I. (1973). Crisis in adaptation in the families of fatally ill children. In E. J. Anthony & C. Koupernik (Eds.), The Child and his family: The impact of disease and death. New York: Wiley.

Gerber, I., Rusalem, R., Hannon, N. et al. (1975a). Anticipatory grief and aged widows and widowers. *Journal of Gerontology 30*, 225–229.

Gerber, I., Weiner, A., Battin, D. et al. (1975b). Brief therapy to the aged bereaved. In B. Shoenberg et al. (Eds.), *Bereavement: Its psycho-social aspects*. New York: Columbia University Press.

Gerstel, N. (1978) *Computer marriage: constraints on spouses*. Paper presented at the American Sociological Association.

Glick I., Weiss R. S., & Parkes, C. M. (1974). *The first year of bereavement*. New York: Wiley.

Goldberg, S. B. (1973). Family tasks and reactions in the crisis of death. *Social Casework* (July), 398–405.

Gove, W. (1972). Relationship between sex roles, marital status and mental illness. *Social Forces 51*, 34–44.

Gramlich, E. P. (1968). Recognition and management of grief in elderly patients. *Geriatrics 23*: 87–92.

Gurman, A. S., & Kniskern, D. P. (1981). *Handbook of family therapy*. New York: Brunner/Mazel.

Helsing, K. J., & Szklo M. (1981). Mortality after bereavement. *American Journal of Epidemiology 114*, 41–52.

Helsing K. J.. Szklo M., & Comstock, G. W. (1981). Factors associated with mortality after widowhood. *American Journal of Public Health 71*, 802–809.

Heyman, D. K., & Gianturce, D. T. (1973). Long term adaptation by the elderly to bereavement. *Journal of Gerontology 28*, 359–362.

Hofer, M. A., Wolff, C. T., Friedman, S. B., & Mason, J. W. (1972a). A psychoendocrine study of bereavement. Pt. I: 17-Hydroxycorticosteroid excretion rates of parents following death of their children from leukemia. *Psychosomatic Medicine 34*, 481–491.

Hofer, M. A., Wolff, C. T., Friedman, S. B., & Mason, J. W. (1972b). A psychoendocrine study of bereavement. Pt. II: Observations on the process of mourning in relation to adrenocortical function. *Psychosomatic Medicine, 34*, 492–504.

Horowitz, M., Wilner, N., & Alvarez, W. (1979). Impact of event scale: A measure of subjective stress. *Psychosomatic Medicine, 41*, 209–218.

Imboden, J. B., Canter, A., & Cluff, L. E., (1961). Convalescence from influenza. *Archives of Internal Medicine 180*, 393–399.

Jacobs, S. C., Kasl, S. V., Ostfeld, A., Kosten, T. R., & Sharpentier, P., *The assessment of grief following spousal loss: I. Item analysis.* Manuscript submitted for publication.

Jacobs, S. C., & Ostfeld, A. (1977). An epidemiological review of the mortality of bereavement. *Psychosomatic Medicine, 39*, 344–357.

Kasl, S. V., Ostfeld, A. M., Brody, G. M et al. (1980). Effects of "involuntary" relocation on the health and behavior of the elderly. *Second conference on the epidemiology of aging.* Washington D.C.: NIH Publication No. 80–969.

Katz J., Weiner, H., Gallagher, T. E., & Hellman, L. (1970). Stress, distress, and ego defenses: Psychoendocrine responses to impending breast tumor biopsy. *Archives of General Psychiatry 23*, 131–142.

Kirkley-Best E., & Kellner, K. R. (1982). The forgotten grief: A review of the psychology of stillbirth. *American Journal of Orthopsychiatry*, (July), *52*(3) 420–429.

Klerman, G. & Izen, J. E. (1977). The effects of bereavement and grief on physical health and general well-being. In *Advances in psychosomatic medicine. Epidemiologic studies in psychosomatic medicine.* Basel, Switzerland: Karger.

Kosten, T. R., Jacobs, S. C., & Mason J. W. (1984). The dexamethasone suppression test during bereavement. *Journal of Nervous and Mental Disease, 172*, 359–360.

Kosten, T. R., Jacobs, S. C., Mason, J. W., Wahby V., & Atkins, S. (1984). Psychological correlates of growth hormone response to stress. *Psychosomatic Medicine, 46*, 49–58.

Kraus, A. S., & Lilienfeld, A. M. (1959). Some epidemiologic aspects of the high mortality rate in the young widowed group. *Journal of Chronic Diseases 10*, 207–217.

Krupp, G. P., & Kligfeld, B. (1962). The bereavement reaction: A cross-cultural evaluation. *Journal of Religion and Health 1*, 222–246.

Lebovits, B. Z., Shekelle, R. B., Ostfeld, A. M., & Paul, O. (1967). Prospective and retrospective studies of coronary heart disease. *Psychosomatic Medicine 29*, 265–272.

Lewis, J. M., Beavers, W. R., Gossett, J. T. et al. (1976). *No single thread: Psychological health in family systems.* New York: Brunner/Mazel.

Lindeman E. (1944). Symptomatology and management of acute grief. *American Journal of Psychiatry 101*, 141.

Lopata, H. Z. (1973). *Widowhood in an American city.* Cambridge, Ma: Schenkman.

MacMahon, B., & Pugh, T. F. (1965). Suicide in the widowed. *American Journal of Epidemiology 81*, 23–31.

Maddison, D., & Viola, A. (1968). The health of widows in the year following bereavement. *Journal of Psychosomatic Research 12*, 297–306.

Maddison, D., & Walker, W. L. (1967). Factors affecting outcome of conjugal bereavement. *British Journal of Psychiatry 113*, 1057–1067.

Markus, R. E., Schuab, J. J., Farris, P. et al., (1977). Mortality and community mental health. *Archives of General Psychiatry 39*, 1393–1401.

Mason, J. W. (1975a). Clinical psychophysiology: Psychoendocrine mechanisms. In M. Reiser (Ed.), *American handbook of psychiatry* (Vol. IV, pp. 553–582). New York: Basic Books.

Mason, J. W. Buescher, E. L., Belfer, M. L. et al. (1967). Pre-illness hormonal changes in army recruits with acute respiratory infections (Abstract). *Psychosomatic Medicine, 29*, 545.

Mathison, J. (1970). A cross-cultural view of widowhood. *Omega, 1*, 201–218.

McNeill, D. N. (1973). *Mortality among the widowed in Connecticut, 1965–1968.* New Haven: Yale University M.P.H. Essay.

Myers, R. J. (1963). An instance of the pitfalls prevalent in graveyard research. *Biometrics 19*, 638–650.

Nixon, J., & Pearn, J. (1977). Emotional sequelae of parents and sibs following the drowning or near-drowning of child. *Australian and New Zealand Journal of Psychiatry* (December), *11* (4) 265–268.

Parkes, C. M. (1964a). Effects of bereavement on physical and mental health—A study of the medical records of widows. *British Medical Journal 2*, 274–279.

Parkes, C. M. (1964b). Recent bereavement as a cause of mental illness. *British Journal of Psychiatry, 110*, 198–204.

Parkes, C. M. (1965). Bereavement and mental illness. Pt. I: A clinical study of the grief of bereaved psychiatric patients. *British Journal of Medical Psychology 38*, 1–12.

Parkes, C. M. (1970a). The first year of bereavement: A longitudinal study of the reaction of London widows to the death of their husbands. *Psychiatry, 33*, 444.

Parkes, C. M. (1970b). The psychosomatic effects of bereavement. In O. Hill (Ed.), *Modern trends in psychosomatic medicine.* London: Butterworths.

Parkes, C. M. (1972b). *Bereavement: Studies of grief in adult life.* New York: International Universities Press.

Parkes, C. M. (1975). Determinants of outcome following bereavement. *Omega, 6*, 303–323.

Parkes, C. M., Benjamin, B., & Fitzgerald, R. G. (1969). Broken heart: A statistical study of increase on mortality among widows. *British Medical Journal, 1*, 740.

Parkes, C. M., & Brown, R. J. (1972a). Health after bereavement: A controlled study of young Boston widows and widowers. *Psychosomatic Medicine, 34*, 449–461.

Paul, N. L. (1967). The use of empathy in the resolution of grief. *Perspectives in Biological Medicine, 11.*, 153–69.

Pugh, T. F., & MacMahon, B. (1962). *Epidemiologic findings in U.S. mental hospital data.* Boston: Little, Brown.

Radloff, L. (1975). Sex differences in depression: The effects of occupation and marital status. *Sex Roles, 1*, 249–265.

Radloff, L. (1977). The CES-D scale. A self-report depression scale for research in the general population. *Applied Psychological Measurement, 1*, 385–901.

Rahe, R. H. (1972). Subjects' recent life changes and their near-future illness susceptibility. *Advances in Psychosomatic Medicine, 8*, 2–19.

Rahe, R., & Arthur, R. J. (1978). Life change and illness studies: Past history and future directions. *Journal of Human Stress, 4*, 3–15.

Raphael, B. (1975). The management of pathological grief. *Australian and New Zealand Journal of Psychiatry 9*, 173–179.

Raphael, B. & Maddison, D. C. (1976). The care of bereaved adults. In O. Hill (Ed.), *Modern trends in psychosomatic medicine.* London: Butterworths.

Rees, W. D. (1971). The hallucinations of widowhood. *British Medical Journal 4*, 37–41.

Rees W. D., & Lutkins, S. C. (1967). Mortality of bereavement. *British Medical Journal 4*, 13–16.

Sachar, E. J., MacKenzie, J. M., Binstock, W. A. et al., (1967). Corticosteroid responses to psychotherapy of depression. *Archives of General Psychiatry 16*, 461–470.

Sanders, C. (1979–1980). A comparison of adult bereavement in the death of a spouse, child and parent. *Omega: Journal of Death and Dying, 10*(4), 303–322.

Shanfield, S. B. (1981). Predicting bereavement outcome: Marital factors. *Proceedings of the American Psychiatric Association.*

Shepherd, D., & Barraclough, B. M. (1974). The aftermath of suicide. *British Medical Journal, 2*, 600–603.

Shoenberg, B., Carr, A. C., Kutscher, A. H. et al (Eds.). (1974). *Anticipatory grief.* New York: Columbia University Press.

Siggins, L. D. (1966). Mourning: A critical survey of the literature. *International Journal of Psychoanalysis, 47*, 14–25.

Stein, M. (1983, March). *Bereavement and lymphocyte function.* Paper presented at the American Psychosomatic Society Annual Meeting.

Stein, Z., & Susser, M. (1969). Widowhood and mental illness. *British Journal of Preventive and Social Medicine, 23*, 106–110.

Stern, K., & Williams G. M. (1951). Grief reactions in later life. *American Journal of Psychiatry, 108*, 289–294.

Tietz, W., McSherry, L., & Britt, B. (1977). Family sequelae after a child's death due to cancer. *American Journal of Psychotherapy* (July), *31*(3) 417–425.

Tunstall, J. (1966). *Old and alone.* London: Routledge and Kegan-Paul.

Walker, K. N., MacBridge, A., & Vachon, M. L. S. (1977). Social support networks and the crises of bereavement. *Social Science and Medicine, 11*, 35–41.

Waller, D. A., Todres, I. D., Cassem, N. et al. (1979). Coping with poor prognosis in the pediatric intensive care unit. *American Journal of Diseases of Children, 133*, 1121–1125.

Ward, A. W. M. (1976). Mortality of bereavement. *British Medical Journal, 1*, 700–702.

Wolfenstein, J. (1966). How is mourning possible? *The Psychoanalytic Study of the Child, 21*, 93–123.

Wolff, C. T., Friedman, S. B., Hofer, M. A., & Mason, J. W. (1964a). Relationship between psychological defenses and mean urinary 17-OHCS excretion rates: Pt. I. A predictive study of parents of fatally ill children. *Psychosomatic Medicine, 26*, 576–591.

Wolff, C. T., Hofer, M. A., & Mason, J. W. (1964b). Relationship between psychological defenses and mean urinary 17-OHCS excretion rates. Pt. II. Methodological and theoretical considerations. *Psychosomatic Medicine, 26*, 592–609.

Yamamoto, J., Okonogi, K., Iwasaki, T. et al. (1969). Mourning in Japan. *American Journal of Psychiatry, 125*, 1660–1665.

Young, M., Benjamin, B., & Wallis, C. (1963). The Mortality of widows. *Lancet, 2*, 454.

Zisook, S., De Vaul, R. A., & Glick, M. A. (1982). Measuring symptoms of grief and bereavement. *American Journal of Psychiatry, 139*, 1590–1593.

12

Behavioral Medicine and the Family: Historical Perspectives and Future Directions

Robert D. Kerns

Dennis C. Turk

The phenomenal growth of the field of behavioral medicine appears to have been facilitated by the endorsement or consideration of several overlapping principles, goals, and theoretical perspectives. These include (a) an interdisciplinary emphasis; (b) consideration of integrative systems models emphasizing the interrelationship among biological, psychological, and social/ecological subsystems; (c) recognition of the contributions of an experimental analysis of behavior, applied behavior analysis, behavior modification, and cognitive-social learning theory; and (d) recognition of historical roots in human psychophysiology and clinical biofeedback. The specific role of the family, however, has not received much emphasis. A brief overview of each of these principles or models for investigation will be presented and we will underscore their links with family issues to help clarify these associations and contributions and to identify future directions for integration and research.

INTERDISCIPLINARY EMPHASIS

In 1977 the Yale Conference on Behavioral Medicine specifically emphasized the importance of interdisciplinary study and clinical efforts (Schwartz & Weiss, 1977). It was suggested that improved communication among representatives of these disciplines should be encouraged not only to foster interdisciplinary collaborative investigation but also to increase the sharing of knowledge across disciplines. Among the disciplines specifically noted were medicine, psychiatry, psychology, anthropology, sociology, epidemiology, education, and biostatistics.

Inconsistencies appear when considering the impact of this interdisciplinary perspective on investigating the role of the family in health- and illness-related issues. One need only review the References at the end of each chapter in this volume to realize that lines of communication across disciplines are present when considering the family. In taking two chapters as examples (Leventhal et al., Chapter 5, and Johnson, Chapter 8), it is clear that relevant work has been published by a wide range of disciplines. In these two chapters alone the following disciplines are acknowledged: psychology (including social, developmental, physiological, clinical, and personality), nursing, genetics, neurosciences, sociology, social work, epidemiology, public health, gerontology, social biology, and a wide domain of medical specialities (e.g., oncology, gastroenterology, neurology, rheumatology, pediatrics, family practice, cardiology, psychiatry, endocrinology, and diabetology).

Closer scrutiny of the cited articles, however, reveals a disappointing finding for those who would encourage interdisciplinary collaborative research. In fact, only a small minority of the empirical papers cited involved significant methodological or conceptual contributions from more than one discipline. Although there are a number of important exceptions to this rule, relatively few truly collaborative interdisciplinary research projects have appeared.

The absence of consideration of the family from interdisciplinary research is further underscored by reviewing recent volumes of the *Journal of Behavioral Medicine* and the program for the fifth annual meeting of the Society of Behavioral Medicine. A review of articles published in the *Journal of Behavioral Medicine* during the past three years reveal that of 87 papers, only six considered the family in any significant manner (Billings & Moos, 1981, 1982; Gross, Eudy, & Drabman, 1982; Jorgensen & Houston, 1981; Margolis, McLeroy, Runyman, & Kaplan, 1983; Schaefer, Coyne, &

Lazarus, 1981). Similarly, of 201 paper presentations, workshops, institutes, and invited addresses listed in the program for the 1984 meeting of the Society of Behavioral Medicine only 12 considered the role of the family in a significant manner. Of these, only four were authored by representatives of more than one discipline (Affonso & Domino, 1984; Fox, Tsou, & Klos, 1984; Litt, Turk, Salovey, & Walker, 1984; Speers, Freeman, & Ostfeld, 1984).

One final example comes from review of the journal *Health Psychology*, a publication developed out of the emerging interest in the behavioral medicine perspective within psychology. Surprisingly, during its first two years of publication, *only one article* (Wallston, Alagna, DeVellis, & DeVellis, 1983) made more than a passing reference to the role of the family in the topic under consideration. In summary, it seems clear that attention to the family within the context of the growth of the field of behavioral medicine has certainly not been emphasized, but rather has been relatively ignored.

The neglect of the family in behavioral medicine is unfortunate when one considers the wealth of information, both conceptual and empirical, noted within many health-relevant disciplines. For example, as clinical health psychologists become interested in the process of adaptation and coping with chronic illness, it is incumbent upon them to look beyond psychological, psychiatric, and psychosomatic models developed to describe and explain the role of the family. Sociologists, epidemiologists, and a range of medical specialties have already derived a wealth of information and continue to pursue alternative models related to these same issues.

Methodological advances, research design, and data analytic procedures that have been initially developed and applied in one area could make significant contributions to another, previously stymied, program of research. For example, the development of structured family assessment strategies by family therapists may be adapted for application in sociological studies. Another important example may be recent developments in longitudinal causal modeling of latent variables, which is an innovative approach to evaluating change in two or more variables over time (Joreskog, 1978; Kenny, 1979). Longitudinal causal modeling has recently been applied in studying the relationships between depression and alcohol use (Aneshensel & Huba, 1983) and between stress, social support and depression (Aneshensel & Frerichs, 1982) over time. This methodologically sophisticated approach may be applied to help uncover important causal relationships between, for example, social/familial support and physical symptomatology, relationships that have up to this time been empirically described only as correlational (e.g., Wallston et al., 1983).

INTEGRATIVE SYSTEMS MODELS

Systems theory (e.g., DeRosnay, 1979; von Bertalanffy, 1968) has been widely cited as an important framework for conceptualization and development of knowledge within the field of behavioral medicine (Schwartz, 1981). Leventhal et al., in Chapter 5, this volume, describe two ways in which this framework may be useful. First, a systems perspective may aid in the description of the relationships between various levels of data. Within this context, for example, knowledge about family structure and function may be integrated with information about psychological functioning of individuals within the family. Second, Leventhal et al. acknowledges that a systems perspective may be useful in articulating the content, organization, and operation of the components at each level of description. A review of the contributors to this volume reveals that both applications of systems theory are at least implicitly endorsed by the majority of the authors.

Family Systems Perspective.   In considering the role of the family in health and illness, the acceptance of a definition of the family that is consistent with a systems perspective is universal (see the chapters by Turk & Kerns; Gochman; Baranowski & Nader). The definitions offered by these authors emphasize not only the component members of the family but also the interaction of these members across varying levels of analysis (e.g., roles, goals, shared resources). Family systems theory (Ferreira, 1963; Jackson, 1957) and its potential application is briefly described in Chapter 1 by Turk and Kerns and in Chapter 5 by Leventhal and his colleagues.

Unfortunately, empirical knowledge derived from within a family systems framework has been limited. For example, in contrast to the relatively abundant literature on the relevance of *structural* variables used to describe the family (e.g., family size, socioeconomic status, religious affiliation) and their relation to the development of health-related cognitions and behaviors among children, few researchers have focused on measures of family *functioning* (see Chapter 2 by Gochman). This failure of investigators to address the possible relationship between patterns of family interaction and the development of health beliefs and behaviors may be one important reason why Gochman concluded that family factors may *not* be primary determinants of children's health concepts. In this area of investigation, at least, assessments of families that are limited to family structure may lead to potentially premature conclusions.

In areas of investigation in which attention has been focused on various aspects of family functioning, only rarely have efforts been made to evaluate family member interaction directly. Instead, researchers have typically relied on self-report measures of family functioning (e.g., questionnaires, interviews). Potential biases inherent in the use of these self-report strategies are repeatedly cited by the authors of the chapters in this volume (e.g., Bohm & Rodin, Chapter 10; Kosten, Jacobs, & Kasl, Chapter 11). The few attempts that have employed observation procedures may serve as important models for future research. For example, Ritchie's (1981) study of problem-solving interactions among members of families of epileptic children versus healthy controls using a structured observation procedure resulted in a specific description of potential problem areas. Application of similar assessment strategies in the childhood epilepsy literature as well as in evaluating family adjustment to other chronic diseases among children will likely yield additional heuristic findings. Other innovative analogue procedures used in the evaluation of family functioning are cited throughout this volume (e.g., Costelli, Reiss, Berkman, & Jones, 1981; Olivieri & Reiss, 1981), but have rarely been applied in the behavioral medicine research.

Several reasons probably contribute to the failure of most investigators to move beyond the assessment of structural family variables and global levels of family functioning. Most obvious is the current lack of specific measures of family functioning with established reliability and validity. Also difficult is the task of developing relatively nonobtrusive and minimally reactive observation strategies. Nevertheless, it is incumbent upon researchers to meet this challenge to clarify the role the family plays both in health and illness and conversely the impact of illness on the family.

An additional shortcoming of the family literature in behavioral medicine is the general failure of researchers to assess more than one member of the family. Typically, a single family member, most often a mother or spouse, is taken to "represent" the family (e.g., Brown, Rawlinson, & Hardin, 1982). This limitation precludes valid interpretation of findings within a family systems perspective.

Biopsychosocial Perspective. Besides the importance of organizing information and principles from a systems perspective for each level of description (e.g., the family system), application of a model that aids in the conceptualization of the relationship between interacting levels of analysis has also been emphasized in this volume. In particular, several authors (e.g., Kerns & Curley; Leventhal et al.) have endorsed aspects of a biopsychosocial perspective for investigation of the interactions between biological and psychological systems and the family (e.g., Engel, 1977).

In the Leventhal et al. chapter, details of the biopsychosocial perspective were outlined and the principles useful in guiding our understanding of the interactions among these levels of analyses were discussed. In the Kerns and Curley chapter, the biopsychosocial model was applied to a review of the literature regarding the role of the family and a specific disease system—neurological disease. Similarly, Leventhal et al. emphasized the importance of considering the family system in interaction with other systems as a dynamic process, subject to critical changes across the life span. Kerns and Curley provided three specific examples of neurological disease—childhood epilepsy, traumatic brain injury, and senile dementia-Alzheimer's type—not only as representing three divergent disease systems but also to dramatize significant differences in the interactions of these disease systems with the family at three relatively distinct points along the life-span continuum.

The biopsychosocial model, as articulated by these authors, appears as a particularly appealing perspective for consideration of the family and its relationship to health and illness issues. Engel (1980), for example, provides an account of potential application of the model in a clinical situation. He discusses the case of a middle-aged man presenting himself to an emergency room with symptoms of a myocardial infarction and contrasts the evaluation and decision making and their implications from a traditional biomedical perspective and the biopsychosocial perspective. Engel argues that the application of the conventional biomedical model is reductionistic in its orientation, leading to exclusion of the social and family interactions of the patient, "except as a matter of compassion and humanity" (e.g., Engel, 1980, p.543). Within the biopsychosocial perspective, information about the family of the patient becomes important in evaluating the patient's symptom presentation, response to intervention, and eventual rehabilitation. Appreciation of the potential disequilibrium in the family in relation to the impact of the heart attack of a family member is similarly viewed as critical in maximizing the adaptive response of the patient. In summary, within the biopsychosocial perspective, the evaluation and the intervention process are broadened to include the family as an important system to be considered.

Attention to the family in health and illness issues probably has little to do with the recent articulation of the biopsychosocial model. The truth of this statement is substantiated by a critical review of the literature cited and an awareness that few studies do more than *describe* the supposed effects of health or illness on the family. Rarely is there a consideration of a transactional model attempting to *explain* the maintenance of health or the process of change in the family as a function of the illness in a family member or, conversely, the impact of the family system on the biological, psychological, and social functioning of a healthy or ill individual (cf. Turk & Kerns, Chapter 1). Consideration of the biopsychosocial model, as a systems model, implies not only consideration of each level of analysis (e.g., the family, the psychology of the individual) as separable systems but also the development of hypotheses to explain the organization and function across these systems.

Two additional perspectives that may be helpful in explaining the process of transduction of information between the family and the biological and psychological organization of an individual family member are social learning theory and psychophysiology. As noted in the introduction to this chapter, each of these orientations has contributed significantly to the clinical practice and science of behavioral medicine. Each will be reviewed briefly in terms of its explanatory potential in relation to the family and health and illness issues.

LEARNING THEORY AND BEHAVIORAL MODIFICATION

Pomerleau (1979) has emphasized the significant role that experimental behavioral sciences, as opposed to other social sciences, has played in the development and proliferation of behavioral medicine. Pomerleau challenges the definition of the field as provided by Schwartz and Weiss (1977) and along with Brady suggests an alternative definition that emphasizes "(a) the clinical use of techniques derived from the experimental analysis of behavior" and "(b) the conduct of research within a behavioral perspective" (Pomerleau & Brady, 1979, p.xii). These authors argue that historical roots in psychosomatic medicine, recent labeling and endorsement of the biopsychosocial model, and, in fact, incorporation of a wide domain of represented disciplines within behavioral medicine have provided the "necessary but not sufficient condition for the development of behavioral medicine" (Pomerleau & Brady, 1979, p. xii). Rather, they propose that the development of behavioral strategies for intervention usefully applied to the health field has provided the critical impetus for the development of the new field.

In considering the role of the family in health and illness issues, it is clear that a behavioral framework has made and will continue to make important contributions both in terms of clinical practice and research. Pomerleau (1979) discusses four principal lines of development that may help organize the present discussion: (a) intervention to modify an overt behavior or physiological response that in itself constitutes a problem; (b) intervention to modify behavior of health care providers to improve the delivery of service; (c) intervention to modify adherence to prescribed treatment; and (d) intervention to modify behaviors or responses that constitute risk factors for disease. (p. 657)

Direct Modification.   Behavior modification and behavior therapy strategies have been applied in a number of areas in which the intervention is conceptualized as having a relatively direct impact on the health problem per se at a pathophysiological or symptomatic level of analysis. The specific rationale for application of these behavioral intervention strategies within classical and/or instrumental conditioning frameworks varies with the specific disorder and the affected individual and his or her family. In most cases, the validity of the theoretical model is tested by means of an empirical intervention trial.

As an example of this model of direct intervention, Johnson (Chapter 8) provides data supporting the efficacy of a behaviorally oriented residential treatment for poorly controlled insulin-dependent diabetic children. Family intervention focusing on education about diabetes, diet, and behavioral management of the diabetic child is provided as a central component of the program. The rationale for this intervention is based on hypotheses that contingencies within the family maladaptively support poor eating habits, insufficient exercise, and a generally high level of emotional stress, all factors that may contribute to poor diabetic control. Interventions designed to alter contingencies within the family are hypothesized to result in improvement in a measure of diabetic control—specifically, glycosolated hemoglobin levels. Indeed, the available data demonstrate such changes.

Flor and Turk (Chapter 9) have discussed an operant model of chronic pain that emphasizes the important role of environmental contingencies in maintaining the experience of pain through reinforcement of pain behaviors (i.e., overt motor demonstrations of pain). These authors discuss the particularly important role that family members play in this regard. Fordyce (1976) has described an inpatient treatment model that focuses on decreasing contingent reinforcement for pain while increasing reinforcement for well behaviors. Fordyce emphasizes the need to transfer the responsibility for continued application of the operant model from the controlled inpatient environment to the family. Unfortunately, little empirical attention has focused on this treatment issue, and no empirical trials of an operantly oriented family treatment for chronic pain have been published.

A third example is cited by Kerns and Curley (Chapter 6). Timming et al. (1980) describe a multidisciplinary treatment program for traumatically brain injured (TBI) individuals. One important component of the program is a social skills training module designed to improve social relations, a particular problem within the family of a TBI individual. An important extension of this program would be to alter family members' behaviors in such a way as to increase their contingent reinforcement of adaptive social skills emitted by the TBI family member. Again, this strategy has the potential advantage of minimizing relapse following discharge from a controlled inpatient environment to a family environment lacking the skills to maintain improvements in the patient's behaviors.

It is also important to consider the reciprocal relationship between the ill family member and other family members. That is, not only does the family help to shape the behavior of the patients but also the patient has the potential to mediate the behavior of other family members. For example, the patient may positively reinforce others through praise in their performing a household chore or personal care task that the patient could otherwise perform. A process of negative reinforcement may also develop in which family members learn to terminate the aversive complaining or demonstrations of frustration exhibited by the patient by taking over the responsibilities of the patient. To the extent that performance of the task would be aversive to the patient, a process of negative reinforcement, or secondary gain, becomes operable as the patient effectively avoids undesirable, but potentially adaptive, tasks associated with rehabilitation efforts. Behavioral family interventions must therefore focus not only on training the family members to appreciate their roles as discriminant cues, sources of reinforcement, and behavioral models for increasing the instrumental behavior of the patient, but additionally, families must be taught strategies to minimize the pitfalls associated with the ill family member's power as a stimulus for other family members' behavior.

It seems clear that the development of intervention strategies designed to alter patterns of contingent reinforcement among family members may have important benefits for maintaining health, enhancing adherence, and for the recovery of adjustment of a physically ill member. Such interventions may be appropriately developed in the context of interdisciplinary treatment of a wide range of health problems where maladaptive family interactions appear to play a contributing role in the development or maintenance of the problem. It is incumbent upon behavioral medicine practitioners to consider the cost effectiveness of behavioral family interventions for directly altering the health problem and for generalizing and maintaining improvements in the home environment.

Indirect Modification.   Attempts to modify the behavior of medical personnel to provide more cost-effective care to the patient or client is a second area outlined by Pomerleau (1979). In many ways the boundary between the previous discussion about direct modification and the possibility of indirect modification is blurred when considering the family. In each case just described, the family is considered the critical health care environment (cf. Baranowski & Nader, Chapter 3; Melamed & Bush, Chapter 7; Litman, 1974). Thus behavioral family interventions may be viewed as indirect strategies designed to alter family members' behavior in order to effect behavior change in the ill member. Alternatively, and more consistent with a family systems model that integrates learning theory, contingencies within the family are conceptualized as factors contributing to the development or maintenance of these health problems (i.e., uncontrolled diabetes, chronic pain, social skills deficits among the traumatic brain injured) (cf. Watzlawick & Coyne, 1980). Consistent with this perspective, behavioral family interventions are appropriately considered direct modification strategies within Pomerleau's (1979) organization.

Adherence.   Dunbar and Stunkard (1977) in a review and discussion of issues related to adherence to drug and diet regimens among coronary heart-diseased patients recommended making full use of the family as a source of social support for adherence. Several authors in this volume have provided specific examples of family involvement in therapeutic interventions designed to improve adherence to prescribed regimens. Literature supporting family involvement was cited for hypertension, cardiovascular disease, and arthritis (e.g., Baranowski & Nadar, Chapter 4), childhood diabetes (e.g., Johnson, Chapter 8), and childhood epilepsy (e.g., Kerns & Curley, Chapter 6) among others.

From a behavioral perspective, family members can serve several roles in attempts to improve adherence to a treatment regimen by another member. First, the family member may provide reminders or cue the recommended behavioral response. Second, the family member may provide contingent positive reinforcement for the appropriate behavioral response. Thus a supportive family member, insofar as he or she is perceived as a source of reinforcement, may function as an important mediator of adherence. Third, family members may alter their own behavior in order to serve as positive models for behavior change on the part of the patient.

Common examples include the spouse who quits smoking or reduces caloric intake as an encouragement or incentive. Family members can also facilitate other guidelines recommended by Dunbar and Stunkard (1979) to improve adherence. Examples include cueing the patient to self-monitor adherence (e.g., attending to weight loss or increased exercise) and tailoring a family routine to meet the demands of the treatment regimen (e.g., changing family dietary habits). However, family members may also interfere with adherence or even create disturbance by being unsupportive, thereby reinforcing inappropriate behaviors and modeling maladaptive responding. It is important to consider both the facilitating and the debilitating potential of the family.

Teaching the family the use of learning theory to improve adherence by a family member makes intuitive sense in most clinical situations. Perhaps most important is the improved likelihood for long-term adherence in the home environment where cueing and contingent reinforcement from health care providers is absent. Unfortunately, little empirical attention has yet to be paid to evaluating potential benefits from family involvement in adherence issues. Furthermore, specific questions related to an appreciation of family variables that may contribute to maximizing adherence have yet to be addressed (see chapters by Baranowski & Nadar; Leventhal et al.)

Prevention.   An impressive literature has evolved in the context of several large-scale epidemiological studies leading to an articulation of a range of behavioral risk factors for the development or at least proliferation of cancer (Sklar & Anisman, 1981) and cardiovascular disease (Jenkins, 1976) among others. Specific aspects of life style, such as diet, physical activity, cigarette smoking, consumption of alcohol, and the type A behavior pattern (Rosenman & Friedman, 1974) have been found to have important effects on morbidity and mortality (Pomerleau, Bass, & Crown, 1975).

Gochman (Chapter 2, this volume) reviewed the literature relevant to the role of the family in the development of health-related attitudes and beliefs (e.g., perceived vulnerability, definitions of health and illness) and Barnowski and Nader (Chapter 3) have reviewed the role of the family in promoting a range of health-related behaviors (e.g., utilization of health services, eating behaviors, smoking, use of alcohol). Parental modeling, in particular, has been implicated as an important determinant.

As with the other areas reviewed, intervention at the family level designed to promote health behaviors and target risk factors for reduction has been limited. However, given the mediation potential of the family in facilitating life-style changes, it seems clear that these efforts will likely increase in frequency. Theoretical models and intervention strategies developed in relation to issues of adherence are likely to be generalizable to issues of prevention. In fact, in many cases, regimen adherence in the form of risk reduction is appropriately conceptualized as secondary prevention (e.g., cigarette smoking cessation or Type A modification among coronary heart disease patients to reduce risk for recurrence of symptoms of ischemia).

In sum, it seems evident that consideration of human models of learning has important explanatory potential for articulating the relationship between the family and physical health and illness among its members. Development of explanatory models based on learning theory within a transactional systems perspective, such as the biopsychosocial model, may have heuristic as well as clinical significance. Development of family assessment and intervention strategies consistent with these explanatory models, and empirical tests of their utility in direct and indirect modification of illness behaviors and in promoting prevention and adherence are goals for future investigation.

PSYCHOPHYSIOLOGY

A fourth important perspective that has contributed significantly to the development of the field of behavioral medicine is human psychophysiology as a research methodology, strategy for assessment, and a clinical intervention strategy in the form of clinical biofeedback. Schwartz, in particular, has helped promote the contributions of psychophysiology to investigations of biobehavioral relationships (Schwartz, 1977, 1979; Schwartz, Shapiro, Redmond, Ferguson, Ragland, & Weiss, 1979).

Consideration of the family within this perspective has been limited. Application of methodological advances in psychophysiology (e.g., continuous, on-line monitoring of multiple physiological parameters) clearly has limited applicability for family assessment. However, application of these protocols for evaluation of individual family members other than the patient may provide answers to a variety of important questions. Use of telemetric procedures that permit measurements at a distance from the subject by recording information transmitted by radio signals (e.g., radio-electrocardiography, radioencephalography) may ultimately be applied with multiple family members in a structured, or even unstructured, environment.

Analyses of psychophysiological reactivity, as opposed to resting or baseline levels of analyses, have proven a more fruitful strategy in a number of areas of investigation (e.g., headaches, hypertension). For example, in the headache literature, assessment of muscle tension reactivity to a variety of laboratory stress stimuli has helped specify the hypothesized relationship between the experience of stress and headaches (e.g., Blanchard & Andrasik, 1982; Haynes, Gannon, Cuevas, Heiser, Hamilton, & Katranides, 1983). In this example the psychophysiological response (e.g., EMG, skin temperature) to specific stressful laboratory stimuli is presumed to reflect the individual's characteristic response to naturally occurring stress experiences and is hypothesized to mediate the development of the headache condition.

In considering a transactional family model (Hill, 1949; Turk & Kerns, Chapter 1, this volume), the family member with a particular health problem may be conceptualized as either a stimulus for provoking a response in other family members or, conversely, may be viewed as the responder to stimuli in his or her environment as, for example, in other family members or family interactions. In this manner, the impact on the family members of a health problem experienced by a single family member may be investigated. Alternatively, the impact of the family on the psychophysiological responding of an individual family member may be evaluated. Two examples may help clarify these perspectives.

Several investigators have similarly hypothesized that psychological or emotional stress may be an important independent risk factor for the development of angina pectoris (e.g., Jenkins, 1976) and may even precipitate episodes of chest pain (Schiffer, Hartley, Schulman, & Abelmann, 1980). Central mediation of autonomic nervous system arousal and associated release of catecholamines are presumed to result in an increased demand for oxygen by the heart under stress conditions. When the demand for oxygen outstrips the supply, ischemic chest pain may occur (Nestel, Verghese, & Lovell, 1967). Empirical validation of this process in naturalistic or laboratory settings has been limited.

Medalie and Goldbourt (1976) have found, in a large-scale prospective study, that report of a high level of family-related stress among healthy male subjects was a powerful predictor of the later development of angina. Application of psychophysiological methodologies such as those mentioned above may significantly contribute to the understanding of mechanisms mediating the relationship between family stress (e.g., aversive family interactions, family conflicts) and coronary heart disease, and specifically angina pectoris. One strategy yet to be employed would be to structure spousal discussions about a particular area of disagreement while monitoring each spouse psychophysiologically. Particular emphasis could be placed on assessment of the cardiovascular system (cf. Cacciopo & Petty, 1983).

Block (1981) investigated the physiological responses of spouses of chronic pain patients to videotapes of their mates, other chronic pain patients, and actors exhibiting "painful" and "neutral" facial expressions. Spouses were found to exhibit greater skin conductance reactivity to displays of pain than to neutral expressions regardless of who they were watching. The findings were discussed in terms of possible implication for the observed frequent development of pain and other psychophysiological symptoms among the members of families of chronic pain patients (see Flor & Turk, Chapter 9; Schaffer, Donlon, & Bittle, 1980). Continued examination of this hypothesized maladaptive "empathic" response of spouses of pain patients and other chronically ill patients (cf. Klein, Dean, & Bogdonoff, 1967) using psychophysiological methodologies is indicated.

SUMMARY AND CONCLUSIONS

This chapter has summarized the contributions of four important influences on the development of behavioral medicine. It has also examined, through references to a number of chapters in this volume, the applicability of these perspectives to investigations of the role of the family in health and illness. Finally, it has articulated several areas for future attention within these perspectives. The contributors described innovative research and detailed a range of areas in need of empirical investigation. Additional perspectives or orientations that have been applied to these same issues (e.g., epidemiological models, social attribution theory, the cognitive-behavioral perspective, psychoimmunology, neuroendocrinology), although excluded from the present discussion, have certainly made and will continue to make significant contributions. Integration of these perspectives leading to the development of empirical models for description and explanation of the role of the family in health and illness and the controlled tests of these models are critical. A rich clinical literature has helped foster an interest in the family in the context of behavioral medicine. It is now incumbent upon researchers to validate and extend this lore in order to significantly advance our understanding of a wide range of important questions and problems. Such advances may ultimately lead to refinement of presently applied clinical strategies and the emergence of more effective alternatives. It is our hope that the material presented here will serve as a stimulus for the integration of the family within the burgeoning field of behavioral medicine. The success of our attempt to focus on the family will be judged by examining future issues of relevant journals and the indexes of future volumes focusing on behavioral medicine.

REFERENCES

Affonso, D., & Domino, G. (1984). *Adaptation and depression following childbirth*. Paper presented at the annual meeting of the Society of Behavioral Medicine in Philadelphia.

Aneshensel, C. S., & Frerichs, R. R. (1982). Stress, support, and depression: A longitudinal causal model. *Journal of Community Psychology, 10*, 363–376.

Aneshensel, C. S., & Huba, G. J. (1983). Depression, alcohol use, and smoking over one year: A four-wave longitudinal causal model. *Journal of Abnormal Psychology, 92*, 134–150.

Billings, A. G., & Moos, R. H. (1981). The role of coping responses and social resources in attenuating the stress of life events. *Journal of Behavioral Medicine, 4*, 139–157.

Billings, A. G., & Moos, R. H. (1982). Social support and functioning among community and clinical groups: A panel model. *Journal of Behavioral Medicine, 5*, 295–311.

Blanchard, E. B., & Andrasik, F. (1982). Psychological assessment and treatment of headache: Recent developments and emerging issues. *Journal of Consulting and Clinical Psychology, 50*, 859–879.

Block, A. (1981). An investigation of the response of the spouse to chronic pain behavior. *Psychosomatic Medicine, 43*, 415–422.

Brown, J. S., Rawlinson, M. E., & Hardin, D. M. (1982). Family functioning and health status. *Journal of Family Issues, 3,* 91–110.

Cacioppo, J. T., & Petty, R. E. (1983). *Social psychophysiology: A sourcebook.* New York: Guilford Press.

Costelli, R., Reiss, D., Berkman, H., & Jones, C. (1981). The family meets the hospital: Predicting the family's perception of the treatment program from its problem-solving style. *Archives of General Psychiatry, 38,* 569–577.

DeGraff, C. D. (1981). Marital interaction among chronic pain patients. *Dissertation Abstracts International, 42,* 762-B.

DeRosnay, J. (1979). *The macroscope.* New York: Harper & Row.

Dunbar, J., & Stunkard, A. J. (1977). Adherence to diet and drug regimen. In R. Levey, B. Rifkin, B. Dennis, & N. Ernst (Eds.), *Nutrition, lipids, and coronary heart disease.* New York: Raven Press.

Engel, G. L. (1977). The need for a new medical model: A challenge for biomedicine. *Science, 196,* 129–136.

Engel, G. L. (1980). The clinical application of the biopsychosocial model. *American Journal of Psychiatry, 137,* 535–544.

Ferreira, A. J. (1963). Family myth and homeostasis. *Archives of General Psychiatry, 9,* 457–463.

Fordyce, W. E. (1976). *Behavioral methods in chronic pain and illness.* St. Louis, MO: Mosby.

Fox, S., Tsou, C., & Klos, D. (1984). *An intervention to increase mammography screening behavior in family physicians.* Paper presented at the annual meeting of the Society of Behavioral Medicine in Philadelphia.

Gross, A. M., Eudy, C., & Drabman, R. S. (1982). Training parents to be physical therapists with their physically handicapped child. *Journal of Behavioral Medicine, 5,* 321–328.

Haynes, S. N., Gannon, L. R., Cuevas, J., Heiser, P., Hamilton, J., & Katranides, M. (1983). The psychophysiological assessment of muscle-contraction headache subjects during headache and nonheadache conditions. *Psychophysiology, 20,* 393–399.

Hill, R. (1949). *Families under stress.* New York: Harper & Row.

Jackson, D. D. (1957). The question of family homeostasis. *Psychiatric Quarterly, 32,* 79–90.

Jenkins, C. D. (1976). Recent evidence supporting psychologic and social risk factors for coronary disease. *New England Journal of Medicine, 294,* 987–994.

Joreskog, K. G. (1978). Structural analysis of covariance and correlation matrices. *Psychometrika, 43,* 443–478.

Jorgensen, R. S., & Houston, B. K. (1981). Family history of hypertension, gender, and cardiovascular reactivity and stereotypy during stress. *Journal of Behavioral Medicine, 4,* 175–190.

Kenny, D.A. (1979). *Correlation and causality.* New York: Wiley.

Klein, R. F., Dean, A., & Bogdonoff, M. (1967). The impact of illness upon the spouse. *Journal of Chronic Diseases,* 241–248.

Litman, T. J. (1974). The family as a basic unit in health and medical care: A sociobehavioral overview. *Social Science and Medicine, 8,* 495–519.

Litt, M., Turk, D. C., Salovey, P., & Walker, J. (1984). *Seeking urgent pediatric care: Causes of appropriateness of patients' decisions.* Paper presented at the annual meeting of the Society of Behavioral Medicine in Philadelphia.

Margolis, L. H., McLeroy, K. R., Runyman, C. W., & Kaplan, B. H. (1983). Type A behavior: An ecological approach. *Journal of Behavioral Medicine, 6,* 245–258.

Medalie, J. H., & Goldbourt, U. (1976). Angina pectoris among 10,000 men: II. Psychosocial and other risk factors as evidenced by a multivariate analysis of a five year incidence study. *American Journal of Medicine, 60,* 910–921.

Nestel, P. J., Verghese, A., & Lovell, R. R. H. (1967). Catecholamine secretion and sympathetic nervous responses to emotion in men with and without angina pectoris. *American Heart Journal, 73*, 227–234.

Oliveri, M. E., & Reiss, D. (1981). A theory-based empirical classification of family problemsolving behavior. *Family Process, 20*, 409–418.

Pollard, C. A. (1981). The relationship of family environment to chronic pain disability. *Dissertation Abstracts International, 42*, 2077-B.

Pomerleau, O. F. (1979a). Commonalities in the treatment and understanding of smoking and other self management disorders. In N. Krasnegor (Ed.), *Behavioral approaches to analysis and treatment of substance abuse (NIDA Research Monograph Series)*. Rockville, MD.: National Institute on Drug Abuse.

Pomerleau, O. F. (1979b). Behavioral factors in the establishment, maintenance, and cessation of smoking. *Smoking and Health: A Report of the Surgeon General.*

Pomerleau, O. F., Bass, F., & Crown, V. (1975). The role of behavior modification in preventive medicine. *New England Journal of Medicine, 292*, 1277–1282.

Pomerleau, O. F., & Brady, J. P. (1979). Introduction: The scope and promise of behavioral medicine. In O. F. Pomerleau & J. P. Brady (Eds.), *Behavioral medicine: Theory and practice.*

Redden, J. (1980). Self-control cognitive modification techniques in the treatment of chronic low back pain. *Dissertation Abstracts International, 41*, 698-B.

Ritchie, K. (1981). Research note: Interaction in the families of epileptic children. *Journal of Child Psychology and Psychiatry, 22*, 65–71.

Rosenman, R. H., & Friedman, M. (1974). Neurogenic factors in pathogenesis of coronary heart disease. *Medical Clinics of North America, 58*, 269–279.

Schaefer, C., Coyne, J. C., Lazarus, R. S. (1981). The health-related functions of social support. *Journal of Behavioral Medicine, 4*, 381–406.

Schaffer, C. B., Donlon, P. T., & Bittle, R. M. (1980). Chronic pain and depression: A clinical and family history survey. *American Journal of Psychiatry, 137*, 118–120.

Schiffer, F., Hartley, L. H., Schulman, C. L., & Abelmann, W. H. (1980). Evidence for emotionally-induced coronary arterial spasm in patients with angina pectoris. *British Heart Journal, 44*, 62–66.

Schwartz, G. E. (1977). Psychosomatic disorders and biofeedback: A psychobiological model of disregulation. In J. D. Maser & M. E. P. Selgman (Eds.), *Psychopathology: Experimental models.* San Francisco: Freeman.

Schwartz, G. E. (1979). The brain as a health care system. In G. Stone et al. (Eds.), *Health psychology.* San Francisco: Jossey-Bass.

Schwartz, G. E (1981). Integrating psychobiology and behavior therapy: A systems perspective. In G. T. Wilson & C. M. Franks (Eds.), *Behavior therapy: Theoretical and experimental foundations.* New York: Guilford Press.

Schwartz, G. E., Shapiro, A. P., Redmond, D. P., Ferguson, D. C. E., Ragland, D. R., Weiss, S. M. (1979). Behavioral medicine approaches to hypertension: An integrative analysis of theory and research. *Journal of Behavioral Medicine, 2*, 311–363.

Schwartz, G. E., & Weiss, S. M. (1977). *Proceedings of the Yale Conference on Behavioral Medicine.* Washington, D.C.: U.S. Department of Health, Education, and Welfare.

Sklar, L. S., & Anisman, H. (1981). Stress and cancer. *Psychological Bulletin, 89*, 369–406.

Speers, M., Freeman, D., & Ostfeld, A. (1984). *Correlates of blood pressure: The role of the spouse.* Paper presented at the annual meeting of the Society of Behavioral Medicine in Philadelphia.

Timming, R. C., Cayner, J. J., Grady, S., Grafman, J., Haskin, R., Malec, J., & Thornsen, C. (1980). Multidisciplinary rehabilitation in severe head trauma. *Wisconsin Medical Journal, 79*, 49–52.

von Bertalanffy, L. (1968). *General systems theory*. New York: Braziller.

Wallston, B. S., Alagna, S. W., DeVellis, B., & DeVellis, R. (1983). Social support and physical health. *Health Psychology, 2,* 367–391.

Watzlawick, P., & Coyne, J. C. (1980). Depression following stroke—brief problem-focused family treatment. *Family Process, 19,* 13–18.

Wifling, F. J. (1981). Psychophysiological correlates of low back pain. *Dissertation Abstracts International, 42,* 2592-B.

Author Index

Subject Index